COMPLICATED GRIEVING AND BEREAVEMENT:
Understanding and Treating People Experiencing Loss

Edited by
Gerry R. Cox, Robert A. Bendiksen,
and Robert G. Stevenson

Death, Value and Meaning Series
Series Editor: John D. Morgan

Baywood Publishing Company, Inc.
AMITYVILLE, NEW YORK

Library of Congress Catalog Number: 00-041426
ISBN: 0-89503-213-9 (cloth)

Library of Congress Cataloging-in-Publication Data

Complicated grieving and bereavement : understanding and treating people experiencing loss / edited by Gerry R. Cox, Robert A. Bendiksen, and Robert G. Stevenson.
    p. cm. - - (Death, value, and meaning series)
    Includes bibliographical references and index.
    ISBN 0-89503-213-9 (cloth)
    1. Grief. 2. Bereavement- -Psychological aspects. 3. Death- -Psychological aspects. 4. Loss (Psychology) 5. Grief in children. 6. Bereavement in children. 7. Children and death. 8. Loss (Psychology) in children. 9. Sudden death. I. Cox, Gerry R. II. Bendiksen, Robert. III. Stevenson, Robert G. IV. Series

BF575.G7 C645 2000
155.9'37- -dc21   00-041426

Table of Contents

Preface

Gerry R. Cox, Robert A. Bendiksen,
and Robert G. Stevenson

As editors, we undertook this project at the request of Dr. John Morgan who annually hosts the King's College Conference of Dying, Death, and Bereavement in London, Ontario, Canada, and who serves as editor of the Baywood series *Death, Value and Meaning*. The topic of complicated grieving and bereavement is of great interest to us as long- term faculty members who teach university courses in dying, death, and bereavement. In this volume, our hope is that this selection of chapters meets the needs of many professional practitioners and academics, and ultimately, through them, those who must face the difficult times associated with complicated grieving and bereavement.

We would like to thank Stuart Cohen, President of Baywood Publishing Company, and his fine staff, including Bobbi Olszewski, Julie Krempa, and Erin Murphy for their aid in this project; Dr. Morgan for his encouragement and assistance; Dr. Jac Bulk, Mary Clements, and our colleagues at the University of Wisconsin-La Crosse for their help and assistance; and other unnamed, but no less important, individuals for their help and assistance in this project whose aim is to improve the understanding and treatment of people experiencing loss.

SECTION 1:
Theories of Complicated Grief

The first chapter by Tom Attig examines the concepts of grief and extraordinary grief and their impact on the ability of the grieving to relearn their world. This chapter establishes the framework for the text.

1

SECTION 2:
Children and Complicated Grief

The second section of the text focuses upon traumatic death and its impact on grieving individuals and families. As individuals face and attempt to manage grief, each may develop a style that allows him or her to cope. Certainly, there are different styles of grieving and any style may have elements that complicate or facilitate coping with loss. For each of us, however, losses may be a turning point where the individual faces personal and social choices. He or she can move forward, maintain the status quo, sicken and/or die, face the loss cognitively and/or spiritually, be active or passive in his/her response, or simply do nothing. While each of us places meaning on our losses, why is it that some make meaningful choices and others do not? Why is it that making no choice at all may challenge our sense of meaning? Do children need "adult" models to be able to cope? Do we "socialize" people too much, and by doing so make their grieving more complicated?

The next two chapters focus upon children and traumatic death. David Adams presents an analysis of the consequences of sudden traumatic death on children. He makes specific suggestions for ways to address the vulnerability of bereaved children and adolescents and offers concrete suggestions as to how adults might be able to help. The chapter offers suggestions for professionals and for families and parents to aid children and adolescents. Paul Clements, Jr. investigates the impact of homicide on children and offers suggestions for aiding children to manage their grief in the face of traumatic death.

Toni Griffith examines the responses of rage, regret, and revenge in children. She suggests that it may be helpful to incorporate programs using puppetry, music, song, and expressive arts as ways to aid elementary school children in loss, grief, and transition. Griffith offers ideas as to how to uncover and assist with children who exhibit such grieving patterns. Kerry Cavanagh presents and analyzes three case studies of children that suggests that children experience long-term effects of bereavement that are often ignored. He examines the dynamics of the family and its impact on that system.

SECTION 3:
Complicated Grief in Special Populations

Larry Darrah examines the impact of grief on families of soldiers who are listed as "missing in action." This particular grief is further complicated by the fact that there is no verification of the actual death of the soldier whether it be World War II, Korea, Viet Nam, or any other war. At what point does the person who is grieving lose hope and accept that the loved one is dead? When does one consider remarriage? Darrah offers practical suggestions for managing such traumatic grief. Antoon Leenaars then examines the complication of grief when suicides occur among Canadian Inuit groups. While his analysis is applied to an isolated geographical group, he offers practical suggestions that would apply to any suicide survivor.

Jane Powell offers insights that might be useful for all who grieve, as she examines the responses of differently-abled people and grief which is complicated by their disabilities. She suggests that each of us can learn from their patterns of grieving. Powell offers seven specific actions to aid people with disabilities to manage their grief. Lynne Martins addresses the impact of grief upon those coping with mental illnesses. To be coping with a mental illness and to have the additional burden of coping with the death of a loved one would indeed complicate one's grieving. Martins offers an in-depth analysis of what the problems might be and specific suggestions offering how to aid the mentally ill individual. Catherine Quinn offers a similar analysis of the problems and possible solutions presented with the grieving of demented individuals including Alzheimer's disease. All three of these chapters offer suggestions for dealing with special populations. Clearly, in examining traumatic death and complicated grieving, special needs must be addressed.

Boyd Purcell examines the impact on grief of spiritual abuse. He suggests that those offering spiritual care may, at times, abuse with their attempts at care.

The next chapters in this section address issues that are not often presented in texts designed to aid professionals. Those who work as professionals in dying, death, and bereavement are aware of a variety of models, theories, and/or strategies for assisting people who are bereaved. These professionals face many challenges, problematic connections, and goals that need to be addressed. It is difficult to assess, direct, and assist people in need, with full assurance that the approach being applied is the "correct" one for the individual(s) being assisted.

Support groups may allow some to normalize their grief, to ventilate their personal issues, to receive support, and to receive suggestions for coping. One wonders why groups work for some and not for others. Most families share emotions, feelings, and grief, but why do some families not share? Death appears, at times, to be unfair and unjust. Sometimes one cannot make sense out of the death. Yet as humans, we engage in meaning-making.

Richard Gilbert responds to the realities of spiritual abuse by offering suggestions for those providing care on how to aid, rather than hurt, people in their spiritual journey and longing. He also suggests help for tracking our own spiritual issues and stories.

Christine Hodgson, Lynda Weaver, and Pippa Hall provide an assessment tool for those who work in a palliative care setting to better assess families who will potentially experience complicated grief. Susan Parker presents the role of personality as a variable in one's grief response. Diane Midland's chapter analyzes the impact of miscarriage that often occurs without interventions that are normally given following a death. All three chapters are empirically based and offer analysis that is grounded on research.

Janis Keyser presents an analysis of death at birth and its impact on the family. She examines research and offers an analysis of journals of grieving mothers.

Hannah Sherebrin discusses the reactions of grief when terrorism occurs. She suggests that, while the grief is ultimately the families' alone, the support of the community (or nation in the case of well-known figures) can greatly aid one's grieving. The sense of community that emerges at times like this might offer a lesson for any town, village, or nation that experiences such traumatic loss.

Richard Paul offers an analysis of viewing the body and its impact on grief from the perspective of a professional funeral director. He critically analyzes the arguments for and against viewing the dead body and makes suggestions for reaching a decision. Robert Stevenson provides educators and parents of school children insights for helping students and those who teach them to manage death in schools. He offers positive interventions and the research to support those interventions. In another chapter that examines grief in family systems, Stephen Hoogerbrugge examines the impact of family systems on grief. He suggests that the family system can be used as a model to aid those experiencing complicated grief. The final chapter by Gerry Cox suggests that care givers consider the use of art in its various forms, music, and humor to aid dying and bereaved children.

SECTION 1

Theories of Complicated Grief

CHAPTER 1

Relearning the World: Always Complicated, Sometimes More Than Others

Thomas Attig

Some time ago I was called by a US television network that was preparing a segment on grief and loss for their news magazine program. The caller began by asking me to tell her my view of "the stages of grief." I said, "I don't believe grieving is as simple as the unfolding of a series of stages. We do not become as much alike when we grieve as that kind of thinking suggests. Nor is grieving something that happens to us; it is what we do in response. We relearn the entire world of our experience." "Well, if it isn't a matter of stages, what is it like then, in your view? Is it like a roller coaster?" she went on. I reiterated, "It really isn't that simple either. It really isn't a very simple matter at all. Relearning a world of experience just doesn't boil down to any such thing." She said curtly, "We'll get back to you," and I never heard from the network again.

They didn't want to hear that grieving is complicated. But any who have been bereaved or who have listened carefully to the bereaved know that grieving nearly always is complicated. "Nearly" because sometimes we grieve moderately: for some who are not particularly close or whose lives are not extensively intertwined with our own. Ordinarily, grieving involves nothing less complicated than relearning the world, including our physical and social surroundings, our place in the greater scheme of things, our selves, and our relationship with the one who has died (Attig, 1996).

Here I do three things: First, I offer clarification of the meanings of "complication." I urge the importance of distinguishing between ordinary and extraordinary complications in bereavement and grieving as a key to estimating when it is more likely that professional support services will prove useful. Second, I show how ordinary grieving as relearning the world is "always complicated" through discussion of how bereavement entails complex suffering and how grieving inevitably involves complex responses to that suffering. Third, I show how grieving is complicated "sometimes more than others" in extraordinary circumstances. In them we encounter "special challenges" that add to the mixture of those we ordinarily face in ways that adversely affect our effectiveness in responding to them. Throughout I consider what the bereaved themselves and their caregivers, including family, friends, and professionals, can do to meet the challenges of relearning the world and overcoming interference in effectively relearning.

ABOUT "COMPLICATED"

The dictionary offers several definitions of "complicated," including "consisting of an intimate combination of parts or elements not easy to unravel or separate; involved, intricate, confused" and "complex, compound, the opposite of simple" (*Oxford English Dictionary*, 1971, I, 729). At most something is complicated when it is a complex mixture or combination. And, correspondingly, a complication is something added that either makes something simple complex or that further compounds already existing complexity.

Given these definitions, we need not hesitate to refer to either bereavement or grieving as complicated. None can deny that bereavement is a complex state resulting from the death of another that affects us in all dimensions of our lives at once. And none can deny that grieving is a complex process of response to our being cast into that state.

None of the dictionary definitions of "complicated" carries the connotation of "additional symptom or pathology" so frequently associated with the term in medical contexts. And it is appropriate to resist this medicalizing connotation when describing bereavement and grieving. Bereavement following the loss of a loved one is a state of deprivation that we all experience many times. It is far less physical than either a disease or a wound and far more like other non-physical deprivations, disruptions, or crises in our lives. Grieving is our normal response to deprivation and loss. In contrast to disease and pathology, effective grieving is functional and adaptive. Bereavement is unusual insofar as it takes us out of the normal patterns of our daily lives and disrupts the smooth unfolding of our life stories. And grieving is a response to the unusual challenges bereavement presents. But neither is unusual in the way that symptoms or pathologies are. There is nothing "wrong with us" when we are bereaved or when we grieve. Bereavement and grieving in themselves are not complicated in this medical sense of the term.

We should also resist the idea that complication entails anything about our need for professional services or their nature when we are bereaved and grieving. In medical contexts, complications are usually cause for alarm and typically rouse professionals to expand or intensify their efforts. The ordinary complications of bereavement and grieving entail no such things. In medical contexts, expanded and intensified professional efforts usually involve the further application of medical treatments to passive recipients, or patients. But none of the ordinary complications of bereavement or grieving are appropriately addressed through the laying on of professional services while we remain passive. Rather, we welcome professional help and benefit from it when it acknowledges that grieving is an inherently active process and when it enables and supports us as we actively respond to what has happened to us (Attig, 1991).

It is, of course, important to identify when those of us who are bereaved or grieving are at risk of unnecessary suffering and more likely to need professional services. And the concern to use limited mental health resources and target services to optimize benefit is legitimate. But referring to complicated bereavement or grieving (as if there were much of either that is not complicated) will not do the work that is required here. On one hand, it would be a mistake to conclude that we will nearly always benefit from professional services because bereavement and grieving are nearly always complicated. We are remarkably resilient and often capable of coming to terms with our suffering and relearning our ways of being and acting in the world in separation from those we love without such services. On the other hand, it also would be a mistake to conclude that we will most likely never benefit from such services because ordinarily we grieve effectively using our own resources and drawing upon the help and support of family and friends. We often meet with challenges that compromise or even block our own effectiveness in grieving, and when we do, we are very likely to benefit from professional services.

A more fruitful question to ask, then, is *not whether* bereavement or grieving is complicated *but precisely how* either sometimes becomes complicated in ways that make it more likely that we will benefit from or even need professional services. Many elements in these experiences are nearly universal (or ordinarily present), and most of us manage to contend with them reasonably well on our own most of the time. Some elements in these experiences that I call "extraordinary complications" are less universal, and they tend to give us more difficulty than we can typically come to terms with on our own. In what follows, I look first at the ordinary complications of bereavement and grieving. Then I offer a categorization of the extraordinary complications that make it more likely that we will benefit from or need professional services.

THE "HURT" OF ORDINARY BEREAVEMENT AND GRIEVING

Too often bereavement and grieving are treated as if they reduce simply to a kind of undifferentiated hurt we experience when someone close has died. As if the experience of emotional pain and anguish were itself without complexity. As if the experiences of bereavement and grieving were entirely emotional in character without equally important psychological, physical, behavioral, social, intellectual, and spiritual aspects and dimensions. And as if the only appropriate help or support for those having such experiences would be listening, comfort, and emotional support.

In focusing on the "hurt" of ordinary bereavement and grieving, I in no way intend to treat these experiences in these simplistic ways. Instead, I intend to describe and analyze the pain and anguish of bereavement and grieving to underscore the complexity of the pain and anguish we typically experience. This analysis serves as a prism through which we can see the complex psychological, physical, behavioral, social, intellectual, and spiritual aspects and dimensions of the experiences that I have described and analyzed more directly in another essay (Attig, 2000a).

Bereavement hurts. When someone we love or care about dies, we are thrust into the state of deprivation we call bereavement. A participant in a workshop years ago perhaps best captured the wrenching character of deprivation when she called bereavement "a choiceless event." It is something that happens to us without our consent. We feel helpless and powerless, at the mercy of, and sometimes victimized by events beyond our control, such as terminal illness, suffering, accident, and death. We may also feel bitter and resentful.

Deprivation also hurts because it entails loss of something precious. We would not experience the death of another as a deprivation or as a loss were it not for our valuing, even cherishing, the living presence that has been extinguished and taken from us. We feel robbed of someone unique and irreplaceable. We experience our lives and our selves as immeasurably diminished and compromised, distant from so much that made life worth living.

When we are bereaved, we suffer a shattering loss of wholeness. The patterns of connections to things, places, other people, experiences, activities, and projects in our daily lives are in tatters. Our individual, family, and community life histories are disrupted and cannot follow the courses we expected them to follow had our loved one lived. Lines of connection to larger wholes and our sense of place in the larger scheme of things within which we find and make meaning are broken, undermined, or threatened. We feel undone, at a loss as to how to go on, anxious, insecure, unsafe, vulnerable. We may also feel abandoned or betrayed.

"Grieving" understood as the painful emotion that accompanies bereavement is itself a complex mode of hurting. We feel the pain of missing those who have died. We long to love and be with them still. The experience of separation from them permeates our experience of the world. Again and again we realize painfully that we will never see or be

seen by, hear or be heard by, touch or be touched by, share daily life with, or walk the world with them. Their absence haunts us. We notice it everywhere. We still carry within us most, if not all, of the desires, motivations, dispositions, habits, expectations, and hopes that shaped and directed our lives while they were with us. We feel sharp dissonance between these things within us and the near constant and often poignant reminders that they are no longer with us. Reality again and again brings us up short. We feel profoundly sad and lonely. We feel the frustration of unfulfilled assumptions, desires, expectations. We miss the satisfactions and fulfillment that only their presence could bring.

Our very souls ache when those we love die. We experience soul pain as we feel uprooted, as if the ground has been pulled out from under us. We feel homesick for the familiar and settled life we knew with those who have died that nourished, sustained, and comforted us. We recognize, and are perhaps ashamed, that we have taken so much for granted. We feel out of place, as if we don't belong anymore among the things, within the places, and with the fellow survivors our loved ones left behind. We are at a loss as to how to reweave familiar threads of caring about these remnants of our lives with those who have died into patterns of daily life without them. We fear that we cannot be ourselves in a world transformed by loss, that returning home and immersing ourselves in life again in familiar ways may no longer bring peace and contentment, that caring again may only lead to more pain.

We are often profoundly dispirited when our loved ones die. We experience spiritual pain as we feel hopeless, mired in sadness and anguish with no visible way out, at a loss as to how we can overcome what has happened and begin moving and striving again. We feel shaken in our faith and fear that life has been drained of its meaning, as if we have been abandoned by higher powers or cast adrift in the greater scheme of things. We feel joyless and fear that we may never again laugh or be happy. We are anxious about what is to become of us. We are daunted by the unknown and unfamiliar future before us. We fear we may be unable to revive hope and find the courage and capacities to meet the unprecedented challenges of giving new shape and direction to our lives.

We experience existential anguish. We feel anxious about our own finiteness and limitations. We feel small and insignificant. Change and impermanence make us feel helpless, powerlessness, without control. Imperfection and fallibility make us feel guilt, if it is our own, or anger, if it is another's. Not knowing, not being able to make sense of things, makes us feel confused, disoriented, abandoned in an unsafe, insecure, chaotic, irrational, and meaningless world. Vulnerability to suffering makes us feel anxious for ourselves and others, fearful of what might happen next.

Our suffering tends to immobilize us. When we suffer, we experience our selves as powerless and helpless, as passive recipients (victims) of blows to our present life patterns, disruptions of our life stories, and separations from larger wholes. We experience our plight as beyond our control, our losses as irretrievable, our present distress and anguish as unending and unrelenting, and our future as hopeless.

Grieving as mourning, the process of coming to terms with bereavement, hurts. It is painful to face and wrestle with challenges. We carry the burdens of relearning the world that none can carry for us: Individually and together as families and communities we struggle to make ourselves whole again. We return home to and try to learn to trust and find meaning again in still viable connections with things, places, events, activities, experiences, and other people (soul work). We endeavor to revive hope as we face the unknown, reshape our daily lives, redirect our life stories, search for a deepened or new sense of our place in the greater scheme of things, and seek new accommodation with the great mysteries that pervade the human condition (spiritual work). We struggle to relearn our relationship with those who have died and make the difficult transition from loving in presence to loving in separation, embracing the legacies of those who have died in individual, family, and community life (Attig, 1996, pp. 163-192; Attig, 2000b). In these ways we work to make ourselves whole again as we endeavor to restore integrity to and find meaning in our daily lives.

As we wrestle with these life transitions, we change in all dimensions of our lives at once. Emotionally, we struggle to find new bases for security and stability. Psychologically, we seek new ground for our self-confidence, self-esteem, and self-identity. Behaviorally, we transform innumerable desires, motivations, habits, and dispositions. Physically, we struggle to meet our biological needs, including our need for closeness. Socially, we shape new patterns of interaction with others at home, at work, and in the community. Intellectually, we question and modify our understandings and interpretations of life, death, and suffering. Soulfully and spiritually, we seek a sense of belonging, a sense of order, a sense of purpose in daily life, a sense that there is reason to go on living, and firmer ground for faith and hope.

We do all of these things while we struggle with the pain of deprivation and loss. It is unrealistic to expect that even the most effective relearning of the world will eradicate the pain of missing those who have died. Nothing can substitute for their living presence. We struggle to learn to carry this residual hurt for the rest of our lives.

As we address these challenges and make these transitions, we feel the weight of hard work. We feel self-doubt about whether we are up to the challenges. We feel anxious and uncertain about what to do. We may become exhausted.

We can do much to mitigate our own hurt in bereavement and grieving. Finding meaningful ways of choosing and doing in response to what has happened to us tempers the pain of deprivation: our feelings of choicelessness, helplessness, and powerlessness. Recovering still viable connections, establishing new life patterns, and giving new direction to our life stories does much to mitigate our pain and anguish. It restores some degree of wholeness to our lives and tempers the shattering hurt of bereavement. As we find our ways back home in our life surroundings and in the experiences and activities of the daily lives we live in them, our soul pain moderates. As we rediscover and revive our capacities for hope, faith, and joy, our spiritual pain moderates.

Learning to love those who have died in separation gives them a new and welcome presence in our lives. We give their legacies places in our memories, practical lives, souls, and spirits. As we do, we realize how much of value in their lives has not been lost. This tempers the pain of missing them, making it unlike the agony of utter deprivation and more like the pain of separation when they were alive.

We can temper our existential anguish as we muster the courage to be. We can work to accept life with human, all too human, limitation. We can endeavor to make ourselves at home in the human condition, the ultimate challenge for our souls. We can rein in discontent rooted in our unwarranted expectations of something more than the human condition affords us while we sustain hope and faith. We can recognize that we are wrestling with mysteries, that is, elements in life, and forces that transcend our grasp and control. We can stop seeking solutions to make it all better. We can realize that our responses to mysteries are at best tentative, provisional, partial, and temporary accommodations. We can recognize that some level of anxiety and insecurity is inevitable. We can resolve to do the best we can, with what we have, where we are, for the moment.

We can cultivate wisdom that the great traditions offer about suffering. They see the tie of our suffering to "desire" and its potential to grip us and undermine our thriving. It is not a recommendation against all desire. It is instead a recommendation to rein in desire and clear our heads of unrealistic expectations. Such expectations take for granted what has not yet been granted and perhaps, or definitely, never will be. Such expectations pretend to know beyond the limits of our knowing. When they do, they become very controlling and demanding. They extend confidence beyond the limits of what we can reasonably anticipate. They are presumptuous.

The wisdom traditions recommend that we avoid reaching beyond the possible, aspiring to transcend the human condition while we remain in it. The wisdom traditions favor hopeful desire over expectation. Hope is neither so pretentious nor so presumptuous as unrealistic expectation. It is more a matter of want and motivation. When we are hopeful, we make ourselves receptive to what might yet be, open to grace. We posture and move ourselves toward the best that life affords. The wisdom traditions encourage us to see that our finite condition is also filled with unforeseen and even surprising possibilities to realize value, find meaning, and know love, including lasting love of those who have died. When we revive hope when those we love have died, we reach through the pain of missing them toward these very possibilities. Realizing them mitigates our sorrow.

Caregivers, too, can do much to mitigate our hurt. Caregivers can only be effective if they respect the uniqueness of our experience of loss and our individuality and recognize the ordinary complexity of grieving: They need to learn how those who have died were individuals who occupied distinct places in our lives. To appreciate how bereavement is itself idiosyncratic and complex in its own ways, encompassing subtly contoured pain and anguish and particular loss of wholeness. To grasp how each of us lives in distinctive life circumstances and has a unique world to relearn. To understand how we make transitions in all dimensions of our individual, family, and community lives at once. To acknowledge how we are, ultimately, wrestling with great mysteries of life, death, suffering, and love from particular perspectives. To be sensitive to our desire to learn to love in separation. They serve us best when they take an active and concerned interest in the details of our lives and experiences.

Caregivers fail us if they harbor illusions about rescuing us from our pain and anguish. They must let go of any desire to eliminate or enable us to entirely overcome our hurt and recognize that much of our grieving is about learning to carry pain. They can offer their presence. In it, they can listen, validate, and normalize the full range of our painful experiences.

Where relearning is complicated in the ordinary ways I have described, caregivers should recognize that relearning the worlds of our experience for us is impossible. Only we can do the work that grieving requires. They should understand that paternalistic intervention (based in presumption about what is "best" for us) is destructive: It fails to respect our autonomy, compounds our helplessness, delays our own relearning, and postpones our returning to thriving again in reshaped and redirected lives. They must appreciate our need to set our own pace and find our own ways in the world again.

Caregivers should be prepared to comfort and support, to be gentle, not demanding. They do best when they reflect about and strive to do what good teachers, mentors, or guides would do to encourage and support us as we face difficult challenges and relearn our ways of being and acting in the world. They can help us to recognize and face the variety of challenges before us, set our own priorities, identify and use our own strengths and other resources, identify and evaluate alternative responses, make and enact choices, and learn from our mistakes. They can be especially effective when they understand how lasting love can motivate our relearning, temper our pain and anguish, and restore our wholeness and that of our families, and communities.

Of course, even when no extraordinary complications are involved, we may welcome and derive great benefit from support groups or professional services. Caregivers often serve us best when they know the value of support groups and are prepared to refer us to them when it appears we could benefit from participation. Family, friends, and members of support groups should know the limitations of their own abilities and the potential of professional services. And they should, when the need becomes clear, do the homework to identify professionals who recognize the ordinary complexity of grieving and have a reputation for promoting our effectively relearning the world.

WHEN BEREAVEMENT OR GRIEVING ARE EXTRAORDINARILY COMPLICATED

Relearning the world is sometimes more complicated when we encounter special challenges. Here I have in mind extraordinary "complications" of the sort that compromise, inhibit, interfere with, undermine, or block the ordinarily quite complex and multi-dimensional journey of the heart and relearning of the world that I have been describing. The point is that we become less effective or even ineffective in grieving when such extraordinary complications are present, not that our grieving itself becomes somehow pathological when they are. When extraordinary complications are involved and our effectiveness in grieving is diminished, the likelihood that professional services will benefit us increases, in some cases to near certainty.

I have in mind three major types of extraordinary complication: Some arise from something between us and those who have died. Some arise from within us. And some arise from circumstances around us.

We are vulnerable to some extraordinary complications that have to do with our relationships with those who have died. Wishing that those who have died were with us is a common aspect of missing them. It is nearly inevitable since our feelings, desires, motivations, habits, and dispositions that took root in the expectation that they would still be with us are not extinguished the instant that they die. Such wishing is harmless and episodic. We do not seriously imagine that such wishes can or will come true.

Preoccupying and fervent longing for their return, by contrast, is dangerous. It hinders or stalls our grieving as it undermines our motivation to reshape and redirect our lives. We "know they are gone." Yet, paradoxically, we desire their return with every fiber of our being. This desire can motivate no action: Nothing can fulfill it since their return is impossible. Such longing frustrates us, induces helplessness, and can paralyze us. It persists as we stay in retreat from a new and frightening reality, dwell in a desire that once held close those who have died, receive secondary rewards for our obvious distress, or fear that we will forget or stop loving those who have died.

We may become preoccupied with unfinished business with those who have died, especially when death is sudden and unexpected. Commonly, we long to share experiences, realize hopes and aspirations for accomplishing something together, utter unspoken words of love and affection, or say good-by. When adults die, the intensity of our anguish over unfinished business depends on our closeness to and the extent of our interaction with them. When children die, parents realize they can no longer watch over and nurture them. The children's very lives seem unfinished when they die prematurely. The greater the burden of unfinished business, as we experience it, the more likely it will distract us from relearning the world effectively.

We are vulnerable to complications in grieving that derive from hurtful or dysfunctional aspects of our relationships with those who have died. Loss of less than fully loving relationships is not less difficult to deal with. Negative ties can bind us more tightly than positive ones and often destructively. We may become caught up in extreme anger for what they did or failed to do or in extreme guilt for what we did or failed to do. We may have been dysfunctionally dependent upon them, or they upon us. We may fervently long for their return to address these issues. This is typically not a loving longing. Resentment, frustration, and bitterness more likely prevail. We struggle even to acknowledge or express these negative ties or feelings. Family and social pressures may reinforce our reluctance.

We are also vulnerable to some extraordinary complications that have to do with our own limitations in ability to relearn. We may lack well developed capacities to relearn but have the potential to acquire them. We may not be up to the emotional, psychological, behavioral, social, intellectual, or spiritual challenges of ordinary grieving. We may lack the physical stamina that grief work demands. Care of the dying through a protracted illness may have sapped our energy. Grief work itself may exhaust us. We may be compromised because we are children, adolescents, or developmentally retarded, or because our coping capacities have been affected by injury, physical illness, or dementia.

We may suffer from any of a wide variety of diagnosable psychological disorders. Some of us have such disorders prior to bereavement. Others may acquire them after bereavement. In either case, they can block, or interfere with, our effectively relearning the world.

We are vulnerable to still other extraordinary complications that have to do with factors in our surrounding life circumstances. Sometimes we must deal with difficult circumstances surrounding the death itself. We may suffer fixating trauma, typically from horrific circumstances of death or experiences where we unexpectedly witness something that overwhelms us. We may be traumatized by multiple deaths that occur all at once or so close together that we experience the challenges of grieving as overwhelming. Such trauma blocks us from dealing with these challenges of relearning the world. The trauma holds our attention. When we experience deaths as preventable or caused by human action, we can become preoccupied with those responsible, mired in legal system and media distractions and interferences, or deeply fearful that we live in a threatening, menacing, and untrustworthy world.

Sometimes we must relearn in social circumstances that seriously interfere with our relearning. Families and community members can hinder or undermine effective individual coping: They can offer bad advice and counsel. They can visit unwelcome expectations or make excessive demands upon us. They can abuse power or authority, attempt to manipulate or control us, or interfere paternalistically in the name of "what is best" as they see it. They can fail to support us when we need support the most. They can discount the significance of our loss or stigmatize our grieving. Families and communities may lack tolerance for individual differences, fail to respect individual preferences, or lack the skills of negotiation, cooperation, and compromise necessary for effective relearning together.

We can do much to help ourselves in coming to terms with extraordinary complications. We can sometimes do remarkably well on our own with even the most difficult of these challenges, especially when we are well supported by family, friends, or members of support groups. We usually avoid allowing simply wishing that those who have died were with us to become fervent longing for their return. Even when we allow it, we are sometimes able to recognize that the desire can lead us nowhere, resist the temptations to dwell in it, and see the possibilities of love in separation as a hopeful alternative. We frequently use our imaginations and take initiatives in addressing and completing unfinished business. Most of even our most loving relationships are ambivalent, and we can often effectively work our way through their negative aspects and avoid becoming caught up in destructive consequences of them. Some of us are quite adept at finding our way through difficult social pressures and impingements on our grieving.

We can recognize when we are becoming overwhelmed by the challenges that extraordinary complications present, when we are becoming frustrated, preoccupied, mired, or stuck. We can sense when we are not prepared for or not effectively addressing the emotional, psychological, behavioral, social, intellectual, or spiritual demands of grieving. We can recognize when we are dealing ineffectively with fervent longing for those who have died, unfinished business, or socially difficult situations. We can honestly acknowledge the likelihood that our own resources will not be sufficient to come to terms with such things as the most powerfully negative elements in our relationships with the deceased, psychological disorders, or trauma. We are often able to recognize when we need help and to take some responsibility for reaching out for it.

Extraordinary complications make it more likely that we will need professional services. Where relearning the world is compromised, hindered, interfered with, undermined, or blocked in any of these ways, friends, family, and volunteers should avoid joining forces with the pestilences, making things worse for us. They should strive to maintain ties with us and embrace us in community. And they should recognize when we are not doing well on our own and are likely to benefit from professional services. They should then encourage and support us as we seek and avail ourselves of them.

Professionals should learn as much as possible about our vulnerability to extraordinary complications in grieving, and how to support us when we are challenged by them. They should learn to recognize when they are out of their depth and refer us when appropriate to others who are specially trained. They should expect that some of us will recognize when we are in trouble and seek their services directly. But they should also expect that many of us will come to them with non-grief-related concerns, and they should be prepared to discern the underlying or hidden issues of compromised grieving. And they should take some responsibility for reaching out and making services available to developmentally challenged populations and survivors of traumatizing deaths.

Professionals can help us address extraordinary complications that arise from something between us and those who have died. They can support those of us who get stuck in fervent longing for those who have died to make the all-important transition from loving in presence to loving in separation. They can help us to identify and embrace the legacies of memory, practical life, soul, and spirit we still have, giving those who have died a new presence in our lives as we do. They can help those of us who become distracted by unfinished business to find ways of doing and saying—literally, symbolically, or ritualistically—what we feel we need to do or say. They are often well prepared to help us when we cannot free ourselves from destructive negative ties that bind us.

Professionals can help us to address extraordinary challenges that arise from something within us. Those with expertise in emotional, psychological, behavioral, social, cognitive, or spiritual areas can facilitate and support us in developing the coping skills we need to effectively relearn the world. Or they can help and support us in ways that compensate for our compromised abilities to relearn on our own. They can also help us to come to terms with psychological disorders and support the still necessary relearning that the disorders compromise.

Professionals can help us to address extraordinary challenges that arise from circumstances around us. Specialists are trained to address the issues of trauma and serious distraction and interference so that we can move on with ordinary grieving. Some can help us individually to understand the social contexts within which we grieve, learn to assert our rights as individuals, learn to respect the rights of others, or learn skills in negotiating our way through troubled social waters. And some can help our families and communities to recognize the shared challenges before us and facilitate and support us as we develop tolerance and the abilities to negotiate, cooperate, and compromise we need to reshape and redirect our collective lives.

CLOSING

So often those who die told us that they "Don't want us to grieve." They very likely mean that they don't want us to become caught up in the ordinary pain and anguish of loss or in any of the extraordinary complications I have described. If they were alive, they would encourage us to seek support from family, friends, support groups, and professionals when we feel we need them. They would want us to do what we need to do to return to life whole. They would want us to remember them and cherish their legacies. They would want us to sense that they still love us. They would want us to find our way back home in life with those who survive with us, embrace life in the human condition, shadow of mystery and all, and keep love for them alive in our hearts.

Effective grieving brings us to these places. We often come to them on our own as we, like so many before us, successfully address the ordinary complications of bereavement and grieving. We are more likely to come to such places through extraordinary complications with the help of skilled professionals. That is surely the point of striving to identify the kinds of extraordinary complications that are likely to compromise, hinder, interfere with, undermine, or block our effectiveness in relearning the world.

REFERENCES

Attig, T. (1991). The importance of conceiving of grieving as an active process. *Death Studies.*

Attig, T. (1996). *How we grieve: Relearning the world.* New York: Oxford University.

Attig, T. (2000a). Relearning the world: Making and finding meanings. In R. A. Neimeyer (Ed.), *Meaning reconstruction and the experience of loss.* Washington, D.C.: American Psychological Association

Attig, T. (2000b). *The heart of grief: Death and the search for lasting love.* New York: Oxford University.

Oxford English Dictionary (1971). New York: Oxford University.

SECTION 2

Children and Complicated Grief

CHAPTER 2

The Consequences of Sudden Traumatic Death: The Vulnerability of Bereaved Children and Adolescents and Ways Professionals Can Help

David W. Adams

Sudden traumatic death can leave bereaved children and adolescents with haunting, vivid memories that may be etched in their thoughts and feelings for the rest of their lives. When tragedy affects the entire family, the ability of parents to nurture, role model, and protect their children is severely compromised by their own grief. This chapter uses case examples to illustrate the vulnerability of bereaved, traumatized children and adolescents; delineates major challenges that confront them; focuses on the impact of sensory stimuli and ways children manage traumatic anxiety; and briefly discusses post traumatic stress disorder (PTSD).

The chapter concludes with a discussion of critical incident debriefing (CISD), the prevention of PTSD, and rules of thumb for professional intervention based on the authors clinical experience.

THE ROLE OF PARENTS IN DEATH EDUCATION OF CHILDREN AND HOW IT MAY BE COMPROMISED

Parents have a compelling need to protect their children from physical and emotional distress. At the same time they are acutely aware of the need to help them to learn and grow so that they are able to cope with the many obstacles and stressors that are part of daily life. Death as a natural part of the life cycle creates a major dilemma. Most parents are aware of the need to help children and adolescents to face death. Yet death is often the least desirable subject for discussion. Death of a family member, friend, or even a pet is accompanied by intense emotions that may be heart rending and begin a prolonged process of mourning. How do parents manage the need to educate and train children to deal with grief when they have an overwhelming desire to protect them?

There is increasing recognition at home and school that for young children in particular, the death of pets or small creatures presents teachable moments. Children can begin to recognize and process some of the characteristics and consequences of death. Teachable moments of this nature are manageable for parents as they tend, in most instances, to cope with the task effectively (Corr, 1995; DeSpelder & Strickland, 1995). When death involves family members or very close friends, the process becomes more difficult. When there is time to prepare, teaching opportunities are exercised more readily than when death is sudden and accompanied by little or no warning. The abilities of children and teens will be governed by a variety of factors such as their cognitive capabilities, the significance of the death, the process of dying, cultural and societal expectations, spiritual beliefs, religious practices, and how constructive the contributions of other important family members, friends, and professionals are in the learning process (Adams & Deveau, 1988; Deveau, 1995). Are children included in the flow of truth about the death? Are they prepared for what they will see, hear, and smell? Are they able to be present at the funeral home and participate in the rituals? Can they openly clarify what has transpired so they can make sense of the death and the behavior of others?

From birth on, all children grieve losses when attachment from loved or familiar objects is broken. It is usually when parental guidance is weak or lacking that children and teens struggle most to comprehend, cope, and learn to live with the significance of an important loss. Often we hear adults assuring the bereaved that they will get over it, that mourning is finite, or mourning is neatly staged in a series of clear emotional segments occurring in a chain reaction. The reality is that although mourning is a natural process and the emotions of mourning are readily identifiable, the patterns of mourning are seldom simple and straightforward. For bereaved children and adolescents, learning to live with a death means revisiting and re-interpreting its impact on their lives at each stage of their development (Adams, 1998). Parental nurturing, role modeling, and willingness to continue to openly share thoughts and feelings about the death over time play a major role in reconciling what has transpired.

Continuance of the teaching process becomes even more difficult for parents when death is sudden, tragic, and impacts heavily on the family. When violence, destruction, mutilation, or multiple deaths are added to the equations, the intensity and complexity of mourning may be amplified for everyone in the family (Rando, 1993). For bereaved children and adolescents often strong attachment to the deceased, close physical proximity to the tragedy, and witnessing the event or its aftermath make them vulnerable to protracted, complicated, and damaging mourning reactions (Frederick, 1985; Pynoos & Eth, 1985).

When the consequences of sudden traumatic death overwhelm parents, and they are preoccupied with their own grief, bereaved children and adolescents may be left on their own to try to understand, adapt to, and make sense of a death. Parental wisdom, guidance, and protection that is usually taken for granted is suddenly absent. When this happens, bereaved children and teens may be simply overlooked. Their needs are lost in the confused aftermath of the tragedy; or adults, other than their parents, see them as requiring less attention than their grieving parents, particularly their mothers. Young children especially may be disenfranchised and sent to stay with relatives or friends (Ellis, 1989). They may be excluded from wakes and funerals at a time when their need for understandable information, emotional support, and family involvement is greatest. Lack of parental guidance makes them especially vulnerable to inaccurate beliefs and perceptions of a death and their responsibilities pertaining to it.

THE VULNERABILITY OF BEREAVED CHILDREN AND ADOLESCENTS

Early in life children are especially vulnerable to grief reactions due to the following:

- limited ability to conceptualize death and comprehend its meaning;
- use of their imagination and magical thinking;
- difficulty communicating their thoughts and feelings;
- dependency on adults for nurturing, role modeling, and protection especially when adults are also mourning;
- lack of emotional maturity and limited capacity to tolerate uncertainty, ambivalence, and vivid death related stimuli; and
- tendency to somatize feelings that are overwhelming (Adams, 1986; Rando, 1995).

Once children at any age emerge from the emotional shock of a sudden tragic death, the impact of the trauma may be so invasive and overwhelming that they are flooded with anxiety-provoking thoughts and difficult emotions. They may regress to behavior common to earlier developmental stages or become passive and helpless. Their ability to cope may be further compromised by their inability to modify the tragic event, to obtain or process information, or to differentiate between life and death, especially if adults forbid them from seeing or touching any part of the deceased.

When left to their own resources the intensity of the loss may prolong shock and postpone or distort mourning. Vivid recall of real or imaginary details of negative effects of the trauma may become etched in their memories and negatively affect their personalities, beliefs, emotions, and conduct for years to come (Everstine & Everstine, 1993; Pynoos & Eth, 1985). The following case examples are snapshots of the legacy of sudden, traumatic deaths faced by children and adolescents.

Case #1

For Tom, no one could compare to his twelve-year-old brother Paul. At age ten, he admired Paul's prowess as a hockey player and constantly sought his company. Their parents, Myra and John, were proud of their boys and the quality of the relationship between them. They were both surprised that both sons still wanted to share a bedroom, play computer games together, and be companions.

In early December, Paul banged his right leg into the boards during hockey. His leg swelled quickly and became extremely painful. Paul and his parents were dismayed when the family doctor admitted him to hospital and arranged to have an orthopedic specialist examine his leg immediately. Tests, x-rays, and further examinations resulted in a diagnosis of osteogenic sarcoma. Paul was devastated when told that his leg might be amputated. Since the age of four he had lived and breathed hockey and his goal in life was to play professionally.

Myra and John were shocked by the diagnosis and distressed at the prospect of amputation. They were relieved that radiation and chemotherapy would be tried first with amputation as a last resort.

Ten days after diagnosis Paul's temperature was elevated. His condition deteriorated rapidly. Within hours he was delirious and died the next morning in his fathers arms. No one, not even the hospital staff, could believe that he would die so suddenly. Tom was devastated. He had remained at home with his grandmother while his parents stayed at the teaching hospital thirty miles away. After shedding tears at the funeral and living through what his parents described as a miserable Christmas for everyone in the family, he became increasingly silent and withdrawn. By mid-April he was failing in school, lashed out and seriously injured another boy in hockey, and became verbally abusive toward his parents. One day in an outburst of anger he accused them of murdering Paul.

Case #2

The fire in the Evan's home began at eleven o'clock on a Saturday evening in November when Douglas, age fourteen, and his friend Robert were smoking in the basement of the old two-storey home. His parents, Beth and Edward, had gone to a late movie leaving Douglas to baby-sit his brother Ira, age nine, and sister Penny, age seven. Both were asleep in separate bedrooms on the second floor.

Douglas and Robert were wrestling when a lighted cigarette fell into a box of cleaning supplies. The fire flared and quickly blocked off the internal stairwell and advanced to the floors above. By the time the boys realized what was happening it was too late to escape except by breaking a basement window, a task made difficult due to protective bars encasing the only remaining route to safety.

A neighbor who saw smoke coming from the frame siding called the fire department.

On the second floor, Penny awoke. Several weeks later she said she knew something was wrong and cried out for her parents, then for Ira and Douglas. Her room was filled with smoke. The door knob was hot and she could not reach Ira's room. Just as the firemen broke her bedroom window and rescued Penny, her room caught fire. She was in shock for several days following. Ira died before he could be rescued.

Douglas was extremely upset. Both he and Robert were severely criticized. His father yelled and screamed at Douglas. Both of his parents were devastated. An angry policeman also chastised Douglas and accused him of killing his brother. This accusation had a profound effect on Douglas and became a dominating influence throughout Douglas' painful, guilt ridden, grief reaction. Five years later at age nineteen, Douglas had dropped out of school, left home, been charged with petty theft and drunkenness, remained unemployable, and rejected all attempts to help him.

Penny was emotionally crushed by Ira's death. She received counseling for the next few months, and gradually began to talk about what transpired, learned to express her feelings and thoughts, and slowly reinvested in life at a new school. Now at age twelve, she says she remembers Ira each day, prays for him and talks to him each evening, and wishes she could be closer to Douglas. Penny and her parents have forgiven Douglas and wish he would return home. His mother says she knows that this will not happen until Douglas learns to forgive himself.

Case #3

The MacDonald household was the noisiest on the street. The neighbors all knew that when Mark began drinking he and Sheila would argue and threaten each other. Their only son Ben, age eleven, was upset that his parents were so unhappy. Deep down he knew they hated each other and on several occasions told his closest friends that he never wanted to go home. Ben was always worried that his parents would separate and stayed in the safety of his room with the family dog when his parents battled. Several times he thought they would kill each other. During the spring semester, Ben's homeroom teacher had noted that Ben seemed sad, preoccupied, and very sensitive to criticism of any kind. She was concerned that he avoided his classmates except for two other boys who lived near him.

One day when the class had completed special outdoor activities, Ben was allowed to go home early. He found his father in the garage with the door closed and the motor running. Mark was slumped over the wheel.

Ben tried unsuccessfully to rouse his father. He shut off the car, opened the garage door, and ran to several homes in the neighborhood. He finally found a neighbor who tried to calm him down long enough to tell her why he was so upset. When she learned what had happened, she called 911 and ran with Ben to his house. Mark was dead when the ambulance, police, and fire department arrived.

At his father's funeral Ben was withdrawn. For several days Sheila could hear him crying in his room and tried to comfort him but he rejected her. In the weeks following he refused to talk with anyone about his father's death, ate very little, and became increasingly preoccupied. Whenever Sheila tried to communicate with him, he retreated to his room. He stopped playing with his friends and could often be found lying on his bed. Eighteen months later, he told a school counselor that he had been planning to kill himself and began to cry incessantly. In therapy, he revealed that he had always believed both parents would have been happier without him. He still believed his mother did not love or want him. However, he thought his father loved him and did not truly want to leave him or hold him responsible for the conflict between his parents. When Ben was suicidal he had believed that the only way to have his father forgive him for causing parental conflict was to join him. However, killing himself was too frightening. Memories of finding his father dead came flooding back and in the counselor's words Ben was "frozen in his misery."

CHALLENGES FOR BEREAVED CHILDREN AND TEENS FOLLOWING SUDDEN TRAUMATIC DEATH

In our case examples, surviving children and teens reflect the array of challenges arising from a sudden, traumatic death. These include 1) intellectual; 2) practical; 3)physical; 4) emotional; 5) social or inter-personal; and 6) spiritual or existential challenges (Adams, 1995; Chesler & Barbarin, 1987).

Intellectual Challenges

When Tom tried to make sense out of his brother's death, the problem was compounded by the reality that even hospital staff were surprised that he had died so suddenly. Tom had great difficulty understanding how a bump on Paul's leg could uncover a more serious, life threatening illness resulting in his death. In his situation, Ben struggled with reasons for his father's suicide. In trying to determine his role in the process he erroneously assumed responsibility for his parents' unhappiness and the final outcome.

Practical Challenges

Because their lives had been so interwoven, Tom missed his continuous contact with his brother. Most of the time Paul had been his advisor, teacher, and role model. At first, Tom had great difficulty sleeping in the room he had shared with Paul as it reminded him of bedtimes when they had laughed or joked or talked about mutual interests and concerns.

For Penny, Ira's death brought major practical repercussions. After the family home was destroyed, her parents could not bear to live there any longer. The loss of familiar surroundings at home, the move away from the neighborhood, and a change of schools midway through the year made Penny's life more difficult at a time when she was least able to manage the changes. In looking back, her parents said they should have remained closer to their old neighborhood and the children's school. Both believed that the move was also difficult for Douglas although he would never admit to anyone that it affected him.

In Ben's life, his father had been his driver and his greatest soccer fan. After he died, Ben ostracized his mother, refused to be driven by neighbors to his games, and stopped playing. Reliance on others was just too difficult.

Physical Challenges

It was several months following his father's death that Ben complained about leg pains that resulted in three trips to the family physician. A careful review of Ben's symptoms revealed that these pains came at bedtime and were accompanied by episodes of choking and complaints that the pain forced him out of bed. Exhaustive medical tests, the nature of the pain, and the characteristics of its onset led the physician to conclude that Ben's symptoms were grief related.

Robert, who had been with Douglas when the fire began and was his best friend, developed severe migraine headaches. In the year following the tragedy, he missed many days of school and required continuous medical attention. It was only when he became part of a bereavement support system that the frequency and intensity of his migraines subsided.

Emotional Challenges

The greatest and most lasting impact of sudden traumatic death is frequently reflected in the extent and duration of emotional trauma. Each bereaved child and teen in our case examples was emotionally traumatized.

Tom's feelings led him to withdraw and become angry. His frustration led him to physically attack another boy and to verbally attack his parents and blame them for Paul's death. Penny, on the other hand, became sad and remained so. Even years later, she cries easily when she thinks about how Ira's death had torn the family apart. Her brother Douglas was overwhelmed with guilt and anger to the point where he rebelled against his parents, the school, and society in general.

Ben's guilt has continued to be a haunting presence in his life. He still feels sad and misses his father; and three years later, he still resents his mother for her part in his father's death and sometimes must remind himself that he is not to blame.

Social or Interpersonal Challenges

When life is difficult to manage at home, when feelings are intense, and regular activities of daily life are disrupted, interpersonal connections may become strained or severed. For instance, Tom was usually quieter than his brother but was well liked by his peers for his modesty at school and his willingness to keep playing hockey even though he was slower and less skilled than most of the team. When he became withdrawn, sullen, and aggressive, his friends left him.

In Penny's life before the tragic fire, neighborhood and school friends were welcome at her home. She had several very close girl friends and loved to mother the younger children next door. The devastation of the family home, relocation to another part of the city, and leaving her school, left Penny feeling lonely and isolated. Despite her parents' encouragement to make new friends, at first it was just too difficult.

Spiritual or Existential Challenges

In the aftermath of a sudden traumatic death the challenges previously cited for bereaved children and teens are often viewed by parents and other significant adults as more important and requiring greater attention than spiritual or existential challenges. Perhaps this is because such challenges are more readily recognized as adult concerns and are more readily fitted into a framework of adult beliefs about life and death. Perhaps parents leave such matters to the clergy as part of religious rituals at the time of the funeral, burial, or cremation; or, perhaps such matters assume little or no importance when spirituality or religion are a low priority in family life (deVeber, 1995).

Regardless of parental priorities, spiritual matters, although heavily influenced by parental beliefs and actions, are seldom completely absent from the thoughts of bereaved children and teens. Sudden death frequently triggers spiritual challenges that may be most difficult for bereaved pre-teens and teens who think in abstract terms and grapple with questions about the meaning of life and death, their identity with the deceased, and their acceptance of their parents' religious practices (Adams & Deveau, 1988; Fleming & Balmer, 1996). Younger children may be more compliant.

For example, at age seven, Penny accepted her parents' belief about heaven and was convinced that Ira was safe there. In her imagination she pictured him up in the clouds, incorporated him into play activities, and kept communicating with him.

Ben was much less certain about where his father went when he died. He was not certain if his father's spirit was safe. He struggled with his desire to be with his father and considered using his own death as a bridge to join him. Ben also had problems with his exposure to the concept of purgatory. In therapy, he said that he would never really know what to believe and rejected the therapist's offer to help him discuss his concerns with the clergy.

Although information concerning Douglas' spiritual beliefs is limited, apparently he was very distressed about Ira's death and tried to reach out to him. In several poems found by his mother after he moved out, Douglas reflected on his "cremation of his brother," and questioned how he could reconnect with his spirit. He wondered if Ira would always be nine years old, and if he would forgive Douglas after Douglas died.

THE SENSORY STIMULI ACCOMPANYING
A SUDDEN, TRAGIC DEATH

When sudden, traumatic death is accompanied by violence, mutilation, or massive destruction, the ability of bereaved children and teens to cope with a range of intense, interconnected challenges may be compromised by sensory recall. Sights, sounds, smells, and tactile stimuli become noxious when they trigger rapid recall of terrifying and devastating experiences that result in immediate distraction and distress (Adams, 1998; Ayalon, 1983; Frederick, 1985; Pynoos & Eth, 1985; Terr, 1985, 1990, 1991).

For example, Penny panics when she smells woodsmoke or hears the crackling of a fire or the sound of sirens. Ben cannot tolerate the smell of automobile exhaust, avoids garages, and has an aversion to touching anything dead, such as meat or poultry.

I have encountered other examples which reflect the intensity of visual stimuli. For example, Monica in her late teens, when discussing the impact of her sister's death ten years previously, said,

> I remember the newspaper picture of my sister's mangled bicycle, her running shoe, and the black puddles on the road. Even as a child I knew the puddles were her blood. I still cannot stand the sight of blood and avoid reading the newspaper.

PROCESSING THE AFTERMATH

Managing Traumatic Anxiety

In their classic works, Pynoos and Eth suggest that there are four psychological methods that children use to manage traumatic anxiety. These include the following:

1. *Denial-in-fantasy* in which children and some adolescents try to revise or modify the outcome of the event in order to lessen the severity of what has transpired.
2. *Inhibitions of spontaneous thought* achieved by avoiding reminders of the event and reducing exposure to mind triggers.
3. *Fixation to the trauma* through an incomplete, detached, objective recounting of the details of the tragedy or repetitive partialization of the severity of the experience demonstrated through expressive media.
4. *Fantasies of future harm* which add new fears that supplant the anxiety generated by the tragic event. (Pynoos & Eth, 1985, p. 25)

In the process of assimilating information when violence is a major contributor to sudden death, children and teens may replay the violent act by assuming the roles of victim, perpetrator, or rescuer. The role of perpetrator for males is the most dangerous as it may trigger uncontrollable rage and intense retribution anxiety (Hendricks, Black, & Kaplan, 1993).

Post Traumatic Stress Disorder (PTSD)

The adult literature warns that tragic events outside of the usual range of human experience may result in symptoms collectively categorized as Post Traumatic Stress Disorder (PTSD). Both adults and children may develop PTSD as a result of homicide, suicide, disaster, war, molestation, rape, abuse, incest, or life threatening illness.

Researchers and clinicians such as Terr, Pynoos and Eth, and Frederick, all suggest that PTSD symptoms of children and adolescents frequently differ from those of adults in frequency and intensity (Ayalon, 1983; Frederick, 1985; Pynoos & Eth, 1985; Terr, 1985, 1990, 1991). Three major components are present in their reactions:

1. Re-experiencing the traumatic event which may include the following:
   - pre-verbal memory of a tragic event that may lead young children to exhibit in play, mannerisms, and feelings associated with distress that are traceable to infancy or early childhood;
   - recurrent nightmares and night terrors especially from toddler stage on;

- visual hallucinatory episodes or feelings of presence experienced by some children particularly in the stages of latency and pre-adolescence;
- integration of thoughts and visions of this tragic event in play or dreams as opposed to suffering visual flashbacks common to adults. I believe that in mid-to-late adolescence flashbacks may be present in keeping with the ability to think in abstract terms. However, the frequency and rationale of this occurrence merit further study.

2. Avoidance of stimuli associated with the trauma or a numbing of general responsiveness include the following:
   - the potential absence of the psychic numbing found in traumatized adults. This process may be manifested more basically by showing lack of feeling;
   - inclusion of residual psychic phenomena in their play including re-enactment of the tragic event;
   - an absence of the vegetative or nervous symptoms displayed by adults.

   Alternatively, children and sometimes teens may exhibit physical distress as a component of phobic reactions or chronic anxiety and may exhibit these signs:
   - regressive behavior common to previous developmental stages;
   - an absence of disavowal or traumatic amnesia. However, I am concerned that a delayed and partial traumatic amnesia with symptoms such as increased arousal, hypervigilance, and panic reactions may surface later in adulthood and be manifested as anxiety disorders.
   - hints that their future may be shortened. Mid-to-late adolescents may parallel adult reactions and be less willing to communicate or be more secretive about such thoughts.
   - differences in time interpretation particularly in pre-latency as young children lack the sense of time and the historical perspective common in adolescence and adulthood.

3. Persistent increased arousal is a common problem that may be manifested through these symptoms:
   - hypervigilance, especially when children are fearful of a recurrence of the traumatic event or are suffering from chronic anxiety;
   - problems getting to and remaining asleep as children frequently engage in reflection at bedtime. Memories of the deceased may be aroused through discussions with a surviving parent or adult; sharing thoughts and feelings with siblings; listening to stories; prayers; or experiencing the loneliness of a darkened room. In some instances, children who wake up in the night may gravitate to

unusual places to sleep in safety such as on a mat close to the family dog or beside a parent's bed or outside of the room of a deceased sibling (Adams, 1998);

• irritability aggravated by sleeplessness, emotional fatigue, a parent's behavior, the absence of the deceased, or major changes in their lives. Underlying rage, accumulation of frustration, and inability to perform regular activities or control peers may result in aggressive outbursts, especially on the playground;

• concentration difficulties manifested in children's restlessness and inability to focus at school. Although Terr suggests that school difficulties are short lived, I believe that for some bereaved children concentration problems are prolonged or delayed. When children remain untreated for PTSD reactions, they may be misdiagnosed by school officials who believe that they have learning deficiencies or attention deficit disorders(ADD) (Adams, 1998).

HOW PROFESSIONALS CAN HELP

Key Components of Intervention to Prevent PTSD

In our work with traumatized, bereaved children and adolescents we must be acutely aware of the need to understand their limits of tolerance. In some instances, older children and adolescents show us that they have reached their limits by changing the subject, becoming angry, or telling us they have had enough. Younger children may require increased sensitivity on our behalf and a willingness to structure sessions and limit content in order to avoid reaching their saturation point. The literature reflects a diversity in the beliefs and practices of professionals who help bereaved children and adolescents to debrief, cope with the impact of a sudden tragic death, and prevent PTSD. However, intervention may enable bereaved children and teens to do the following:

1. reduce avoidance of the details of the sudden traumatic event and its impact;
2. describe and discuss such details and have their questions answered honestly in terms they understand;
3. incorporate activities and rituals that have meaning for them;
4. express their thoughts and feelings through puppets, dramatic play, or other expressive modalities such as art, creative writing, or poetry;
5. re-live the experience and be desensitized in vivo. Bereaved children and teens in this process are re-introduced to the site and the sensory stimuli of the tragic event under the supervision of highly skilled therapists. This process is not favored by some

clinicians as it may cause psychic numbing that further complicates grief reactions;

6. manage their thoughts, feelings, and physical symptoms. Mastery may help rebuild self-confidence;
7. increase their awareness of noxious stimuli that can trigger outbursts of intense emotions, particularly anger, that may result in aggression and destruction (Adams, 1998).

Intervention Methodologies

Group Critical Incident Debriefing

Both group and individual intervention can be effective in debriefing bereaved traumatized children and adolescents and preventing PTSD. Group intervention following the Mitchell Model for adult debriefing focuses on seven phases through which critical incident victims are guided (Mitchell & Everly, 1994) . These include the following:

1. introduction of the intervention team, ground rules, and process (Introduction Phase);
2. a description of the facts from each participant's perspective (Fact Phase);
3. sharing participants' cognitive reactions (Thought Phase);
4. discussion of the most important aspects of the event (Reaction Phase);
5. identification of personal symptoms of distress (Symptom Phase);
6. education by the intervention team concerning normal reactions and adaptive coping mechanisms. The team provides a cognitive anchor and facilitates stress management (Teaching Phase);
7. clarification of ambiguities and preparation for closure (Re-entry Phase).

A modified version of this process may be applied when bereaved children and teens have had the opportunity to rest and begin to recover from the initial impact of the tragedy. For instance, children in a classroom or recreational group who have witnessed tragedies may, with careful preparation and guidance, benefit from debriefing in the company of peers (Terr, 1985, 1990). Facilitators who apply group debriefing techniques must be aware of the fragility of some children or teens and provide other alternatives for victims who should not wish to be part of this process. For those who are capable of participating, skilled group debriefers who are sensitive, patient, and willing to let children and teens express their thoughts and feelings over one or several group sessions can be extremely effective. Modifications in applying the Mitchell model in this context may include limiting discussion to one or two phases, with repetition of a brief introduction and a process for closure at each session. Another approach may involve continuing a discussion which involves all or most phases over several days. Often a less rigid but structured format that includes the use of non-verbal techniques to facilitate expression works best. Fundamental to intervention with traumatized bereaved children and adolescents is the need to allow them to use their creativity, to have adequate time for discussion and diversion as needed, and to help them find ways to help each other cope. Children usually demonstrate much more capability than adults to connect with and help each other.

Individual Debriefing and Prevention of PTSD

In some situations, group debriefing is inappropriate, too difficult to introduce, or a second choice to individual debriefing sessions for traumatized bereaved children and teens. Individual debriefing may be less threatening, easier to manage, and more personal. For this purpose, a useful and effective methodology was developed by Pynoos and Eth. Their approach involves a ninety-minute interview for assessment and debriefing that has been proven effective with children ages three to sixteen who are prone to PTSD. I appreciate the flexibility in the timing of the application of their technique. It can be used for both debriefing and therapeutic intervention when PTSD symptoms are entrenched (Pynoos & Eth, 1986; Pynoos, Frederick, Nadar et al., 1987). The process includes three phases:

1. *Engagement or Validation* in which children and teens recount their story and draw relevant pictures. This process links their inner concerns to the event.

2. *In-depth exploration* focusing on perceptions and affect in order to facilitate release of emotions. The therapist leads the child or teen through a process that includes discussion, enactment, or illustration of each part of the traumatic experience. Subjects are encouraged to include specifics of what happened, their observations, perceptions, and the worst moment. This phase includes confrontation of accountability issues; fantasies about preventive or modifying action that could have changed the outcome; expression of anxiety and the potential for punishment and retaliation; acknowledging fear of recurrence; discussion of previous traumatic experiences and dreams; and concerns about impulse control.

3. *Closure* involves a review of the session; acknowledgment of normalcy and legitimacy; an outline of future expectations; reinforcement of self-esteem; and evaluation of the interview.

Pynoos and Eth found that the interviews brought immediate relief and improvement. Traumatized children and adolescents were most willing to accept further assistance and stated that the discussion of revenge fantasies helped them most.

Although one interview may bring considerable relief and result in permanent, positive adaptation, it is important to recognize that in some instances, further therapy may be in order. In my practice, I may pursue the content of each phase in greater detail in interviews held weekly over two or three months. Much depends on my assessment of their needs, based on their limitations and vulnerability. Several rules of thumb apply. These include the following:

1. Debrief as early as possible once initial needs for safety, security, nurturing, and rest have been met. Traumatized bereaved children and adolescents need to be able to discuss and manage what they think and feel. Even brief discussions may be taxing for some children. Careful evaluation is a necessity.
2. Provide individual follow-up after each debriefing whenever feasible and definitely when participants appear to be vulnerable to progressive complicated mourning reactions.
3. Provide sufficient time for the use of age-appropriate expressive techniques.
4. If intervention is extended, expect some regressive behavior and help children and teens to manage it.
5. Welcome doll and cuddly animal partners. The security of a doll or toy may facilitate indirect expression of thoughts or feelings in pre-latency and latency children in particular.
6. Remember that trust is the cornerstone of successful intervention. Children and teens need to feel secure, to have their confidentiality and privacy respected, and to be clear about the process and content of interviews.
7. Establish routines that are readily identifiable and non-threatening.
8. Consider linkage to other therapists for longer term or more skilled therapy when needed. Consider the use of bereavement support groups as an adjunct to or extension of intervention.
9. Remember that children and adolescents are an integral part of a family system and are guided and protected by parents. They may need our assistance to express their thoughts, feelings, and needs to parents or to advocate with their permission on their behalf. The ground rules for parental contact and involvement need to be established at the beginning of the process so that everyone is clear about the flow of information and the potential for parents to communicate and reinforce gains made in individual or group debriefings or therapy.

IN CLOSING

As professionals we are privileged to be granted the opportunity to help bereaved children and adolescents manage the sequelae of sudden tragic death and avoid the complications that result from memories festering beneath the surface for years to come. Our availability, sensitivity, honesty, and clinical skill can ensure that they are able to face what transpired. We can help them examine their thoughts, feelings, and behavior, work through the process of mourning, and learn to live with their losses.

Our relationship may also enable us to assume the roles of educator and advocate so that children and teens are supported appropriately by significant adults. We may help to stabilize the living environment; facilitate family communication; coach parents to meet the needs of their bereaved children and teens; advocate for their involvement in adult rituals; and help adults to avoid blaming them for the tragedy or allocating inappropriate roles and responsibilities. Marty, age ten, summed up the potential benefits of involvement when he told me the following:

> I felt awful when Cathy (his sister age twelve) was killed. I couldn't talk about it. My Dad was angry and Mom just kept crying. I didn't want to come here (to my office) but I guess I needed to. It still hurts but I can talk about her now. My Mom and Dad talk to me too . . . it's better now for all of us . . . we will be OK.

REFERENCES

Adams, D. W. (1986). Understanding sibling grief and helping siblings to cope. In G. H. Paterson (Ed.), *Children and death*. London, Canada: King's College.

Adams, D. W. (1995). The suffering of children and adolescents with life-threatening illness: Factors involved and ways to help. In D. W. Adams & E. J. Deveau (Eds.), *Beyond the innocence of childhood: Helping children and adolescents cope with life-threatening illness and dying* (Vol. 2). Amityville, NY: Baywood.

Adams, D. W. (2000). Children's exposure to sudden traumatic death: Bereavement, post-traumatic stress disorder and the case for early intervention. In J. D. Morgan (Ed.), *Meeting the needs of our clients creatively*. Amityville, NY: Baywood.

Adams, D. W., & Deveau, E. J. (1998). How the cause of a child's death may affect a sibling's grief. In M. A. Morgan (Ed.), *Bereavement: Helping the survivors*. London, Canada: King's College.

Ayalon, O. (1983). Coping with terrorism. In D. Meichenbaum & M. Juremko (Eds.), *Stress reduction and prevention*. New York: Plenum Press.

Chesler, M. A., & Barbarin, O. A. (1987). *Childhood cancer and the family*. New York: Brunner/Mazel.

Corr, C. A. (1995). Children and death: Where have we been? Where are we now? In D. W. Adams & E. J. Deveau (Eds.), *Beyond the innocence of childhood: Factors influencing children and adolescents' perceptions and attitudes toward death* (Vol. 1). Amityville, NY: Baywood.

DeSpelder, L. A., & Strickland, A. L. (1995). Using life experiences as a way of helping children understand death. In D. W. Adams & E. J. Deveau (Eds.), *Beyond the innocence of childhood: Factors influencing children and adolescents' perceptions and attitudes toward death* (Vol. 1). Amityville, NY: Baywood.

Deveau, E. J. (1995). Perceptions of death through the eyes of children. In D. W. Adams & E. J. Deveau (Eds.), *Beyond the innocence of childhood: Factors influencing children and adolescents' perceptions and attitudes toward death* (Vol. 1). Amityville, NY: Baywood.

deVeber, L. L. (1995). The influence of spirituality on dying children's perception of death. In D. W. Adams & E. J. Deveau (Eds.), *Beyond the innocence of childhood: Helping children and adolescents cope with life-threatening illness and dying* (Vol. 2). Amityville, NY: Baywood.

Ellis, R. R. (1989). Young children: Disenfranchised grievers. In K. Doka (Ed.), *Disenfranchised grief: Recognizing hidden sorrow*. Lexington, MA: Heath and Company.

Everstine, D. S., & Everstine, L. (1993). *The trauma response: Treatment for emotional injury*. New York: W. W. Norton & Company.

Fleming, S., & Balmer, L. (1996). Bereavement in adolescence. In C. A. Corr & D. E. Balk (Eds.), *Handbook of adolescent death and bereavement*. New York: Springer.

Frederick C. F. (1985). Children traumatized by catastrophic situations. In S. Eth & R. S. Pynoos (Eds.), *Post-traumatic stress disorder in children*. Washington, D.C.: American Psychiatric Press.

Harris Hendricks, J., Black, D., & Kaplan, T. (1993). *When father kills mother*. London: Routledge.

Mitchell, T., & Everly Jr., G. S. (1994). *Human elements training for emergency services, public safety and disaster personnel: An instructional guide for teaching debriefing, crisis intervention and stress management programs*. Ellicott City: MD: Chevron Publishing Corporation.

Pynoos, R. S., & Eth, S. (1985). Children traumatized by witnessing acts of personal violence. In S. Eth & R. S. Pynoos (Eds.), *Post-traumatic stress disorder in children*. Washington, D.C.: American Psychiatric Press.

Pynoos, R. S., & Eth, S. (1986). Witness to violence: The child interview. *Journal of the American Academy of Child Psychiatry, 25*, 306-316.

Pynoos, R. S., Frederick, C., Nader, K., Arroyo, W., Steinberg, A., Eth, S., Nunez, F., & Fairbanks, L. (1987). Life threat and post-traumatic stress disorder in school-age children. *Archives of General Psychiatry, 44*, 1057-1063.

Rando, T. A. (1993). *Treatment of complicated mourning*. Champaign, IL: Research Press.

Rando, T. (1995). Anticipatory grief and the child mourner. In D. W. Adams & E. J. Deveau (Eds.), *Beyond the innocence of childhood: Helping children and adolescents cope with death and bereavement* (Vol. 3). Amityville, NY: Baywood.

Terr, L. (1985). Children traumatized in small groups. In S. Eth & R. S. Pynoos (Eds.), *Post-traumatic stress disorder in children*. Washington, D.C.: American Psychiatric Press.

Terr, L. (1990). *Too scared to cry*. New York: Basic Books.

Terr, L. (1991). Childhood traumas—An outline and overview. *American Journal of Psychiatry, 110,* 10-20.

CHAPTER 3

Homicide Bereavement: Scary-Tales for Children

Paul T. Clements, Jr.

Every day on television networks across the United States, news reporters inform the public of yet more homicides. Exposure to violent crime, and more so to violent death and murder, has dramatically increased over the past decade. Murder is the unlawful taking of human life.[1] It is a behavioral act that terminates life in the context of power, personal gain and brutality (Douglas, Burgess, Burgess, & Ressler, 1992). "The weapons of murder are as manifold as the unlimited human imagination: shotguns, rifles, pistols, knives, hatchets and axes, meat-cleavers, machetes, ice picks, bayonets, hammers, wrenches, screwdrivers, crowbars, pry-bars, two-by-fours, tree limbs, jack handles, building blocks, crutches, artificial legs, brass bedposts, pipes, bricks, belts, neckties, pantyhose, ropes, bootlaces, towels and chains" (Maples & Browning, 1994, p. 119). Homicide is a public health problem in the United States, resulting in a catastrophic impact upon not only the actual murder victim, but those left behind in the aftermath. This is an especially unique and painful burden for children to bear.

CASE EXAMPLE #1

In November, as a cold Autumn rain pelted Fayette Street in Philadelphia, a man wearing a wolfman mask attacked a woman and her seven-year-old daughter as they returned from an after-school center. After parking the car, the mother and child approached the back door to their home as part of their daily routine. The masked man approached from behind and ordered them both inside.

---

[1]Although the literature makes distinctions between the legal definitions for homicide, murder, and killing, for the purpose of this chapter these terms will be used interchangeably.

Once inside, he forced both the mother and the daughter upstairs, where he tied the girls' hands and feet with shoelaces and left her lying in the second-floor hallway. The little girl, named Danielle, told police that a short time later she began to hear loud noises, noises that investigators believe were three gunshots. Danielle reports that she kept her eyes closed tight out of panic and fear. Around midnight, roughly six hours after the ordeal began, Danielle managed to free herself, and fled the house with a tale of horror that turned out to be true: her mother lay dead, shot to death, on the bathroom floor. She immediately phoned her grandmother in West Philadelphia, who called the police. Officers who arrived at the house found Danielle's mother in the shower of the basement powder room. She had been shot at least once in the left temple and was pronounced dead at the scene. The man behind the wolfman mask still lurks somewhere in the city (Gammage, 1995; Gibbons, 1995).

CASE EXAMPLE #2

On a warm June evening in a quiet town, seven-year-old Seth played in the aisles of the small mini-mart store where his mother worked. As he played, his mother, Tammy, made preparations to close the store for the night as she had done for many years. Across the street, Tammy's "friend" Christian was sitting in his truck, waiting to take her and Seth home. After locking the glass doors to the store, Tammy and Seth were quite terrified as Alex, her estranged husband, used a sawed-off shot-gun to shatter the door, announcing loudly to Tammy: "Honey . . . I'm here. . . ." Alex approached as she was trying to use the checkout counter as protection, and proceeded to shoot her repeatedly. As Seth watched with horror, he begged his father: "Please daddy!!! Don't hurt mommy!!" Subsequently, Seth watched from a distance of less than 10 feet as his father repeatedly pelted his mother's body with bullets.

As Seth lay crying over his mothers lifeless body, Alex walked out of the store and across the street to where Christian was still waiting in his pick-up truck. Totally unaware of what had just happened, Christian was not expecting the appearance of Alex in his truck window, with subsequent gunshots to the face, head, and torso; his mission complete, Alex climbed into his car and disappeared into the night. In the meantime, Seth picked up the store phone and dialed the one number he had committed to memory: his grandmother's. As reported by the police, when they arrived at the store, Seth was sitting on the curb in front of the store with his head in his hands. His mother's lifeless body behind him and that of Christian slouched onto the steering wheel of the truck across the street, both in clear view.

That night, Alex called the police to give an account of the crime as he expressed a desire to preserve the accuracy of the events. The next day he was found hanging from the large arm of a front loader by several landfill site construction workers. He apparently had committed suicide. In less than twenty-four hours, Seth had lost the three most important people in his life to the grip of violent death. The three people upon whom he depended for day-to-day love, support, and belonging.

SCARY-TALES FOR CHILDREN

The above vignettes are not lines from some movie script or book; rather, they are accounts of two tragic but true murders experienced by children. Tales such as these are becoming all too common in our country. In cities all around the country, children are hearing gunshots inside and outside their homes, witnessing shootings, stabbings, and other assaults What action must be taken to respond to these surviving children of a murdered loved one? What are their needs? How can we ensure that these children who are survivors of a murdered loved-one will receive the compassion, care, and support that will help them rebuild their lives?

Before any action can be taken to address the needs of these survivors of murder victims, it is critical to have a clear understanding that these children are more than just traumatized individuals. Indeed, they are victims as well, resulting from the sudden and traumatic loss accompanying a homicide. Unfortunately, all too often, the attention of the media and the shocked community is on the murder victim and the murderer. This is presented, not to say that it is necessarily wrong or abnormal, rather, to bring forth the fact that the survivors, especially the children, are typically lost in the shadows of all the surrounding trauma. Stereotypically, children are thought to be resilient and able to withstand such traumatic events by "bouncing back." However, these children are probably more significantly traumatized than anyone could imagine.

Homicide is the sudden and deliberate taking of another's life. The homicide victim represents the loss of a father, mother, sibling, or other significant person. The effects of homicide are not limited to the death of the murder victim. While the victim's violation and suffering ends with the death, the child's trauma, victimization, and grief begins with the death. The process of grieving that occurs after the homicide of a loved one is referred to as "homicide bereavement." There is no escape from the severe pain and multifaceted aspects of victimization associated with homicide. For the bereaved, homicide creates a uniquely painful new existence: life without hope of ever again being in the presence of the lost loved one. Coping with this new life in the absence of the loved one represents one of the most difficult and immediate tasks in homicide bereavement.

Although there is a paucity of literature surrounding children who are exposed to homicide, this type of death represents a significant and serious trauma and threat to their biopsychosocial development (Brazino, 1998; Clements, 1996; DeSpelder & Strickland, 1996; Redmond, 1989). Researchers have explored responses in traumatized children, and these studies have contributed toward the identification, description, and understanding of symptoms related to trauma responses for a number of stressors, such as sexual abuse (Burgess, Hartman, & Clements, 1995; van der Kolk, 1989, 1988), exposure to violence (Burgess, 1975; Eth, 1989; Eth & Pynoos, 1994; Eth, Silverstein, & Pynoos, 1985; Pynoos & Eth, 1984), and the death of a parent (Finklestein, 1988; Terr, 1991). However, studies of the traumatic effects in children who have lost a loved one to homicide are few.

Loss of a loved one to homicide is a serious problem, especially for children (Clements, 1998; Henry-Jenkins, 1993; Van Epps, Opie, & Goodwin, 1997). Pynoos and Nader (1993) related that exposure to trauma such as homicide may be particularly challenging for children since the child must integrate the experience into a new inner model of the world by imposition upon a model already undergoing constant revision. This can provide a significant challenge to a child's development and ability to cope (Burgess & Clements, 1997; Burgess & Roberts, 1997; Stevenson, 1996). In spite of the lack of statistics for children, the number experiencing this type of bereavement in the United States is conceivably vast and only a conservative estimate can be presented. Above all else, it is critical to understand that any child exposed to this type of traumatic loss is at significant risk for Post-Traumatic Stress Disorder and for complicated and potentially ineffective grieving (Clements, 1998; Picket, 1997; van der Kolk, 1988, 1989).

The brutality with which homicide is committed snuffs out the life of the victim and devastates the senses of the survivors. It is the ultimate crime of human design; the purposeful taking of one person's life by another, which makes it even more uniquely painful and complex. From the moment of the act, the child is faced with the fact that someone violently and intentionally extinguished the life of another; the life of someone they loved—a life that was taken that can never be returned.

Homicide can produce myriad emotional responses in child survivors. According to Burgess (1975), surviving family members experience emotions that are either victim-oriented or self-oriented. They are enraged that a loved one has been killed and at the same time fearful for their own lives. The unexpected transgressive loss evokes intense anger, rage, and feelings of retribution.

Homicide also initiates an unanticipated bereavement (Henry-Jenkins, 1993; Rando, 1993; Redmond, 1996). Children never imagine the day when someone will tell them that a loved one is gone and can never come back. This message is then eventually compounded with the details surrounding the traumatic mode of death. The fact that the act is transgressive and has permanently taken their loved one away, generates the secondary victimization of the trauma, loss, and emotional upheaval. There is shock and typically disbelief. Questions without answers compound the disbelief, confusion, and anger. "How could someone do this to a person I love?" "Can they really never come back?" "Will I really never see them again?" and "I didn't get to say goodbye!" are all typical responses from children in such a situation.

Grieving under normal circumstances is difficult, and is only made more intense after a homicide. There are many reasons that survivors experience such great stress which may lead toward a disruption in functional grieving. These include the transgressive mode of death, the accompanying burden of a legal inquiry, interface with members of law enforcement, the experience of the medical examiners office, sensational and sometimes inaccurate coverage by the news media, and the complexities of the criminal justice department. Contact with each of these agencies is an ongoing reminder of the murder, and subsequently it potentially deepens the sorrow and the suffering of the survivors. It can ultimately result in the grief process being delayed or abandoned. The dynamics of interface with each of these agencies will be presented. It will demonstrate how the aftermath of homicide is a complicated and multifaceted process which predisposes the surviving individuals to complicated grieving which can lead to Post-Traumatic Stress Disorder, manifest in depression, addictions, mental illness, aggressive behavior, and possibly exacerbate pre-existing medical conditions.

LAW ENFORCEMENT

Police officers and homicide detectives are among the first officials with whom survivors must interface. Frequently, it is the duty of the police to bring the news of the murder to the next of kin. Many families are in total shock when the policeman gives the death notification. Often they are unable to process the words and the information being imparted to them. Typically the initial response to the news is anger, which is often focused and projected onto the police officer; the messenger. Having talked with many families about when they were "told," a common theme arises that, in reality, there would have actually been no "good" or "better" way for the police to "tell" them of their loved one's murder. One mother told me "It's not really 'how' the news is delivered, it's just 'that' the news is delivered; news that nobody ever wants to hear!" An additional factor that compounds the delivery of the news is the double-edged sword of the accompanying information. Naturally the first things a family will want to know are: Who did it? What happened? How did the death occur?

Where? and Have any arrests been made? Answers to these questions may or may not be given by the police officer based on the current progress of the investigation and the final determination of the cause and manner of death as a result of a forensic autopsy. Often, families feel like they are told their loved one has been murdered, but then they are "kept in the dark." One father expressed his rage at the police, stating: "They [the police] asked me a hundred questions about my son, like I was on trial, but I answered them. But then, every time I asked the Police a question, they kept tellin' me that they couldn't tell me nothin' because it was 'pending further investigation.' I told them I didn't care about no damn pending investigation. My son was dead, shot like a dog, and I wanted answers! But all I kept getting was the run around. But they acted like they didn't even hear me and asked me more questions!"

The police investigation can take a long time and the hours of inquiry may become very traumatic for the survivors. In fact, children who were witnesses to the murder, or who were nearby, are often questioned, and this frequently occurs at the police department. This can be significantly distressing to a child. Actually, after being questioned by police, some children have expressed feeling as if they were suspects, and they become distrusting of the law enforcement officials. Additionally, many children often feel guilt and responsibility for not being able to prevent the murder, a dynamic which can be inadvertently reinforced if the questioning is not structured in a way as to avoid the misperception of inferring blame. Furthermore, this can become a re-surfacing issue later if no one is apprehended, arrested or charged with the homicide. Children who lose someone to homicide are already victims and can be easily re-victimized by the investigation.

MEDICAL EXAMINERS OFFICE

In most states, the law demands that all deaths which are the result of a homicide or suspected homicide must be investigated by the medical examiner or coroner. An integral part of a homicide investigation is the Medical Examiners Office (MEO). The Medical Examiners Office is responsible for facilitating positive identification of the murder victim, investigating the related circumstances, and determining the cause of death. The murder victim's body usually must be identified by two immediate family members after the autopsy is completed. In essence, the murder victim's body has now become a piece of forensic evidence, and although the MEO attempts to be timely in their examination, there are cases when release of the body is delayed, and therefore the family's grieving rituals are also delayed. Additionally, for most family members, an autopsy is yet another violation of the deceased loved-one's body, and accepting the procedure is often made more difficult since the family actually has no choice or control in approving it. Frequently, children accompany adults to the MEO for the identification of the body. Some family members feel it necessary and important to share the experience with the children; others are unable to find suitable babysitting. As a result, the children can be exposed to the information surrounding the murder, including information gleaned from the crime scene, the circumstances surrounding the death (such as violence, torture, or rape preceding the actual murder), and may also see the deceased body on the viewing screen or in the identification room. Often, the body will still be in the same condition as at the time of death, including bruises, blood stains, and mortal wound sites (gunshot wounds, stab wounds, or wounds from blunt trauma). This visual and experiential information will add stress to the grief and trauma already set in motion by the recent death notification.

NEWS MEDIA

When someone is murdered, it becomes news. This occurs because it is a crime and an act against the commonwealth of the people. In other crimes, many of the victims are treated with confidentiality. This is not true with murder victims. Along with the murder victim, the family members are thrown into the public view, and there is a loss of a great deal of privacy for grief and stabilization in the family system. There is no parity, however, in media publicity. Some homicides receive a great deal of exposure, and others receive little or none. As counterintuitive as it may seem, some family members may be angered by both levels of publicity based on their own need for others to know their plight. For children, there is no escape from other children at school or the neighborhood to know the details of their loved-one's death. The child may feel embarrassed or different from his peers as a result of the murder, especially if death revolved around a crime, such as drug trafficking, and especially if this is announced on the news day after day. Furthermore, homicide is never painted in a positive light; the media coverage is a frequent reminder that their loved one was murdered, and the horrible details with which the death occurred.

CRIMINAL JUSTICE SYSTEM

Once any facet of the criminal justice proceedings start, families are frequently enraged to learn that they are merely spectators and their deceased loved one is almost nothing more than evidence. As with the news media and the law enforcement officials, the criminal justice system wants to understand the circumstances surrounding the murder. Yet, it is through learning about the details of the murder that significant stress can be added to the family system, potentially leading to the disruption of grieving in the surviving members. Family members have often expressed that within the Defense Attorney's attempts at doing a good job in representing their client, that the victim, their loved-one, is all but portrayed as being responsible for their own homicide. Even though the family members of the victim may be outraged at such a portrayal, they are forbidden from any outbursts of disagreement or emotion in the courtroom; otherwise, they are threatened with expulsion by the judge.

Another traumatic factor to consider is a description of the details of the victims last moments of life, which may be reflected in the testimony of bystanders, or of the Medical Examiner. Dolores, whose son was murdered on Thanksgiving Day, did not know until the courtroom testimony of the Medical Examiner almost a year later, that her son most likely laid in the street, alive for another thirty minutes after being shot, eventually bleeding to death from his wounds. Dolores found herself completely re-traumatized with the helpless thoughts of knowing that her son lay dying for nearly a half-hour, and that she could not do the one thing every mother does by instinct: rush to his side and comfort him. As with Dolores, families often leave the courtroom feeling additionally victimized, which adds yet more stigma to their own sorrow and suffering. They can experience intense bitterness and a profound sense of isolation and loneliness.

HEALTH SERVICES

Grief and trauma from the loss created by the murder will be inter-twined, and the surviving family members may seek assistance from their physician to assist their children with emergent symptoms such as sleep pattern disturbances, dietary disruption, or significant avoidant or aggressive behavior patterns. They may seek help from or be referred to mental health agencies. Often, they are medicated with various medi-cations to address their symptoms, but the grief and trauma issues are not explored. This can lead to protracted grieving, especially in children, who cannot understand why the "pill" has not made the grief and fear from the murder "go away." Although survivors do need support from mental health agencies and perhaps a medical professional, it is critical to work on the grief and the traumatic symptomotology simultaneously in order to attain effective and adaptive results. One easy way to help children understand the grieving process is to explain that grief is not something that one can "run away" from. It cannot be "gone around," nor can one climb over it. Grief is something that everyone must go through. True, it will be painful, and will be scary, and we all would really rather not do it, but it is healthy and the sadness will lessen in time. It is critical to help children understand that the goal of healthy grieving is not to "forget" the person or what happened to them. The goal is to be able to wake up every morning, and, in spite of the loss, continue to live a fulfilling and productive life. Some children have admitted that they feel "guilty" for doing things that bring joy and pleasure, such as playing, or talking to friends on the phone, and going to the mall. The perception, or rather the misperception, becomes that "If I am having fun, I really must not be sad" about the loved one who was murdered. These misperceptions must be explored and combated in order to facilitate healthy and effective grieving.

MYTHS AND STEREOTYPES

There are several myths and stereotypes associated with homicide which must be confronted by the survivors on a regular basis. One such stereotype promotes the belief that only certain people are murder victims: African-Americans, gang members, criminals, ghetto dwellers, and "bad" people. These categories of "victims" are commonly discussed on the streets and even in academic settings. Although statistics reflect increased representation by certain demographic characteristics, caution must be used before making cause and effect statements.

Additionally, there is a stigma by which society causes additional pain and suffering by attributing partial blame for the death to the victim and/or the surviving family members, for example, someone who is murdered in a "drug deal that went bad." The victim may be blamed with statements such as "Well, he shouldn't have been dealing drugs," or "If you play with fire you get burned." Although the person may have indeed been killed while engaged in illegal activity such as drug trafficking, murder is never justified. Compounding this type of situation, parents may additionally be confronted with stray statements from friends in the community, and even in the church, such as "Well, where were his parents?" or "If that were my child, he wouldn't have been out there in the streets selling drugs in the first place." This represents yet another way that family members are re-victimized, by feeling as if the family now has a reputation of being "bad" or "dirty."

There can also be a shift in the social support provided to the surviving family members. Since people are afraid to "upset" the survivors with questions or actions, they tend to avoid the subject completely. This sends a mixed message to the surviving family members. Although the "good intentions" of friends and family is to avoid upsetting the survivors, it is often interpreted as lack of support or overt indifference. Children may never be asked about their experience or feelings. Often, it is believed that this is a topic that should not be discussed with children because of the graphic nature. This stance totally eliminates ventilation of feelings, validation of the pain and the loss, and creates major blocks in adaptive coping and grieving. This can create an environment for survivors to interrupt their grief and suppress the emotional pain in order to remain an accepted part of their social setting.

SUMMARY

Loss of a loved one to homicide is a unique and painful experience, and successful grieving is a complex process as a result of the many issues which are encountered in the aftermath of the trauma. As simplistic and altruistic as it may sound, survivors of homicide have three primary needs: to bury their dead, to face the trauma of being a survivor, and to reach grief recovery (Henry-Jenkins, 1993).

For children, this may be a difficult task, because the very essence of being a child precludes exercising individual control in many areas of life. It is critical for parents, church and community members, law enforcement and criminal justice officials, and healthcare professionals to be aware that children have the same needs as adults in homicide bereavement, and to subsequently facilitate effective and adaptive passage through these tasks. We must ensure that children are no longer the silent victims. We must encourage children to express their feelings and their fears after the murder of a loved one, recognizing that experiencing and displaying grief is a healthy and normal response. We must avoid the myth that "not by talking about it" we will avoid upsetting the children. It is safe to say that whether spoken about or not they are already scared and upset! It is through exploring the loss that a child can place the event into the appropriate place in their life history, and then begin to once again re-invest in living.

REFERENCES

Brazino, J. (1998). Nurses on the crossroads of children and violence: Portrait of violence through a child's eyes. Gannett Satellite Information Network, Inc., *The Nursing Spectrum, 7*(16), 4-5, 23.

Burgess, A. W. (1975). Family reaction to homicide. *American Journal of Orthopsychiatry, 45,* 391-398.

Burgess, A., & Clements, P. (1997). Stress, coping, and defensive functioning. In A. W. Burgess (Ed.), *Psychiatric nursing: Promoting mental health* (pp. 77-90). Stamford, CT: Appleton & Lange.

Burgess, A., Hartman, C., & Clements, P., Jr. (1995). The biology of memory and childhood trauma. *Journal of Psychosocial Nursing, 33*(3), 16-26.

Burgess, A., & Roberts, A. (1997). Violence in families. In A. W. Burgess (Ed.), *Psychiatric nursing: Promoting mental health* (pp. 484-489). Stamford, CT: Appleton & Lange.

Clements, P., Jr. (Fall, 1998). "Why did my dad kill my mom?" Homicide bereavement for children. *On the Edge: The Official Newsletter of the International Association of Forensic Nurses, 4*(3), 5-6.

Clements, P., Jr. (1996). *Trauma response patterns of juveniles exposed to homicide: A concept analysis.* Unpublished manuscript, University of Pennsylvania.

DeSpelder, L. A., & Strickland, A. L. (1996). *The last dance: Encountering death and dying* (4th ed.). Mountain View, CA: Mayfield Publishing.

Douglas, J., Burgess, A. W., Burgess, A., & Ressler, R. (1992). *The crime classification manual.* New York: Lexington Books.

Eth, S. (1989). The adolescent witness to homicide. In E. Benedek & D. Cornell (Eds.), *Juvenile homicide.* Washington, D.C.: American Psychiatric Press.

Eth, S., & Pynoos, R. (1994) Children who witness the homicide of a parent. *Psychiatry, 57,* 287-306.

Eth, S., & Pynoos, R. (1985). Interaction of trauma and grief in childhood. In S. Eth & R. Pynoos (Eds.), *Post-traumatic stress disorder in children.* Washington, D.C.: American Psychiatric Press.

Eth, S., Silverstein, S., & Pynoos, R. (1985). Mental health consultation to a preschool following the murder of a mother and child. *Hospital Community Psychiatry, 36,* 73-76.

Finkelstein, H. (1988). The long-term effects of early parent death: A review. *Journal of Clinical Psychology, 44*(1), 13-19.

Gammage, J. (1995, November 16). Nightmare in Cedarbrook. *The Philadelphia Inquirer,* B1, B3.

Gibbons, T., Jr. (1995, November 15). Mother slain, child escapes house. *The Philadelphia Inquirer,* B1, B4.

Henry-Jenkins, W. (1993). *Just us: Overcoming and understanding homicidal grief and loss.* Omaha: Centering Corporation.

Maples, R., & Browning, M. (1994). *Dead men do tell tales: The strange and fascinating cases of a forensic pathologist.* New York: Doubleday.

Picket, M. (1997). Loss, grief, and bereavement. In A. W. Burgess (Ed.), *Psychiatric nursing: Promoting mental health* (pp. 239-257). Stamford, CT: Appleton & Lange.

Pynoos, R. S., & Eth, S. (1984). The child as a criminal witness to homicide. *The Journal of Social Issues, 40,* 87-108.

Pynoos, R. S., & Nader, K. (1993). Issues in the treatment of posttraumatic stress in children and adolescents. In *International Handbook of Traumatic Stress Syndromes.* New York: Plenum Press.

Rando, T. (1993). *Treatment of complicated mourning.* Champaign, IL: Research Press.

Redmond, L. M. (1989). *Surviving when someone you love was murdered: A professional's guide to group grief therapy for friends and families of murder victims.* Clearwater, FL: Psychological Consultation and Education Services, Inc.

Redmond, L. M. (1996). Sudden violent death. In K. Doka (Ed.), *Living with grief after sudden loss: Suicide, homicide, accident, heart attack, and stroke.* Washington, D.C.: Hospice Foundation of America.

Stevenson, R. (1996). The response of schools and teachers. In K. Doka (Ed.), *Living with grief after sudden loss: suicide, homicide, accident, heart attack, stroke* (pp. 201-213). Washington, D.C.: Hospice Foundation of America.

Terr, L. (1991). Childhood traumas: An outline and overview. *American Journal of Psychiatry, 148,* 10-20.

van der Kolk , B. (1988). The trauma spectrum: The interaction of biological and social events in the genesis of trauma response. *The Journal of Traumatic Stress, 1,* 274.

van der Kolk, B. (1989). The compulsion to repeat the trauma: Re-enactment, repetition, and masochism. *Psychiatric Clinics of North America, 12*(2), 389-405.

Van Epps, J., Opie, N. D., & Goodwin, T. (1997). Themes of bereavement experience of inner city adolescents. *Journal of Child and Adolescent Psychiatric Nursing, 10*(1), 25-36.

CHAPTER 4

The 3 R's . . . Rage, Regrets, and Revenge— Uncovering and Assisting with the "Dark Side" Feelings of Children's Grief

Toni Griffith

In 1995, a program was started using the expressive arts of puppetry, music, and song to work with elementary school students in loss, grief, and transition (Caputo, 1993; Carter & Mason, 1998; Levin, 1994; Linde, 1997; Pillow & Henderson, 1996; Tortorella, 1993). Funding for two years came from the Soros Foundation, Project on Death in America. During this time we have been able to work in 150 schools in the Southern New Jersey area. We have given 400 presentations and held workshops with almost 7000 students. We have two presentations, *Good Grief, It's Sky Blue Pink!* and *Birds of a Feather Learn About HIV/AIDS Together.* The presentations have been done in school libraries and classrooms in the inner-cities and in suburban and rural areas.

We have worked with diverse ethnic and cultural populations (Tubbs, 1992). Our target populations are third and fourth grades for grief management, and fifth and sixth grades for HIV/AIDS and grief. We have also processed grief with HIV/AIDS infected and affected children and adults in New Jersey; Washington, DC; Randolph County, NC; and Sao Paulo, Brazil.

The puppet presentation *Good Grief, It's Sky Blue Pink!* is also used to assist professionals in processing grief due to patient deaths in hospices and pediatric hospices. One song from the presentation which is included in the music album, "Songs for Survivors," deals with the fact that sometimes *Life Is Cruel* and recognizes that many things that happen in life are not fair (Bies & Tripp, 1997). We use this song along with a technique called *visionary vengeance* that is described in detail later in the chapter to assist young grievers with complicated grief issues.

The characters in the puppet presentations are large, thirty-six-inch hand puppets that are animals. We find animal puppets less threatening and culturally and ethnically acceptable to all student populations. (There are Native American and Native Canadian cultural taboos against certain animals and we do research before going into an unknown area in order to be culturally sensitive.) The saddest elements in the production are dealt with musically and assist with processing the fears and feelings that often are under the surface in grieving. The script, songs, and music are all original compositions. The presentation is pre-recorded and copyrighted.

Following the presentation there is an interactional workshop that allows for group participation and interaction. Feelings of loss and grief are processed by the students in a group setting which adds to the support given (Eisenberg & Fabes, 1997). Many times feelings surface that have not been heard by parents, teachers, or counselors. *Jealousy* because my Dad died and Tommy's Dad is still alive. A painful disclosure that helps other classmates to understand how complicated grief can be for children and adults. *Relief* because he was mean and cannot hurt me anymore. Sometimes this type of disclosure sparks the discussion that leads to the understanding that not everyone who dies is the "Loved One." *Shame* because he was shot while buying drugs (Wurmser, 1994). Confusion, rejection, abandonment, guilt are just a few of the twenty to twenty-five feelings that can emerge in a workshop session.

RAGE

The first commandment of therapeutic helping is to be where the client is (Goldstein, 1983). For social workers and other therapeutic helpers, this injunction is where we begin our work (Hepworth & Larsen, 1990). Alan Wolfelt, Ph.D., speaking at the Association of Death Education and Counseling conference in Chicago, March 1998, invites us to be companions in grief; to walk the path with our clients and to "companion them on their soul-journey of grief" (Wolfelt, 1998). When we work with children and begin to uncover some of the dark side feelings of grief, the use of both standards becomes of paramount importance: to be where they are, and to be their companions as their grief unfolds.

Why does the therapeutic helper have such difficulty being able "to be where" the enraged nine-year-old is? Why does the therapeutic helper feel so uncomfortable with those strong gut-level emotions of rage, regrets, and revenge that may be emerging in screams and/or physical manifestations of the pain that the young griever is feeling (Sanville, 1987; Stringham, 1995)?

One thought to consider is that therapeutic helpers have taken many years and many paths to get to the place of helper. We have studied many models, practiced many ways of helping, and then formulated our own styles of helping. We have studied and learned ways of confronting, and non-confronting, passive and aggressive ways of coping with our own business of life. Most of the time we do not overtly fly into a rage, kick and scream and demand attention. When our young grievers do just that, kick and scream, we become uncomfortable with the outward manifestations of what we in our *adult* world consider improper behavior. We feel it is certainly not a *grown-up* approach that they are bringing to their grief. For us to get in touch with those feelings means to let the *gut feelings* that we have learned to control or ignore or stifle come to the surface and to allow ourselves to once again feel what they are like . . . those searing hot feelings that always seem to get us into trouble (Blavier & Glenn, 1995). Does that mean we have to become enraged? Certainly not. It means that we have to become more comfortable with displays of strong emotions, displays that we may not allow ourselves, for whatever the reason, to exhibit (Nadelson, 1977; Schrag, 1989).

When dealing with the *dark side* feelings of grief, we often assign a judgment value to these emotions. It is not *nice* to fly into a rage, to want to take revenge, or think about getting even—vengeance. These are often considered strong *wrong* feelings. We give our young grievers the message, either above or below the line, that these feelings are not nice, morally wrong, or they will get you into trouble, so get rid of them (Bosworth & Hammer, 1995; Logan & Chambers, 1987). What we as therapeutic helpers need to understand is that getting the *dark side* feelings to surface is a step toward companioning our young grievers through their grieving process. The feelings themselves, although not pleasant to witness, bring with them the pain and sometimes deeper feelings that the griever is trying to hide or is having difficulty confronting (Rando, 1993).

The therapeutic helper's role is to be where the client is (Logan & Chambers, 1987; Pilsecker, 1994) and to allow those gut level feelings to be expressed without feeling the discomfort of a judgment (Hepworth & Larsen, 1990). If we can provide a safe place for strong feelings, if we are willing to contract (Hartman & Laird, 1983) with our young grievers for their safety and ours, we will be able to offer them the opportunity to work on the areas of grief that sometimes lay under the surface, eat at the soul of the young griever, and often do tremendous damage before surfacing again in adulthood. (Studies confirm that unresolved parental loss surfaces in many complex grieving patterns years into adulthood (Rando, 1993).) Contracts can be made with five, six, and seven year olds, that if they need their time to punch the wall and scream that entitles us to so many minutes of quiet work time with them. Also boundary issues are important:

1. You cannot hurt yourself
2. You cannot hurt others—people and animals
3. You cannot damage property (unless marked for damage) (American Academy of Bereavement, 1992)

Buttons and hats for our clients to wear can tell us what to expect. A button that says "Leave me alone I'm angry" is a good warning device. It can also come with a time limit "Leave me alone for five minutes." A hat worn backwards can be the signal that I'm having a good or bad day. A chair, or a book, or toy flung across the room or at your head is not acceptable and is not within the boundaries as stated above. Emotional storms can engulf young grievers and the role of the therapeutic helper is also to stay out of the way of the debris of the human physical storm. Remember, if you get hurt (physically or emotionally), you cannot help (Collins & Bell, 1997; Cramerus, 1990).

Let us take a look at rage and what the young griever is trying to tell us, but cannot seem to put into words, only into those intense physical actions. What is the actual cause for the rage that is going on inside and outside? What are the circumstances of the grief? Death leaves most grievers—adult and children—feeling out of control, so the young griever feels especially angry and fearful that fate, that God, that the world, that everything is out of their control. Often classmates and school situations only reinforce that feeling of being somehow not normal, "Nobody in my class has had their Dad die!" Supportive peers, teachers, and counselors can help with a young griever's feelings of being different (Moore, 1989). Current statistics tell us that by the age of eighteen, one out of six students will lose a parent (US Census Bureau, 1996). In any given fourth- or fifth-grade classroom 90 percent of the students will have had a death loss of a relative, friend, or pet. Grief feelings are not unusual. They are just not always recognized as grief. Parents often try to shield and protect their children from the pain of grief, not realizing that death has already touched them in many ways. Children need an understanding of grief and the feelings that go with the grieving process so that they can increase their coping skills. Loss is a lifelong experience, as is the coping and adjusting that follows it.

What are the other strong unspoken feelings that often lurk below the surface of rage? What is it that drives the anger? Is it fear? Fear of not being able to live without the person? The first question that children ask in grief is, "Who will take care of me?" What changes are occurring in the young griever's life? Do they have any control over those changes? Is there any recourse to rage? Other questions asked are if this happened to Dad, "Can it happen to Mom?" "Can it happen to me?" Confronting you own mortality is a fearsome task for adults, even more so for young grievers (Wolfelt, 1991). Who do we talk to about our fear of death? Certainly not to our non-understanding peers. Who mentions this unspoken but awesome fear? We, as therapeutic helpers, need to help the young griever be able to verbalize this fear. Getting it out in the open helps to keep it in perspective and helps us to begin to understand why we feel so uneasy. Confronting our own mortality is difficult and uncomfortable for many adults as well as children of any age. It has often been said, *There is the letter I in the word DIE.*

What is the feeling that sometimes is buried even deeper than fear? GUILT (Schwartz, 1986). Often unspoken, often unacknowledged, but eating away at the young griever is the feeling that something was done *wrong*, that something was not done, something was not said, was left out, something happened because. . . . What is the question in children's grief that needs the most assurance? "Did I do anything to cause the death?" Was it my fault?

We watched one fourth-grade student assume the burden of guilt because she and her friend were bicycle riding and the friend fell off her bike and died. The young griever fully believed it was her fault for coaxing the friend to go riding that day. The fatal aneurysm that took her friend's life was beyond the comprehension of the fourth-grade student. She just knew that her other friends did not want to play with her or go bike riding with her anymore, so it must be her fault. The fact that she was a member of an ethnic group that her classmates were not wholly comfortable with had more to do with the isolation than the accident. When this was discussed in the classroom with many of her classmates present, they were able to tell her, amidst tears and hugs, that they did not think she did anything to hurt her friend or make her have an accident. They began playing games with her in the classroom and schoolyard and helped her to regain her place and a new sense of belonging.

We see children in support group situations who appear to carry the weight of a particular death on their shoulders. They say, "I know that my Dad died because I left the skateboard on the steps and he fell and he was never right after that." Often other children in the group will help process the facts and will work together to help everyone understand that it was the disease not the skateboard that took Dad's life. You can almost see the burden of guilt lift off the shoulders of the child—guilt that would have lain like a ton of stone on those shoulders if it had not been shared and dealt with by the young griever and the group (Zenter, 1993).

Sometimes guilt has a rational foundation in fact: the young griever who set fire to the house where his mother and his sister died because they were unable to get out. This young griever *knows* that he is responsible for the fire. No protestations from the group can come forth to help him. It is difficult enough for him to admit to what has happened, and there is no way to soften or rationalize what has happened. Is there nothing that we can do to help the grieving process and to work toward some adjustment of the situation? What can be said to help with this burden of guilt? We can't say, "Don't think like that, you really didn't do anything wrong." He knows the truth and our words do not and will not ring with conviction. How do we start the healing process? We can start by examining our right as human beings to be imperfect. We have flaws. Each one of us has different flaws. We human beings do stupid, ugly, thoughtless, selfish things. Can we ask forgiveness? (Enright, 1998). Forgiveness by the person whom we have wronged. Forgiveness from ourselves for being human? What penance must be paid out in order to gain forgiveness? What tasks will help us obtain that forgiveness from others and from ourselves? It is within the scope of the therapeutic helper to assist with finding the tasks and the ways to forgiveness. It is not our role to judge or to forgive. Our judgment can short-circuit the openness of our therapeutic helping and *our forgiveness* is meaningless because we are not the ones wronged. We need to provide the opportunity, the safe place and some options for forgiveness, but not the answers. They will be more effective coming from the young griever who is actively involved in their own grief work, with assistance from the therapeutic helper.

REGRETS

Regrets are the unfinished business of grief: "I didn't get the chance to say;" "If only I had"; "We were supposed to go"; "I didn't"; "I needed to, but I didn't. . . ." That special sadness that many young grievers feel is due to the fact that they did not get a chance to say good-by to the person who died (Nader, 1989). Either they did not know the person was dying or they were not allowed to see them. They were afraid to go see them in a sick condition, and then the person died and they did not say good-by to them. Sometimes people are separated by circumstances not within their control. Divorce often creates a complicated grief when one of the parents dies separated emotionally as well as by great distance and sometimes living with another family of spouse and children (Tessman, 1996). We know that grief for an ambivalent relationship is often complicated by grief for what might have been or what should have been (Rando, 1984). Young grievers may not have the ability to put into words what they are feeling about the death of Dad, whom they have not seen in five years, who has another two children that he has been with, and who has not contacted, talked to or seen the young griever in all that time. There is sometimes the feeling, "Now we will never. . . ."

How can we assist with saying those difficult, painful words of good-by? How can we do it within the control of the young griever, or with the help of a family member? Can they write a letter and take it to the cemetery? Can they plant a tree or a bush or a flower in memory of the person. Can they, like the families of the TWA flight and the Swiss-Air flight, take flowers to the ocean and send them out into the waves to say good-by. Helping to find rituals to say good-by is a task for the therapeutic helper to suggest (Imber-Black, 1988). Often the young griever will be able to think of or consider something that would be especially meaningful for themselves to do. Elapsed time between the death and the good-by is not a significant thing. A good-by is always possible.

Music, especially for pre-adolescents and teenagers, is an important component in helping to say good-by. There are many current singers and groups that deal with death in their songs and music. Ask any group of young and teenage grievers to do a search of songs, and they can easily find twenty to fifty recordings. Teenagers use music for comfort and for understanding. They can put together thoughts and find a way to say good-by through *their* music. Encourage teenagers to give us one song they think says what they are feeling, and the therapeutic helper has a strong base to start working with the grief process.

Regrets are so painful. One young griever at ten years old waited one year to tell us that he felt guilty because he did not think he told his mother often enough that he loved her before she died. We asked if he had helped with her care, and he had. He brought her water whenever she needed it, came in with her food tray, and helped her while she ate. We assisted in letting him see that every act of helping was for him, and for his mother, a way that he said I love you, and by being there with her, she knew that he loved her. Did he ever say I love you? He said it many times, and he showed it even more by his physical help. Yes, he was there for her, to help her, to care for her, to love her. *SHE KNEW.* And now he knows that she knew.

The regrets of omission are always the strongest regrets that follow us through life into old age (Hattiangadi, 1995). The message that therapeutic helpers can give is an important one: we are *still able to do,* or *redo,* or *do for another,* or *be better for the experiences.* The legacy of honoring the dead person by doing special things that they have held as important is a part of Worden's last task of reinvestment in life (Worden, 1991).

A task that young grievers can use is a goal-oriented direction for their life. What better way for them to honor the one who died than by doing well in school, graduating, and becoming a productive person. That was something the dead person wanted the most to see, and that is what the griever can do while working through their grief. That positive *influence* will be that part that stays always. Their memory can live on in what I do now and as an adult. There is in the young griever, and in all of us, that area that uses magical thinking to propel us to do things that we really never expected that we would or could do. That magical thinking in the grief process can cause guilt (It happened because I said I wanted it to happen), but it can be used to assist with the emotional legacies that enable us to work through the immense changes that death can cause.

REVENGE

Following a session at a grief conference in 1996, a question was raised to Ken Doka, Ph.D., concerning the feelings of revenge in grieving children (Doka, 1996). This section is devoted to what we have seen and how we have attempted to work with young grievers who powerfully feel the need to avenge a wrongful death or seek vengeance on a world full of unfair circumstances.

What is the first thought that enters the therapeutic helpers mind when faced with the young grievers words of revenge? Is it, "don't think it, don't do it, it's something that will just get you into trouble. . . ." Religious messages concerning vengeance and revenge seem to not only vary, but to be contradictory:

> Vengeance is mine says the Lord
> An eye for an eye, a tooth for a tooth
> Turn the other cheek
> A soft answer turneth away wrath

On one hand, there is an acknowledgment of crime and punishment, vengeance, and retribution; on the other hand, is an admonishment to be forgiving and not to provoke a confrontation. Which do we choose? Do we have an inner, inherent need for revenge, for vengeance to right the wrongs of death? Is revenge and vengeance evil? Is humankind inherently evil? (Baumeister, 1996). Are we to stand silently by and say and do nothing when we so desperately are feeling the call to action to right a wrong and the need for justice? Based on their limited abilities and assets, what can young grievers do to restore balance in an acceptable way? Will that acceptable way be sufficient to ease the pain of grief and the injustice of the death?

The concept of justice has and is undergoing a change. Since the 1980s there has been a movement throughout the world to understand and to include *restorative justice* and mediation in our judicial systems (Allen & Abril, 1997; Griffiths, 1996; Umbreit, 1994; Van Ness & Ashworth, 1993; Zehr, 1993). Most judicial systems are and have been based on a *retributive justice* that metes out punishment for the crime committed. So many months or so many years in prison for a crime when a guilty verdict is rendered. The sentence served by the criminal is meant to be the answer to the crime and the balm that heals the victim or the survivors (Allen & Abril, 1997; Marshall, 1990; Umbreit, 1994, 1995).

Restorative justice admits that a grave injustice has been done and that the self-esteem of the injured party must in some way be restored. It means acknowledging that an injustice has happened and has caused great suffering. Considering the Holocaust, or the slaughter of the Armenians by the Turks, there is no way to make full restitution to the injured or dead. The admission that the events have happened *AND ARE WRONG* gives validation to the pain and sorrow of the grief to the survivors or the surviving nation (Griffiths, 1996).

Archbishop Desmond Tutu of Africa has spoken out at the injustice of apartheid and the pain of separation and denial of rights (Tutu, 1986, 1990). Now, in his latest writings about restorative justice and forgiveness, he makes the distinction that retributive justice alone cannot give back the self-esteem and repair the damage that a whole nation of people have felt. *Revenge* will always be the aftermath of retributive justice. People who have been so terribly treated by such injustices will seek ways to have what has been taken from them restored (Tutu, 1998).

Bullying within the school system, in the classroom, lunch room, and school yard, is a cause of violent revengeful behavior for pent-up rage that can be defused by teachers, classmates, counselors, and administrators using restorative justice to right the wrong. The first step is to acknowledge to the injured party that it has happened! (Chiland & Young, 1994; Kim & Smith, 1998; Levin, 1994).

Restorative justice, gives by the acknowledgment of grievous wrong, validation to the courage, the strengths of survival, the pains of torture and death, and the torments of mind, body, and soul that happen because of an injustice. It seeks to restore by recognition of the personhood of the victim of injustice (Tutu, 1998).

Death in the mind of a young griever is just such an injustice (Caputo, 1993; Carter & Mason, 1998; Levin, 1994; Linde, 1997; Pillow & Henderson, 1996; Tortorella, 1993). Sudden violent death brings with it circumstances that include the unfairness of life, the injustice of murder, as well as the unanswerable WHY? The unfathomable suicide, the senseless auto accident, the mutating virus of AIDS, or the rampage of Hepatitis C make death not only less understandable and more fearsome, but also the grieving process much more complex. How does the young griever make sense of the senseless, the unknown, and the uncontrollable?

Revenge is a strong feeling that gets pushed into the interior of grief (Kim & Smith, 1998; Parks, 1997; Regush, 1997). It is a feeling that carries a judgment. "Don't think like that, it will get you into trouble. . . ." It is there, like a burning hot feeling in the pit of a young griever's stomach. Violence and violent death are often a part of the complex grief package that awaits work today (Holbrook, 1997). With the young griever there is often the need to right the wrong of a wrongful death. The following words come from some of our sessions.

- *The drive-by shooting* . . . where the young griever said, "I want to get a gun, and go out and shoot them, the way they shot my brother." "I'm afraid that they'll come back and shoot me. too." "I want to kill them, kill them like they did my brother, and before they kill me."
- *Rape and murder* . . . the brother who knew who raped and killed his older sister and said, "I want to hunt him down and rip him apart."
- *AIDS* . . . the daughter who told us, "I hate the man who sold her the drugs. He also gave her the virus, but I can't do anything to him because he died with it too, like my Mom, but now I hate the virus and everyone who has it because they're giving it to other innocent people" (Reamer, 1991).
- There is the young man who hates himself because he saw his father kill his mother and people tell him he is just like his father, and he has

contemplated the ultimate Freudian revenge on his father by considering his own suicide (Litman, 1996).

Faced with words of such searing pain, such deep and heartfelt feelings, the therapeutic helper is for the moment at a loss for an answer to the depths of despair and hatred that can explode because of the ugly, unthinkable, unfair occurrences that too often today are a part of life. We can begin by acknowledging that the death or that the circumstances of the death are wrong. Reading a recent newspaper clipping that tells of the shooting death of a mother in front of her eight year old son, it states that the son received no injury (Comegno, 1998). No physical injury, yes, but what of the reaction to an abusive man who has just shot and killed his mother? Will there be no psychological scaring? When the shock wears off, what will be the grief reactions? What are the legalities that will now go on for the next two or three years while there is a trial *and perhaps* a guilty verdict or *perhaps* an acquittal? (Getzel & Masters, 1984). What needs to be immediately affirmed for the young man's grief is that what occurred is WRONG. If the words of revenge surface, do they need to be repressed, or acknowledged with a statement of, ". . . that is an understandable way to feel under the circumstances."

A technique we use to help process revenge is called *visionary vengeance*. The one absolute and clear rule is that it takes place ONLY IN THE MIND. It began to emerge in group work when young griever's were asked to describe what kind of bird they wanted to be and why. The brother of the raped and murdered sister wanted to be an eagle who would hunt down the man, catch him, and rip him apart. We had the entire group work out a play scenario with puppets and allowed the griever to do just that. Another griever wanted to be a seagull to fly low over the people who did not understand her grief and "s_ t," on them! Not all revenge is violent (Levin, 1994; Linde, 1997). When a robber took candy that a Brownie Scout group was to sell for a trip, one young Brownie said, "I hope they get cavities!" Delicious revenge. A young man, dying of AIDS, threw imaginary cream pies in the faces of those who stigmatized him because of the disease.

There is a wonderful scene in the movie *The Great Race*, with Tony Curtis, of a pie-fight which takes place in the royal bakery. The only one not hit is Tony Curtis in his pristine white duster, and you ache to be the one who hurls that final pie that splatters in his face and on his coat (*The Great Race*, 1965). A cream pie in the face has wonderful healing properties in visionary vengeance. Another griever, in his imagination, was armed with a sword, a light saber, and dispatched the man who had killed his dog and fed the pieces of the man to the hungry dogs in his neighborhood. A teenager who had witnessed his mom die in pain because his father withheld medication, had a scenario, IN HIS MIND, of his father having prostate cancer and in terrible pain, of his standing in front of him with a needle and instead of giving his father the medication, shooting the pain killer up and into the air, while the father screamed in rage and pain. As the teenager finished processing this scenario, he wept and said that it was so powerful, he was not sure he would ever be able to do that to another human being, but it gave him the validity of feeling his own justification for the need to "get even with his father for his mother's pain," and to see his own inherent good as a merciful person (Cramerus, 1990).

Visionary vengeance allows us to envision, through fantasy, revenge *without hurting* anyone. Imaginary restorative justice takes place while validating the circumstances of complex grief. It gives the griever a way to achieve acceptance and forgiveness by acknowledging the need for retaliation (Tutu, 1998). It can be used in conjunction with an imaginary protective device, such as the light-saber which not only slays the dog-killer but protects the dog-owner, and also sometimes a musical theme. The protective device can be something that the young griever carries with them, such as a magic stone that becomes a cloaking device, or something that once belonged to the person who has died which gives them protection. Musical themes allow young grievers to feel the scenario anytime they hear the music played. For teenagers the music is one of the most important elements of the scenario. During group work, one group used a large alligator puppet which became for the young griever the avenger who ate the drunk driver who killed his mother. The alligator was hiding in the backseat of the driver's automobile. The musical theme that they assigned was the song *Alligator Rock,* and every time the young griever heard it, it allowed him to think about the alligator eating the drunk driver. The protective device was a book of alligator stickers that the young griever could use to mark his things and keep them safe.

It is important to understand that this technique is not useable with those children who exhibit sociopathic tendencies. One therapeutic helper described them as the "hollow souls" of society. The technique is for those young grievers who understand that this is imaginary . . . , it happens only IN THE MIND. It has no power to help if used in reality. . . in the "real" world.

The therapeutic helper is involved in explaining the rules, and the boundaries, but not in creating the scenario. That should be the creation of the young griever. The process works better when the griever is able to voice what they need for healing. The therapeutic helper's role is not to be judgmental. No scenario is too gruesome or too violent. The scenario is what it needs to be in order to restore justice to an unjust situation. We do need to reinforce that the fantasy is just that . . . fantasy.

Scenarios have been sent from all over the country detailing how young grievers have been able to process some of their most difficult grieving situations. The rule of imagination is that anything is possible, nothing is illogical or impossible in my mind. Therapeutic helpers understand magical thinking. The technique of *visionary vengeance* extends the borders of the use of this powerful tool in assisting young grievers to process their grief and often their need for restorative justice in dealing with death.

Death will always remain the great mystery of life. But to begin to accept that death is a part of life is the first real goal of grief work (Worden, 1991). Challenge begins when that acceptance is for a personal death that touches ME in the many ways that death touches us all (MacGregor, 1988). The circumstances may be varied, and are often unfair. The feelings that arise in the griever, especially the young griever, will usually encompass one or all of the three R's. As a *companion on that soul-journey of grief* (Wolfelt, 1998), the therapeutic helper and all who would help need to walk with the griever and listen, not judge, as the words of pain pour out. Once that space inside is empty, it is then free to be filled again with the spirit of life.

REFERENCES

Allen, H., & Abril, J. (1997). The new chain gang: Corrections in the next century. *American Journal of Criminal Justice, 22,* 1-12.

Baumeister, R. (1996). *Evil: Inside human cruelty and violence.* New York: W. H. Freeman and Co.

Bazemore, G., & Umbreit, M. (1995). Rethinking the sanctioning function in juvenile court: Retributive or restorative responses to youth crime. *Crime and Delinquency, 41,* 296-316.

Bereavement Facilitator Certification Program (1992). Tucson, AZ, January 17-21.

Bies, R., & Tripp, T. (1997). Chapter at the breaking point: Cognitive and social dynamics of revenge in organizations. In R. Giacalone (Ed.), *Antisocial behavior in organizations.* Thousand Oaks, CA: Sage, 18-36.

Blavier, D., & Glenn, E. (1995). The role of shame in perceptions of marital equity, intimacy, and competency. *The American Journal of Family Therapy, 23,* 73-82.

Bosworth. K., & Hammer, R. (1995). *Urban middle school students responses to anger situations.* Paper presented at the Annual Meeting of the American Educational Research Association, San Francisco, California.

Caputo, R. (1993). Using puppets with students with emotional and behavioral disorders. *Intervention in School and Clinic, 29,* 26-30.

Carter, R., & Mason, P. (1998). The selection and use of puppets in counseling. *Professional School Counseling,* 50-53.

Chiland, C., & Young, G. (1994). *Children and violence.* Northvale, NJ: Jason Aronson.

Collins, K., & Bell, R. (1997). Personality and aggression: The Dissipation-Rumination Scale. *Personality and Individual Differences, 22,* 751-755.

Comegno, C. (1998). Man shoots wife in head, kills himself. *Courier Post,* Gannett Group, Cherry Hill, NJ, October 24.

Cramerus, M. (1990). Adolescent anger. *Bulletin of the Menninger Clinic, 54,* 512-523.

Doka, K. (1996). *Transformative grief: Empowering growth.* New England Center for Loss and Transition annual conference, Stamford, CT.

Eisenberg, N., & Fabes, R. (1997). Contemporaneous and longitudinal prediction of children's social functioning from regulation and emotionality. *Child Development, 68,* 642-664.

Enright, R. (1998). *Exploring forgiveness.* Madison, WI: University of Wisconsin Press.

Galway, B., & Hudson, J. (1990). *Criminal justice, restitution, and reconciliation.* Anthology of 19 papers, and (1996) *Restorative justice: International perspectives,* Anthology of 30 papers.

Getzel, G., & Masters, R. (1984). Serving families who survive homicide victims. *Social Casework, 65,* 138-144.

Giacalone, R. (1997). *Antisocial behavior in organizations.* Thousand Oaks, CA: Sage.

Goldstein, B. (1983). Starting where the client is. *Social Casework, 64,* 267-275.

Goldstein, B. (1994). *Ego psychology and social work practice.* New York: The Free Press.

Griffith, A. (1996). *Good grief. It's sky blue pink,* puppet presentation; (1997) *Birds of a feather learn about HIV/AIDS together,* puppet presentation.

Griffiths, G. (1996). World criminal justice. *International Journal of Comparative and Applied Criminal Justice, 20,* 195-355.

Hardy, K. (1995). Therapy with African Americans and the phenomenon of rage. *Session, Psychotherapy in Practice, 1,* 57-70.

Hartman, A., & Laird, J. (1983). *Family centered social work practice* (pp. 224-226). New York: The Free Press.

Hattiangadi, N. (1995). Failing to act: Regrets of Terman's geniuses. *International Journal of Aging and Human Development, 40,* 175-185.

Hepworth, D., & Larsen, J. (1990). *Direct social work practice* (pp. 6-135). Belmont, CA: Wadsworth.

Holbrook, M. (1997). Anger management training in prison inmates. *Psychological Reports, 81,* 623-626.

Imber-Black, B. (1988). *Rituals in families and family therapy.* New York: Norton.

Kim, S., & Smith, R. (1998). Effects of power imbalance and the presence of third parties on reactions to harm: Upward and downward revenge. *Personality and Social Psychology Bulletin, 24,* 353-361.

Levin, D. (1994). Teaching young children in violent times: Building a peaceable classroom. In *Educators for social responsibility,* Cambridge, MA.

Lewicki, R. (1997). *Research on negotiation in organizations.* Greenwich, CT: Jai Press, Inc.

Linde, D. (1997). *Prosocial problem solving techniques for conflict resolution in the kindergarten classroom.* Master's Final Report. Nova, Southeastern University.

Litman, R. (1996). Chapter Sigmund Freud on suicide. In J. Maltsberge (Ed.), *Essential papers on suicide. Essential papers on psychoanalysis.* New York: University Press.

Logan, S., & Chambers, D. (1987). Practice considerations for starting where the client is. *Arete, 12,* 1-11.

MacGregor, M. (1988). *The sky goes on forever.* Kapaa, Hawaii: MM Press.

Maltsberge, J. (1996). *Essential papers on suicide. Essential papers on psycho-analysis.* New York: University Press.

Marshall, T. (1990). *Criminal justice, restitution and reconciliation.* Monsey, NY: Criminal Justice Press.

Moore, C. (1989). Teaching about loss and death to junior high school students. *Family Relations, 38,* 3-7.

Nadelson, T. (1977). Borderline rage and the therapist's response. *American Journal of Psychiatry, 134,* 749-151.

Nader, K. (1989). *Childhood post-traumatic stress reaction: A response to violence.* Dissertation, DSW, Tulane University.

Parks, J. (1997). The fourth arm of justice: The art and science of revenge. Chapter, In *Research on negotiation in organizations,* R. Lewicki. Greenwich, CT: Jai Press, Inc..

Pillow, B., & Henderson, A. (1996). There's more to the picture than meets the eye: Young children's difficulty understanding biased interpretation. *Child Development, 67,* 803-819.

Pilsecker, C. (1994). Starting where the client is. *Families in Society, 75,* 447-452.

Rando, T. (1984). *Grief, dying and death.* Champaign, IL.: Research Press.

Rando, T. (1988). *How to go on living when someone you love dies.* New York: Bantam Books.

Rando, T. (1993). *Treatment of complicated mourning.* Champaign, IL: Research Press.

Reamer, F. (1991). AIDS, social work, and the "duty to protect." *Social Work, 36,* 56-60.

Regush, N. (1997). *The breaking point: Understanding your potential for violence.* Toronto, Ontario, Canada: Key Porter Books. Ltd.

Romeo, F. (1998). The negative effects of using a group contingency system of classroom management. *Journal of Instructional Psychology, 25,* 130-133.

Sanville, J. (1987). *Theories, therapies, therapists: Their transformations.* Smith College Studies in Social Work, *57,* 75-92.

Schrag, B. (1989). Inching toward interdependence: Social work and social policy affecting infants, toddlers, and their families. *Child and Adolescent Social Work Journal, 6,* 5-17.

Schwartz, B. (1986). Grief work: Prevention and intervention. *Social Casework: The Journal of Contemporary Social Work, 67,* 499-505.

Stringham, P. (1995). What is known about changing violence. *Smith College Studies in Social Work, 65,* 181-189.

Tessman, L. (1996). *Helping children cope with parting parents.* Northvale, NJ: Jason Aronson, Inc.

The Great Race (1965). Warner Bros. A Time/Warner Co., Burbank, CA.

Tortorella, H. (1993). *Teaching human diversity in the middle school.* Paper presented at the Annual Meeting of the National Council of Teachers of English, Pittsburgh, PA.

Tubbs, J. (1992, August). *Cultural diversity and creativity in the classroom.* Paper presented at the Meeting of the World Organization for Early Childhood Education, Flagstaff, AZ.

Tutu, D. (1986, November). *The Nobel Peace Prize lecture.* Papers of the Phelps-Stokes Fund.

Tutu, D. (1990). *Crying in the wilderness: The struggle for justice in South Africa.* New York: Eerdmans.

Tutu, D. (1998, January). Without memory there is no healing, without forgiveness, there is no future. *Parade Magazine.*

Umbreit, M. (1994). Crime victims confront their offenders: The impact of a Minneapolis mediation program. *Research on Social Work Practice, 4,* 436-447.

Umbreit, M. (1995). Holding juvenile offenders accountable: A restorative justice perspective. *Juvenile and Family Court Journal, 46,* 31-42.

Van Ness, D., & Ashworth. A. (1993). New wine and old wineskins: Four challenges to restorative justice. *Criminal Law Forum, 4,* 251-306.

Van Ness, D. (1990). *Restorative justice.* Monsey, NY: Criminal Justice Press.

Wolfelt, A. (1991). Central reconciliation needs of mourning in the bereaved child. *Bereavement Magazine.*

Wolfelt, A. (1998, March). *Companioning versus treating: Beyond the medical model of bereavement caregiving.* Speech at the ADEC annual conference, Chicago, IL.

Worden, W. (1991). *Grief counseling & grief therapy.* New York: Springer.

Wurmser, L. (1994). *The mask of shame.* Northvale, NJ: Jason Aronson.

Zehr, H. (1989). *Justice: The restorative vision.*

Zenter, E. (1993). Pseudo-guilt: Defense, transaction, and resistance. *Journal of Analytic Social Work, 1,* 29-47.

CHAPTER 5

Children's Experiences of Death: Three Case Studies

Kerry Cavanagh

Working with children can be fun and rewarding but, more often than not, it is difficult and challenging. They are often constrained by their level of development, their family dynamics, their inability, and even their unwillingness to talk about their difficulties. Because of these factors it is imperative that the practitioner takes as broad a view as possible of each presenting problem. To take a uni-dimensional view is to place unwise restrictions on oneself as a practitioner as well as limiting one's effectiveness with the client group. Similarly, the practitioner with a uni-dimensional view is in danger of missing vital information because it cannot be seen and is also in danger of missing the deeper significance of information because the depth provided by a multi-dimensional view is missing in a uni-dimensional view. It can be likened to monocular vision as opposed to binocular vision. An individual with sight in only one eye is able to see enough to get by fairly well most of the time, but there are certain drawbacks to having monocular vision; for example, some objects can only be seen if the head is moved to place them in view or if they suddenly appear in view. If the individual is unaware that the head must be moved, information is in danger of being lost unless it is pointed out by someone else. The most significant drawback, however, is the limited perception of depth. When information from both eyes is combined, a new perspective becomes available, namely depth of vision (Hayes, 1991).

Issues around death and grief can be particularly difficult to address with children because of the associated intense emotions. Their understanding of it depends on many factors, including their developmental stage, the degree to which they have been included or excluded from the mourning rituals, and the effect the death has had on the family. Children are sometimes denied the opportunity to work through their loss because parents and family may believe that dealing with death is beyond their comprehension.

This chapter presents a multi-perspective approach to grief therapy, as it relates to children. It contains dimensions informed by developmental theory, grief and bereavement theory, and family systems theory. Three case examples are presented which demonstrate how this theoretical framework intersects with clinical aspects.

CASE 1: TANIA

Jim and Anne were a married couple in their thirties from a middle class background. Jim ran his own electrical business and Anne worked part-time as a secretary. Tania, who was nine years old, was their only child. They had brought her to see me because of her behavior. They told me that at home she was rude to her mother and at school she was being bullied.

Jim had made a particular point of coming along to the session with Anne and Tania because he was very concerned about the fact that the two women in his life were not only arguing all the time with each other, but were also engaged in fisticuffs with each other. He said his peace and quiet was being shattered and he felt helpless about it. After a hard day's work in the office he wanted to be able to come home and unwind as he used to before this problem began. Instead, he was coming home from work and having to act as a referee for Anne and Tania. Anne, too, was concerned about the violence and aggression and wanted it to go away. She expressed surprise that she and Tania were behaving like this and said that it seemed to come out of nowhere. One minute they would be having an argument about something, and then the next minute one or the other of them would be hitting each other. Sometimes it was Anne who initiated the hitting and sometimes it was Tania. Anne's explanation for this behavior was that it was Tania's way of debriefing from the bullying at school. Both parents requested that I help them find a positive way of dealing with the violence and aggression at home.

Tania went to a private elementary school where she was being bullied by two boys in her class. She had spoken directly to one of them; and he had stopped bullying her but, because she disliked the second boy, she had not spoken to him about his bullying so he continued doing it. Although Tania had spoken to her teacher about the bullying, nothing was being done about it on the school front and the fights between Tania and the boy had escalated to the point of often ending in him hitting her. This pattern appeared to be repeated at home with Tania and Anne having arguments which only ended when one of them hit the other. It seemed that this behavior at home had begun about two years previously and had been getting worse over that time. When I asked what else had happened two years ago, Anne became very emotional and told me that her mother had died, after a long struggle with cancer.

Anne had enjoyed a close relationship with her mother. They were best friends who saw each other regularly and had frequent telephone conversations. Jim was often away from home on business, and Anne had relied on her mother for help in parenting Tania whom she found to be difficult and demanding. Tania told me that she, too, had been very close to her grandmother whom she called "Mumma," and, like Anne, had never talked to anyone about how much she missed her. Mumma had been diagnosed as having cancer around the same time as Tania was born, so Tania had never known her when she was well. Both she and Anne were concerned because the only memories Tania had of Mumma were of her being sick.

This case raises a number of important clinical and theoretical ideas which need to be explored in order to understand what was happening to Tania. In the first instance there was what was happening developmentally for her and how appropriate her behavior was in light of her age and stage of development. There was also the question of attachment and the extent to which Tania was attached to her mother and her grandmother. Another critical theoretical idea was that of grief. Tania's behavior could have been more related to her own grief about the loss of Mumma, or it may perhaps have been more related to her mother's grief. There was a marital question about the part Mumma had played in balancing the relationship between Jim and Anne. Because Jim was away so often, he was not as involved in parenting Tania as Anne was; Anne, because of Jim's absence and the fact that Tania could be quite difficult, had co-opted her mother to help her parent Tania. In a sense, Mumma had become the other parent and wittingly or unwittingly, this was reflected in Tania's name for her—"Mumma" instead of Nana or Grandma. It may have been that Tania's behavior was connected with trying to get her father more involved in parenting her to help fill the hole that had been created by Mumma's death. Tania's behavior could also have been directly related, as Anne suggested, to the bullying at school.

Of these ideas the one I most favored, although not to the exclusion of the others, was the notion that the aggression between Anne and Tania was connected with Mumma's death and possibly was a sign that neither of them had dealt with their grief. I based this choice on the following ideas. In developmental terms, Tania was at the stage where her thinking and understanding were logical and flexible, but she was not able to deal with abstract concepts. In terms of grief theory this means that, although she had a growing understanding of the concept of death, especially the idea of it being permanent and irreversible, she still needed the help of adults close to her to make sense of her loss. Denial, as a way of coping, is a feature of children at this stage of development and can appear as though they do not care about the death. This behavior can lead adults to think that the child is not affected to any great degree by the death, and they, therefore, do not give the child the comfort and explanations that are needed (Nagera, 1970). When family members deny their grief, children do not have the opportunity to talk their feelings through and can resort to expressing their sadness through aggressive behavior (Raphael, 1984).

As a systemic therapist, I understand the family as an inter-active system in which every person's behavior affects everybody else's behavior and so it was reasonable for me to suppose that Anne's grief was impacting on Tania. It is difficult for children to deal with their own grief, especially if it is their first experience of it; but it is also hard for them to deal with their parents' grief and see them acting in ways which show that they are upset and vulnerable and not in charge of their emotions. My task, as a systemic therapist, was to find out how this aggression, which I saw as the symptom, fit into the system that is the family. As I began checking out my hypothesis, I paid particular attention to the dimensions of secrecy, aggression, Tania's age, Mumma's death, and the effect this had had on Anne and Tania.

The patterns of interaction connected with the aggression went something like this. Anne and Tania appeared to have difficulty talking about emotional issues, tending to be rather secretive and silent about things. Tania was not able to talk to the school bully about his behavior, and neither was she able to talk about it at home. Instead, she would bottle things up for days and then let off steam by fighting with her mother. Anne behaved in a similar fashion, getting upset with Tania's behavior, resenting Jim being away so much, and feeling angry toward her mother for dying and leaving her to parent Tania by herself. She, too, would bottle this up and let off steam by fighting with Tania. The theme of secrecy was further extended because the aggression was kept a secret from everyone else. It appeared that Anne was having difficulty with her own grieving process and, therefore, was not in a position to help Tania work through her grief. In addition, Anne was also upset by the fact that she and Tania did not have the same relationship that she had enjoyed with her own mother; and, with things the way they were, it looked to her as though that would never happen.

At the end of the session I talked to Tania about collecting some memories of Mumma that were not connected with her illness and suggested she interview people who had known her before that time, such as her grandfather, parents, aunts, and uncles. She could then put these memories into a book that she could look at whenever she felt like it. Anne thought this was a good idea and said she would like to do one for herself.

Stages of Grief

We can look at this intervention in terms of William Worden's (1991) mourning process and the tasks that are involved. He believes there is a four stage process that must be gone through in order for the mourning to be completed so that the person can successfully adapt to the loss of the deceased. The first of these tasks is to accept the reality of the loss. The death, its permanence and significance to the bereaved must be confronted so that denial cannot be used as a coping device. Anne and Tania appeared to be unable to talk about their grief at losing Mumma. This may have been because they were using denial as a coping device, or it could have been because each was protecting the other from the pain they knew would be caused by talking about such a difficult matter. In any case, suggesting that Tania write a book of memories would give her an opportunity to talk about Mumma within a given structure which centered around happy memories. It would also involve connecting her to her mother in a way that was far more positive than their previous connection through verbal and physical aggression. By talking about their loss I believed Tania and Anne would be better able to face the reality of their loss and the significance it had for each of them.

The second task demands that the emotional, physical, and behavioral pain of the grief be experienced so that it is not manifested at a later date through other symptoms. The intense emotions evoked by the loss of someone close can be overwhelming, especially for children experiencing bereavement for the first time. What appeared to be happening in this case was that Anne and Tania's grief was not being openly expressed, perhaps in their desire to protect each other from further pain, but it was being manifested through their patterns of interaction which involved verbal and physical aggression.

Worden's third task involves the bereaved in adjusting to an environment in which the deceased is missing. This can mean developing new skills and redefining life goals as well as searching for meaning in the loss so that the individual can regain a measure of control over his or her life. Anne, in particular, was finding it difficult to adjust to the fact that her mother was dead. Life at home still went on with Jim going away often and leaving Anne to parent Tania, this time without Mumma's help. Anne also said that she felt she had been parenting her father. He, however, was getting married again soon; and, although Anne was happy for him and glad to be released from looking after him, she found it difficult to accept that he could move on so quickly. To her it seemed disloyal to her mother to move on too quickly. It may have been out of loyalty to Mumma that Anne and Tania found it so difficult to move on themselves. In getting Tania to talk to her wider family, I was hoping she would be able to see how other members of her family were dealing with their grief; and how they were coming to terms with their loss, hopefully in the process seeing a range of responses to Mumma's death. Children need help in dealing with their own grief but they also need to see how adults deal with their grief, and being exposed to a range of responses has a far greater educative value than being exposed to a single response.

Worden's final task requires the individual to find an appropriate place for the deceased in his or her emotional life and to move on with the business of living. Some children can find it painful to be reminded of the deceased person, and what tends to happen in these cases is that they throw away the happy memories along with the sad ones. They then find themselves in a bind; they are afraid to remember things because they trigger intense emotions, but they are also afraid that they will forget things. Children need permission to remember, especially the good things. In doing this they form a new connection to the deceased which helps them find an appropriate place for that person in their life.

Two weeks later, Anne and Tania came back to see me. We had no sooner got into the interview room when Tania pulled a project book out of her bag and thrust it into my lap. She told me she had spoken with members of her wider family, either in person or on the phone, and asked them to write down their memories of Mumma. They had then sent these to her together with some photos of Mumma taken in happier times. Anne also had some letters that Mumma had written to her which she gave to Tania. Tania copied out all the letters into her book, and pasted in the photos. Each person's recollections had a page of writing and a page of photos. Tania also did some drawings of things she had remembered. There were photos of four generations of women in Tania's book—herself, her mother, her mother's mother, and her mother's grandmother. There were happy photos of Mumma's wedding, Anne as a little girl with Mumma, Christmas when Tania was a baby, and holiday times interstate and overseas as well as happy family anecdotes. The book became a family history record of the women in this family that can now be passed on to Tania's children in years to come. When Tania finally stopped talking about her book, Anne told me that she, too, had written her own book of memories. She said it had been a difficult experience for her, but in terms of dealing with her grief had been extremely helpful because it got her to face up to her mother's death. Anne also reported that Tania was now more able to talk about the things that were bothering her instead of bottling them up, and she felt that one important factor influencing these changes was letting the secret (their fighting) out of the bag.

CASE 2: JESSICA

Jessica was a pretty little three-year-old with fair hair and an air of inquisitiveness about her. She was extremely lively and had turned the waiting room upside down in the space of the few minutes it took me to walk downstairs to greet her and her mother, Monica. Monica was a woman in her early forties who had a defeated look about her. She admitted that, even though she was a school teacher, she needed help in dealing with Jessica's behavior.

As I listened to the story, it certainly seemed as though Jessica had the upper hand in this family. She kicked Monica when she tried to dress her, refused to take medication when she had a cold, had regressed in her toilet training, was wanting to go back to her pacifier, pulled Monica's hair and hit her, and never wanted to get dressed in the mornings, especially when Monica had to go to school. She played up in child care and also when her grandmother took her to ballet.

Monica's view about Jessica's behavior was that Jessica had inherited her stubbornness and her father Robert's difficult temperament. Other people had suggested that she might have Attention Deficit Hyperactivity Disorder (ADHD). Monica's parents were now refusing to look after her because of her tantrums so, in desperation, Monica had gone to her local doctor for help. The doctor's view of the whole matter was that Monica needed to take more control of Jessica; and if she needed help in doing this, she had better see a psychologist. And so, Monica had come to see me so that I would "sort this child out."

In the middle of this catalogue of Jessica's repertoire of difficult behaviors, Monica casually said "Her father died ten months ago but I don't think her behavior is related to that. She's always been difficult." She did, however, admit when I questioned her that Jessica's behavior had become much worse after her father's death. Monica then told me the sad circumstances around Robert's death.

He had been diagnosed with a malignant brain tumor when Jessica was fifteen months old and had died about a year later. Monica had taken time off work and cared for him at home. Because of this Jessica had seen him having seizures and becoming more and more physically weak.

Monica appeared to blame herself for Robert's death saying that she had nearly died in childbirth and that Jessica had to be resuscitated at birth. For some time after the birth, the doctors thought that Jessica may have suffered brain damage. Monica had read somewhere that cancer can be caused by traumatic events, and she thought that the events around Jessica's birth, together with a strong family disposition to cancer, had led Robert to an early death.

In addition, Jessica and Monica had lost four family pets since Robert's death. Robert was a great animal lover and had brought three cats and four dogs to the marriage. One of the dogs was very attached to him; and as Robert became blind, so did the dog. Monica had it put down soon after Robert's death together with a cat which had gone, as she described it, "mental." A few months later the other two cats had been given away because Monica could not cope with them.

Robert died in the hospital, having gone there a few days before his death. Jessica had not seen him since he left home. Monica had told her that Daddy died and would not be coming back anymore; but as Jessica was so young, she did not go into a detailed explanation because she thought she would not understand. She also did not want Jessica to see how distressed she was. Since Robert's death, Monica had not spoken to Jessica about him.

My thinking around this case revolved quite significantly, given Jessica's age, around developmental aspects. Some of her behavior, for example, the tantrums, could be seen as developmental. At three, the fact that she had regressed in her toilet training and was wanting to go back to her pacifier, could have been a signal that all was not right developmentally and perhaps she had experienced some sort of brain damage at birth. She may well have had ADHD, and perhaps the doctor should have referred her to a pediatrician to have this checked out. On the other hand, perhaps she had just inherited this difficult temperament; and she and her mother were doomed to clash for a long time yet.

However, to my mind, a more reasonable hypothesis about Jessica's behavior was that it was directly connected to her father's death and the aftermath of it. One of the things that strongly influenced my thinking along these lines was the way in which Jessica conducted herself during the first session. When Monica and I talked about Jessica's behavior and the battles that had ensued between them as a result of it, Jessica began talking loudly and throwing toys and pencils around the room. She openly defied her mother when Monica told her to stop it and sit down quietly; but when Monica and I talked about Robert, Jessica became very quiet and maneuvered herself closer to us.

Jessica had been through an enormous number of very big changes in her short life, none of which she had the capacity to make sense of by herself. We know, from Piaget's work on stages of cognitive development, that children in Jessica's age group, the preoperational stage, only see things from their own point of view and believe that everybody else has the same point of view (Santrock, 1992). They also do not have the cognitive capacity to link up a chain of events. Although Monica and I, as adults, were able to see the picture of change in this family as a series of related events, Jessica's view of it would have been one of a series of unconnected and unrelated events not making much sense. In addition, because of her stage of development, she lacked the linguistic capacity to ask the questions that would give her the information she needed, not only to make sense out of what was happening in her world but also to explain to others how she was feeling.

In terms of grief theory, what this means for very young children is that they take things literally. For example, being told that Daddy has gone to heaven or that he has gone away for a very long time may leave the child feeling that Daddy will come back. The child may believe that heaven is a place where people go to stay just as Toronto and Niagara Falls are places that people go to stay, but people also return from these places; and the child may spend a lot of time waiting for the deceased person to return. If the child has not had the opportunity to view the dead body, attend the funeral, or visit the cemetery, the concept of death as being a permanent state is much harder for them to comprehend. Young children like to ask lots of questions about all sorts of things including death. They soon find out that asking questions about death can cause adults to become very sad and even cry. They can be left feeling guilty when they see that significant adults in their life are upset by their questions and they can also have feelings of anxiety seeing those same significant adults in a vulnerable and unfamiliar state.

The question of attachment is a central consideration in thinking about this case. Berk (1989) defines attachment as ". . . the strong affectional tie we feel for special people in our lives that leads us to feel pleasure when we interact with them and to be comforted by their nearness during times of stress" (p. 440). Robert's death occurred at a time when Jessica, at two and a half, was still developing secure attachments to her parents. We know, from attachment theory (Bowlby, 1969, 1977) that, until the attachments have become secure, the child suffers separation anxiety when away from the primary caregiver for any length of time, reacting as if the separation was permanent. The greater the threat the more intense will be the reaction. A child suffering the loss of someone from his or her world can be affected directly by the death, especially if the child has a strong attachment bond to the deceased. Monica had told me that she thought Jessica had not been too attached to Robert because he had been quite ill for a long time and had not been able to do the things that fathers do, like bath, dress, feed, and play with her. Having seen the way Jessica reacted to hearing her mother talk about Robert, I was not sure that Monica was right about this. As well as suffering the direct effects of a death, small children, like Jessica, can suffer severe separation anxiety around the surviving parent. On the one hand, because her only understanding of her father's death appeared to be that he had left her and had not come back, it is highly likely that she was afraid that her mother would do the same thing which may explain the tactics Jessica used to try and keep Monica from going to work. On the other hand, rather than being comforted by her mother's nearness during this stressful time, her behavior appeared to drive Monica away from her, thus leaving her more anxious. So the pattern of interaction between Jessica and Monica became a vicious cycle.

At the end of the first session I suggested that Monica and Jessica negotiate a task that would connect them with each other over the death and their grief. Because she was only three, her memories of her father would soon be lost if they were not reinforced; and so I encouraged Monica to go home and begin talking to Jessica about the memories they had of Robert and for Jessica to develop her own book of memories. As children of this age make symbolic representations of their world through drawings, I suggested she draw the things she liked doing with him. She and Monica could also find suitable photos and stories that Monica could transcribe about her and Daddy. This task would give both Monica and Jessica permission to talk about Robert. It would help Jessica to find a place in her life for a new relationship with her father; and, hopefully, it would draw Monica and Jessica closer together thus changing the vicious cycle.

When they came back for the second session, Monica said that whenever she and Jessica had spent time on the book, Jessica became quiet and thoughtful and loved doing drawings of Daddy. This seemed to mark the turning point in Jessica's behavior; and, although she reacted to Monica's distress from time to time, things gradually became more manageable. The last time they came to see me Monica was pleased that Jessica was showing an interest in toilet training.

Constraints to Children's Grieving Process

Jessica's grief had not been addressed for a number of reasons. Monica thought she was too young to understand what had happened and so did not explain the situation very clearly to her. Because Jessica had not seen Robert after he died or been to the funeral or the cemetery, she was not able to make any connection between Robert going off to the hospital and never coming back. In fact, he had often gone off to the hospital during the course of the year, but had always come back. Monica, herself, was struggling with her own grief and tried hard not to let Jessica see it and the only way she could manage that was not to talk about Robert, either to other people in front of Jessica or to Jessica herself. Jessica soon learned without really understanding why, that talking about Daddy, especially to Mummy, was not advisable. Children of this age usually ask many questions about death and dying, and Jessica was not able to do this because it upset her mother too much. A second vicious cycle had been inadvertently set up whereby Monica protected Jessica both from her own grief and from the pain associated with Robert's death, and Jessica protected Monica by not talking about Robert because she knew it upset Monica. According to Furman (1974), death is an easier concept for children of this age to grasp if it is not associated with the loss of someone dear to them.

Monica had decided that the best way of getting over Robert's death was to get on with her own life and had started going out with other men. She expected Jessica to allow her to do this and was very angry when Jessica's behavior frightened one man off and was succeeding in doing the same with the next one. For Jessica, it must have appeared as though her father had never existed. On top of all this, Monica had had two of the pets put down and given away another two. Jessica had been fond of the pets and knew that her father had been also. It was no wonder she was angry with her mother and pulled her hair and hit her. Although Monica was well-meaning in everything she did, there was no way Jessica could know this because of her still developing cognitive capacity. Jessica could only deal with things as she saw them and may have thought that Monica had got rid of Daddy just as she had with the pets. Because of her limited linguistic capacity, she was not able to talk to Monica about what was troubling her and so communicated through her behavior.

CASE 3: ROBYN AND KELLY

Helen was a single mother in her late thirties whose youngest daughter, Judy, had died of leukemia six months before Christmas, at the age of twelve. She brought her two other daughters, Robyn and Kelly, with her because she felt that they needed someone to talk to about Judy's illness and subsequent death. Robyn (16) told me she was worried about her mourning process and some of the symptoms she was experiencing. She said she was dismayed by the level of anger she felt and alternated between depression and "biting people's heads off." Kelly (14) told me that she was also worried about her mourning process. The thing that most worried her, she said, was the fact that she was not able to cry. She described it as the sadness welling up from the pit of her stomach but the tears somehow being trapped in her throat; and, no matter how hard she tried to cry, the tears would not come any further. Kelly said she felt different from Helen and Robyn because they were both able to talk about Judy, play her favorite music, and cry openly. She described Robyn as a drama queen who had no qualms about crying in public and obviously found it helpful to do so.

During the first session the family shared with me the history of Judy's illness. She had been diagnosed with leukemia about a year before she died and had appeared to be responding well to treatment. Robyn had been a bone marrow donor for her and was recovering from this when Judy took a sudden turn for the worse and died. Although Helen and Richard had been divorced several years earlier, they had remained friends and the girls were very close to him. Helen told me that Richard had taken Judy's death very hard, becoming severely depressed about it. She then told me about the many inexplicable things that had happened to them, and other people who had known Judy, after her death. The most poignant of these happenings was experienced by a friend of the family who woke up suddenly one morning at about 3 A.M. to find Judy standing at the foot of her bed holding a noose and saying "Dad should either get on with it or forget it." The woman was somewhat frightened by this experience and was unsure what she should do about it. By six o'clock in the morning she decided to ring Helen and talk to her about it. Helen sensed immediately that something was wrong with Richard and rang to see if he was alright. He was, in fact, deeply depressed and told her that he had been seriously contemplating hanging himself in the shed a few hours earlier.

During the second session it became clear to me, as I listened to Kelly and Robyn speak, that Kelly admired the way Robyn and her mother were able to deal with their grief so openly while Robyn admired the emotional control Kelly displayed. They said they were all very worried about Richard's reaction to Judy's death and made sure they had daily contact with him. Helen told me that she was also worried about Kelly who had been sleeping with her since Judy's death and, although she was encouraged to cry, seemed unable to do so. Helen had also noticed that whenever she and Robyn were talking about Judy or playing her favorite songs, Kelly would employ a range of strategies from changing the subject to behaving in distracting ways such as throwing her pencils around the room if she happened to be doing her homework at the time. Kelly, herself, had been unaware of her behavior and protested strongly that she did not behave like this. She did, however, acknowledge that she found it very hard to listen to Helen and Robyn talking so freely about Judy and crying as well.

On the face of it this seemed to be a straightforward case dealing with grief. The girls, being teenagers, were old enough to have a reasonable understanding about death. They had not been shielded from it in any way, quite the contrary in fact, and had been able to talk openly with Judy about death. She, too, had been very open with them, and had discussed her funeral and how she wanted it to be. During the first session I had spoken with them at some length about the various emotions they could expect to encounter during their grieving process and also the different stages of the process. It seemed to me that, given the circumstances, it was no great surprise that Robyn was alternating between anger and depression and crying a lot. Kelly, I was not so sure about. It could have been that she was simply dealing with her sister's death in a way that was different from other family members' grief. As a family therapist, however, I was curious about how this "problem" of Kelly's fit into the system.

The Family as a System

A systems perspective sees the family as an interactive system with individual members as an integral part of this system interacting with each other rather than as separate individuals with no context. As such, the family system has its own unique structure, rules, and goals (Robinson, 1980). A systems perspective of the family means that we must have a circular view rather than a linear view. It also means that we would not look for pathology within the family or a particular member of the family but, rather, would look at the patterns of interaction within the family around the symptom or presenting problem. To put it simply, we will look at how the symptom is connected with the rest of the system.

In relation to Kelly, I could have seen her apparent inability to show grief in an overt way as a sign that she was stuck at some point in her grieving process and that this was undesirable because it could lead to future problems with unresolved grief. However, because of my systemic focus, I looked for a way in which it may have had a positive connection with the rest of the family.

At the end of the second session, I believed that I had found this positive connection to the family and gave it to them as a systemic intervention known as a positive connotation. I told Kelly that I thought she was right to be so controlled in her grief and not give way to tears because it was clear to me that she was protecting her family. Everyone else in the family had, to a certain extent, "lost it." Her father had become so depressed that he had almost killed himself, and she was now sleeping with her mother to keep an eye on her and make sure she did not attempt the same thing. In addition, her mother and sister appeared to have no control over their emotions, so it was no wonder that she could not allow herself to cry and probably would not until she was sure that everyone else was going to be all right. Kelly had difficulty understanding this idea, but her mother thought I was on to something. She had thought Kelly slept with her because she was not able to sleep on her own and needed the company; but, on reflection, she said she thought it was very interesting that Kelly, who normally would not be woken up even if a bus was driving through the house, was awake in a flash whenever Helen began crying softly during the night.

In the third and final session, Kelly told me that she had thought a lot about my explanation for her seeming lack of grieving behavior and thought I was right. She was indeed waiting until her family was out of danger before she allowed herself to grieve. She also admitted that she was particularly worried about her mother in case she became depressed and suicidal just as her father had. Since I had last seen the girls, they had attended a Canteen camp for bereaved siblings which Kelly had found very helpful. Robyn and she had been in the same group of children who had lost siblings to cancer. Robyn had not found it very helpful to talk about her experience of Judy's death, but, she said that Kelly had talked and talked and cried and cried. Kelly admitted that this had been so and that she had been feeling much better ever since.

This case is a good example of how members of the same family deal with grief differently but are also affected by each other's grief. It also shows that we must be respectful of individual ways of grieving even if they do not seem to follow the tasks and prescriptions set down by the "experts." The important thing to keep in mind is the way the different processes fit together within the family. Kelly's inability to grieve in the way her mother and sister grieved seemed a tragedy to her, but it was, in fact, serving a very important purpose in preserving the equilibrium of this family. She felt that, if she allowed herself to "lose" it, she may well have lost her parents to suicide and so it was important that she delay her own process until she was sure that the rest of the family was going to be alright.

CONCLUSION

Death can be seen as a developmental process, although, as Marris (1975) says, it is the one for which we are least prepared. We live in a society where death is dealt with in a minimalist fashion and its impact is often negated. People usually die in the hospital, not at home, and so death is removed from our everyday lives. In Western culture the pressure from society to "get over" one's grief is enormous. The display of strong emotions is discouraged and the tacit messages people get are to grin and bear it or to keep a stiff upper lip. This is the culture around death to which children are exposed.

Children's experience of death is mediated by many factors, including age, developmental stage, and family dynamics. The younger the child, the more difficult it will be for him or her to make sense of the death. If they are unable to talk about the death, ask questions and have them honestly answered, not only will their understanding of it be impeded, but their mourning process may be impeded as well, leading to behavioral difficulties that, on the face of it, appear to have no connection to the death. Children must be able to see adults grieve in order to know how to do it themselves.

These factors may continue to exert a powerful influence on the child long after the event of death has occurred. As children get older and move into more advanced developmental stages, they may be faced with trying to make sense of something that has taken on a meaning it was never meant to have. If children are to make sense of the loss and move on with their own lives, the loss, with all its ensuing sadness, sorrow, fear, anger, and other intense emotions, must be faced fairly and squarely. This process is enhanced by families who are able to face their own grief and work through the mourning process. As practitioners, our work with grieving children is enhanced by having a multi-dimensional view rather than a uni-dimensional view—one that looks at the child and the symptom from a range of perspectives, thus adding depth and breadth to our interventions.

REFERENCES

Berk, L. (1989). *Child development.* Boston: Allyn and Bacon.

Bowlby, J. (1969). *Attachment and loss: Vol. 1 Attachment.* New York: Basic Books.

Bowlby, J. (1977). The making and breaking of affectional bonds, I and II. *British Journal of Psychiatry, 130,* 201-210; 421-431.

Furman, E. (1974). *A child's parent dies.* New Haven: Yale University Press.

Hayes, H. (1991). A re-introduction to family therapy: Clarification of three schools. *Australian & New Zealand Journal of Family Therapy, 12,* 27-43.

Marris, P. (1975). *Loss and change.* New York: Anchor Press/Doubleday.

Nagera, H. (1970). Children's reactions to the death of important objects. *Psychoanalytic Study of the Child, 25,* 360-400.

Raphael, B. (1984). *The anatomy of bereavement.* London: Hutchinson.

Robinson, M. (1980). Systems theory for the beginning therapist. *Australian Journal of Family Therapy, 1,* 183-194.

Santrock, J. (1992). *Life-span development.* Dubuque, IA: William C. Brown.

Worden, W. (1991). *Grief counselling and grief therapy.* London: Routledge.

SECTION 3
Complicated Grief in Special Populations

CHAPTER 6

Camouflaged Grief: Survivor Grief in Families of Soldiers Still Listed as MIA

Larry R. Darrah

General Sherman said that "War is Hell." While he was referring to the Civil War in the United States between 1860-1865, his statement could apply to all wars. That "hell," however, often extends far from the field of battle. Soldiers who return home after combat are often affected. Also, families who remain at home are affected as well. This is especially true of those who have loved ones still listed as missing in action (MIA). It is the grief-related issues of these individuals that I will address in this chapter. I will focus on why their grief is complicated and why many of them are forced to "camouflage" their grief. It should be noted that my research and experiences are from the Vietnam war. I realize there are still individuals who have loved ones listed as MIA from Korea and World War II. Perhaps their grief is somewhat different, but I suspect there are many similarities.

The American Heritage Dictionary defines camouflage as "A means of concealment." I have chosen this word to describe MIA survivor grief for the following reasons:

1. Their grief is a direct result of a military experience and camouflage is usually a military term.
2. More importantly, their grief-related issues are often not validated or even recognized by society (especially now that the war has been over for 25 years), and they are forced to camouflage their true feelings and emotions.

This camouflage is often so effective that, after a while, even they do not attribute certain thoughts, feelings, actions, and reactions to unresolved grief. Thus the camouflage is extremely effective and ultimately to the detriment of the individual.

BACKGROUND

My interest in this area began in 1976. I had just completed my schooling with the Air Force in Texas. I was a Pediatric Nurse Practitioner in the United States Air Force. Some of the mothers of the children I was seeing in my office began confiding in me about their husbands never coming home from Vietnam. Worse than that, they were officially listed as MIA, so the family had no way of knowing if their loved one was still alive or dead. My background before re-entering the Air Force was in Psychiatry; and although somewhat limited, I was naturally interested in listening to their stories. I had worked some with grieving individuals before and was somewhat knowledgeable about "normal" grief. It was clear that there were elements of grief that I was unfamiliar with that were being shared. While I did not understand what made these women's grief reactions different, I became very interested. Since I was going to make the Air Force a career, I decided to start my own research. It should be noted that the field of grief and bereavement was in it's infancy then, so my resources were not as abundant as they are today.

Over the next thirteen years (I retired from the Air Force in 1990 after 20 years of military service), it became clear that not only were the wives affected, but the children as well. Often they presented with somatic complaints without organic basis, and I began to attribute these to grief. The remainder of this chapter will be addressing the effects prolonged absence and no knowledge has on the loved ones left behind. Truly, these are the hidden casualties of war.

Someone once said that "grief is grief," and while there are certain elements of grief universal to all who grieve, there are clearly some individuals whose experience has dictated a more difficult pathway through grief. I personally believe that all grief is complicated and some is more complicated than others. This is certainly true of the MIA wife.

Certainly, there were aspects of her grief common to all grieving situations, but I will focus on what makes her grief unique, and why it is perhaps more complicated than most. Let me create a hypothetical scenario of what life has been like for the typical MIA wife. It will contain those elements of grief experienced by all the women I interviewed. Each case was, of course individual; but the following discussion accurately summed up life for most.

These women were in three groups:

1. Those who had been told their husband was a prisoner of war (POW).
2. Those who had not heard from their husband for an extended period of time.
3. Those who already had been told their husband was MIA.

All of the women felt the end of the war would bring about some measure of closure. Those in group one knew he would be returning. Those in group two felt the same. Those in group three felt he would either be returning or at the very least, they would know his fate. All three groups would be sadly disappointed.

The first group was now being told their husbands were not among the returning POWs and they were now MIA. Those in the second group were now being told the same thing. Those in the third group were now informed their loved one's status had not changed.

It should be noted that my first contact with any of these women was some four years after the end of the Vietnam war.

Each of these wives, regardless of the group they were in, would now embark on a lifelong journey through grief that would be filled with stumbling blocks rarely seen in the "typical" grieving situation. For each of them, the war clearly was not over.

As stated earlier, I will focus on what makes their grief unique. First of all, many of these wives now felt ostracized by both the military and civilian communities. Before their husband's disappearance, they were very much a part of the military community and felt connected to other military wives. They shopped together at the Commissary and BX (military stores). Many lived on the base, so all of their neighbors were military. When the wives got together for social events, they felt a common bond with their neighbors and their conversations were usually focused on military events or circumstances.

Suddenly, the MIA wife found herself in an uncomfortable position. She was permitted to remain on the base for an extended period of time; but that once common bond and feeling of connectedness with her neighbors had now been shattered. Things she used to look forward to, like shopping at military stores, now became a dreaded task. Also, they now felt out of place in the circle of wives they once felt comfortable with, because their husbands had not returned.

They often stayed to themselves, fearing the questions and comments of others. Many told me they did not know what to say and did not want to appear vulnerable by crying, so they simply avoided social contact altogether. They told me they no longer felt like a military wife, and one told me she did not feel like a wife at all.

Some chose to return to their extended families early; and eventually, all had to return to the civilian community. Some related they knew everything would be all right once they were back with loved ones, but for most, this was not a reality.

Many had been part of a military family for a long period of time, some soon felt as an outsider in a place she once called home. Many of her old friends had married and moved away. Even if there were still old friends present, they soon discovered they had little in common and avoided them for some of the same reasons they avoided their military friends.

While many were able to benefit from the love and support of family members, they failed to realize these individuals were grieving as well.

After all, it was their son, son-in-law, brother, grandson who was missing, and they each had their own unique grieving issues to confront. It is often difficult for different individuals grieving the same loss to be a comfort to others. As Earl Grollman states, "It's like two bankrupt people trying to get a loan from each other. It isn't going to happen."

In addition, some members of the community further added to their pain. Many had been opposed to the war and had very little sympathy or empathy for the MIA wife. One woman told me her neighbor told her, "It serves you right for marrying a war-monger in the first place."

So, in a relatively short period of time, many of these women went from a feeling of belonging to both a military and civilian community, to not belonging to any community. All this was because of circumstances beyond her control. No wonder many had to camouflage their grief.

In the women I worked with, three dilemmas were presented to all:

1. Stay on base, return home, or go to a completely new site.
2. Seek employment or return for more schooling.
3. Remain a wife in waiting or seek a new mate.

There were no easy decisions regarding any of these tasks. Regardless of their choice, problems followed and neither choice in each dilemma offered much satisfaction.

We have already discussed the first dilemma. Seeking employment or returning to school created new problems either way. Her funds were certainly limited as she now received only a portion of the money she received prior to her husband's disappearance. Most often, she chose to go to work; but often, with a limited education, she could not find a good job. Going back to school meant she needed money to do that. In addition, many had small children, so some kind of work was their only real option.

The third dilemma certainly posed many problems as well. If she remained a wife in waiting, how long could/should she wait? If she entered into a new relationship and her husband returned one day, what would she do then.

I know of one instance where this actually happened. In 1969, a woman was informed her husband's plane crashed and burned. There were no remains found except for some bone fragments. In 1972, she remarried and in the spring of 1973, her husband returned. He had been a POW since 1969. Although I never heard how the story ended, just imagine the profound grief of all involved.

Perhaps the overwhelming thought that ran through the minds of most MIA wives was reported in an article that appeared in a military journal called *Family Separation and Reunion,* in 1975. The article was titled, "Waiting: The Dilemma of the MIA Wife" (Benson, Dahl, McCubbin, & Hunter, 1975). No matter what else they struggled with, the prevailing thought was "He's probably dead, but he just might be alive."

With this thought came another dilemma. If she viewed him as dead and sought new relationships, conflicts arose with her in-laws. Also, dating or remarrying in the absence of conclusive proof often produced overwhelming guilt, which further compounded their pain. One woman who was struggling with this told me, "I remember my wedding vows: 'til death do us part. Has death really parted us?"

If she felt her husband was probably alive and decided to wait, problems arose anyway. One told me she was presented with "reality checks" from her friends and family. She often heard comments like, "You're only kidding yourself," and "It's been too long. I'm trapped," she said. "If I listen to them and try to start over, I would soon be hearing comments like how could she do that. She doesn't even know if he is dead or not. It's too soon." It was obvious to me that if she finally ceased being a wife in waiting, she would eventually be faced with the same problems as one who early on decided her husband was really dead. She was indeed trapped.

So what problems do these MIA wives face today, some twenty-five years later? My last real contact with any of these women was five years ago, but I believe my research has revealed enough to give me some understanding.

Many are still struggling with the problems I have listed earlier. Some remain in waiting and many have remarried. For both, however, I do not believe there has been true reconciliation. This is because of the absence of one key ingredient in grief reconciliation—closure.

Closure for these women remains difficult, if not impossible. There has not been a body produced. We all know that one of the main functions of the funeral and viewing the body is that it facilitates closure. This has been impossible for the MIA wife. I will discuss some possible interventions later in this chapter that may help bring about closure.

My contact with these women has revealed one certain conclusion: most have not been able to experience closure and still feel trapped in a vicious cycle. This is summed up in my grief wheel (see Figure 1).

Let me go over this wheel and further explain the cycle. First, the wife knows that her husband is missing. This often happens before official notification. There is, of course, hope for his return. Even after a period of time following the war's end (this will vary with individuals), hope for a successful reunion continues.

Gradually, however, the thought that he could possibly be dead creeps into their minds. They do not let this thought dominate, however; so they continue to feel he is probably alive and will return someday.

After another extended period of time, there is a shift. Now the predominate thought is that he is probably dead. Still, there is some hope that he is still alive.

More years pass and this back and forth, roller-coaster ride of emotions, begins to take its toll. Now they do not care whether he is dead or not. They just want a definitive answer.

The next phase of the grief cycle is predictable: overwhelming guilt. They say to themselves, "How could I say I don't care if he's dead? I just want to know!" I do not need to elaborate on the effects of guilt. We all know what that produces.

Finally, their long and painful journey seems to be lessening a bit and there still is a shred of hope. "Maybe, just maybe," they think. They keep hearing of sightings of POWs still alive. The media reports of teams still searching; and, indeed, some of the MIAs have been accounted for. So, "Maybe. Just maybe," they will soon know something.

But then, the cycle returns to where it started years before, and around the wheel they go. There has been no relief by making it around the wheel.

Their husband is still missing and just like years before, there is no news of his fate.

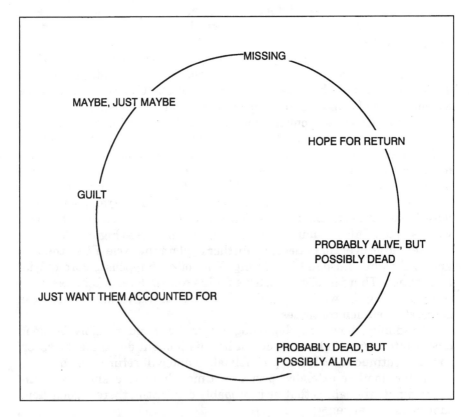

Figure 1. The vicious grief cycle of the MIA family.

As mentioned above, some of these men have been accounted for. Perhaps as years go by, others will become accounted for. On the surface, one would think this issue would finally be over for these wives if they just knew for sure, but that is not the case. While this would indeed be a huge step in the grief reconciliation process, it often would not bring true closure. My research involved four women who did receive notice that their husband was proven to be dead, but it really did not solve much for them.

For one thing, anger toward their government often intensified. One told me, "I feel betrayed and abandoned." Another said, "I still don't believe he is dead. They lied to me before, so they could be lying again!"

One woman's response remains vivid in my mind. She said, "I'm no longer proud to be an American. Look at what my government did. They lied to my husband, me, and all the American people as well. They continued to lie throughout the war and prolonged our involvement when they knew it was hopeless. They lied again, telling me he was a POW and then said he was missing. Now they tell me he is dead and they expect me to believe them. I am considering moving to another country and denouncing my citizenship."

McCubbin, in his article in *Family Separation and Reunion* (Benson et al., 1975), identified a process he called "re-grief." He shared the experiences of some women who did receive notification of their husband's fate after a period of being listed as missing in action. These women erroneously believed that once they knew for sure, they could then initiate rituals of closure and get on with their lives. He reported that these women were "hopelessly unprepared for the new emotions the new status dictated."

My research revealed the same thing. While the ones who finally knew were able to break out of the wheel I described earlier, they experienced new problems with new feelings that kept them fighting the war at home.

The main issue was anger. It was usually directed at the United States government and they simply did not believe the reports. It was almost like they were being forced to grieve all over again. For years, they had to endure the pain of not knowing; and now, even though they were told he was dead, their grief continued. Issues of unresolved grief usually carry over into new grieving situations, and this was the case with these women. The grief of not knowing now shifted.

Larry Knapp, in his book *Beyond Endurance* (Knapp, 1986), coined the phrase "shadow grief." While he was using this phrase to describe grief associated with perinatal loss, I feel it applies to part of the pain of the MIA wife. Shadow grief refers to grief that can never be completely reconciled. This does not mean that the intense pain continues to dominate their lives as it once did, but the loss and attending feelings remain for years and perhaps for the rest of their lives.

Listen to what one woman said. Her husband had been listed as MIA from World War II. She remained a wife in waiting and now, some fifty years later said, "When will my pain end? When I die and not a day sooner." Certainly, some issues with the MIA wife will remain forever.

Sometimes, the phrase "shadow grief" can have a more literal definition. I remember one MIA wife telling me, "I just can't seem to shake my husband's shadow. It's everywhere I go. Even now, when I am driving my car, he's in the backseat."

There is yet another occasional happening that adds to the pain of the MIA wife. This comes from the media. Even now, twenty-five years after the end of the Vietnam war, there are occasionally reports from someone who states they have seen Americans alive and still in captivity in Vietnam. While this has some effect on all MIA wives, it has the most effect on those small number of women whose husbands were known to have been taken captive or whose pictures or voices were seen or heard on film, but never returned.

Even if such reports are false, as long as they persist these MIA wives will continue to grieve and there seemingly is no way for their losses to become reality.

While most of this chapter is devoted to the MIA wives, it is obvious this issue affects many other individuals. These men had parents, siblings, grandparents, and many had children of their own when they left for war. Space does not permit discussing each of these individuals in any depth, but I would briefly like to make some general statements about unique grief factors found among them.

If the soldier who left for war and did not return had children, they were of course affected. How they reacted was basically determined by two factors: 1) Their age; and 2) How their mother reacted.

Children understand death and loss according to their chronological age and their emotional maturity. There is a wealth of information now available on this, so I will not spend much time on it.

The second factor, how well the mother reacted, was the most notable factor influencing the children I saw in my practice. Their reactions usually paralleled the grief reactions of their mothers. If she was able to "carry on" with all the tasks confronting her in a somewhat calm and positive manner, the child usually did quite well.

If, however, the mother seemed totally overwhelmed by the entire situation, the child reacted quite differently. Often these mothers would bring the child in reporting numerous physical symptoms. Most commonly they reported temper tantrums, sleep problems (night terrors and bad dreams), bed wetting, diarrhea, and behavior problems. Often no organic etiology could be found. A large part of my treatment plan involved focusing on how the mother was doing and then helping her better adjust to the behavior of her child. Over time many of these symptoms and behaviors lessened or disappeared completely. This happened only if I was able to help mom with some of her issues. If not, the behaviors of the children rarely improved, no matter what treatment regimen I used.

Many authors have reported that children grow up with their grief and this was certainly the case with the children I was privileged to follow for several years (7 at the most). With each new age group came new understanding and perhaps new problems, but again, how well the child did was directly proportional to how well the mother did.

Parents of a son who is still listed as MIA have their own unique grief issues to deal with. While initially they were not faced with the same dilemmas as the MIA wife, their pain was just as intense. While there is much written about parental grief, rarely does any work deal with this type of parental grief. While my research in this area was somewhat limited, I was able to interview some MIA wives who told me about their parents.

Men and women grieve differently, so each parent reacted differently to their son's status. As with most grieving situations, guilt and anger dominated.

The mothers struggled most with guilt. Many felt they had failed in one of the unwritten responsibilities of a parent to protect your child. They told me they should have stressed college more or come up with other measures to keep their son out of the military. Their life seemed dominated by guilt, regret, and "if only."

Fathers reacted somewhat differently, at least initially. Many were proud to say they had a son fighting in Vietnam. Some had fought in Korea and World War II and felt it was a man's duty to fight for his country, even if that meant giving his life.

As time went on, however, the father of a son listed as MIA often changed in his viewpoint. This pride turned to anger. History has shown many negative aspects of the war in Vietnam, and many now have intense anger at the United States government. Perhaps many of their beliefs can be summed up by the comments of one father I know personally. He said, "It was different when I went to war. We knew what we were fighting for and who the enemy was. Our country was in danger as well as our freedom. Our government lied to us as to why we were there and who the real enemy was. When we came home, there was a real sense of victory. In Vietnam, there was no victory and our men came home to a country that hated them." His anger has not diminished much overtime.

So, it's clear the MIA issue affects numerous individuals. How many is not actually known. In 1995, the National League of Families stated there were 2,248 U.S. servicemen still unaccounted for from the Vietnam war. There are more than that still listed missing from Korea and from World War II.

The exact number is not the important issue. The fact remains that there are thousands of Americans who continue to fight their own private battles, and who have become, as Edna Hunter states, "casualties of war who remained at home (Hunter, 1975).

As was stated earlier, the issue of non-closure is central for all of these people. Since loss and separation are facts of life, the grieving process in relation to that loss or separation can be called "normal." During the resulting grief process, growth is achieved until the bereaved achieves what Alan Wolfelt (1990) calls a "new normal." That grief process had then become a growth-producing experience.

While reconciliation or this "new normal" is the goal of most grief situations, it often does not happen for survivors of men listed as MIA. Without closure, the loss never becomes a true reality and, thus, cannot be growth-producing or reconciled.

Attempts to bring closure often fail as these individuals are forced to grieve alone. Many authors have said that "grief shared is halved, and grief experienced alone is doubled." There is no debating this fact, but where can these individuals go to share their grief? The usual support groups are not very helpful for these people.

Let's look at some factors that force them to camouflage their grief. Many grieving people join support groups which allow them to share their grief. This is not a reality for survivors of men listed as MIA. Which groups would they go to? In most groups, the fate of the deceased is known. Right up front, these survivors tell me that they felt out of place when they entered.

Some would say they could form their own support group. This is not feasible either, as most survivors are widely scattered across the country and rarely are there even a few in any given area.

Grieving alone is often the only choice they have and is often supported by some family, friends, and society in general. Even if unspoken, the message is "Get over it and get on with your life. It's been too long. He's dead and he's not coming back."

My research has shown that the above mentioned factors force these individuals to suffer in silence. All of the negative "stuff" cannot be expressed, so they put on their camouflage to let others feel they are doing all right. But camouflage only hides what is really there. It does not change what is under it. Silently, these individuals continue spinning along the grief wheel described earlier, with no hope of ever getting off.

As hopeless as all of this seems, there are some things that those affected by war in this way, can do to bring about some acceptable measure of closure and gain some reconciliation. While my research did not uncover any "magic bullet" or sure-fire fix for these people, it did reveal some things which did help many when they were instituted. It should be noted that not all things work with all people, because grief is a highly individual experience and each who suffers must find their own meaningful tools, but all is not lost for MIA victims. The following may help them find their own meaningful tools. These are some I have found helpful for many of the individuals that I worked with.

1. *A Memorial Service*—This may seem obvious and some will say "it won't work." This memorial service should be conducted as a regular funeral. It can be done in a funeral home, private home, church, or anywhere for that matter. The important point to remember is that it should be done in accordance with the customs and rituals of one's community and faith. Conduct the service as closely to the way you would conduct it if there was a body present. Take considerable time to organize it. Invite all your family, friends, and members of the community.

2. *Forgiveness*—This is perhaps the most crucial thing needed to bring about some measure of closure. It sounds easy but it will take work. Just as grief is a process, so is forgiveness. It involves forgiving all those who need forgiving: friends, the government, your missing loved one, and even yourself. When I suggested this to one woman, she gave some typical responses as to why she could not completely do this.

First of all, she said, "I can forgive my friends or family who may have contributed to my grief. As a matter of fact, I've already done that. But I will never forgive the government for sending him to that war. Also, why should I forgive myself? For what? It wasn't my fault he had to go or turned up missing. Finally, why do I have to forgive my husband? It wasn't his fault either."

Let's look at these responses a little closer. Being able to forgive their government is crucial. I reminded her of something that I heard about forgiving. I said, "Perhaps you're right. The government may not deserve to be forgiven. But you don't forgive them because they deserve it. You forgive them because you do not deserve to carry around all this anger. Do you really think you are hurting them by continuing to hate them? You are the only one being hurt by this anger." She had to admit that I was right.

Also, she could not see why she had to forgive herself. I reminded her that it is very common for grieving individuals to say, feel, or think something they later feel guilty about. I reminded her saying to me, "I don't care if he is dead, I just want to know," and how she expressed guilt to me later about that. All of us who grieve need to forgive ourselves. Take some time to think back and identify those things. Write them down, look at them often, and then find ways to forgive yourself.

Finally, she was angered to suggest that she needed to forgive her missing husband. Again, I reminded her of how she talked with me about how angry she was at him for enlisting in the military and on two occasions told me she "hated" him for leaving her in such a mess. I asked her if her camouflage had not even deceived her as she had repressed this. Again she admitted that she had a lot of anger she had not dealt with concerning her missing husband. This is not only "normal," but common.

It is important to again be reminded that forgiveness is a process. It is not accomplished by simply saying "I forgive . . . . While much is written on how to go about forgiving, journaling is the main tool that I have found helpful for myself and for the women that I worked with. Write everything down and refer to it often. I encouraged them to be as blunt and honest as they could. It was only for them. They could share it with others, but what they did with it was entirely up to them.

In addition, seek the advice of clergy if you are a person of faith. At the very least, know that God forgives you and you too can forgive. It will not be easy, but believe that it will happen and it will.

Finally, others have asked me what they can do to help someone who still suffers from a loved one who never returned. I always refer them to a poem by Janetta Hendel. I do not have any background on it, but if it was not written by an MIA wife, it could have been.

Don't tell me that you understand,
don't tell me that you know.
Don't tell me that I will survive,
and that I will surely grow.

Don't tell me this is just a test,
and that I am truly blessed
to be chosen for such a task,
apart from all the rest.

Don't come at me with answers
that can only come from me.
Don't tell me that my grief will pass,
and one day, I'll be free.

Don't stand in pious judgement,
of the bounds I must untie.
Don't tell me how to suffer,
and don't tell me how to cry.

My life is filled with selfishness,
my pain is all I see.
But I need you, I need your love,
unconditionally.

Accept me in my ups and downs,
I need someone to share.
Just hold my hand and let me cry,
and say, "My friend, I care."

(*Don't Tell Me* (1991), publisher unknown)

In closing, I do not claim to have all the answers or be any kind of expert in this field. I am just one ex-military person who was privileged to have contact with some of those hidden casualties of war. These women were the real experts and they taught me a lot.

It is my sincere wish that all who continue to suffer may one day be able to break free of their pain and remove their camouflage.

My biggest wish would be for an end to all wars, but this is not a reality. I believe, however, that we should heed the *words shared* by Frank Kautzman in his book, *MIA: WW II* (Kautsman, 1992). He said, "Each of us, those who knew war first hand and those who were thankfully innocent, must carefully substantiate the truths of our aggressions. If we shirk this responsibility, we will be damned to repeat the mistakes history should have taught us to avoid."

REFERENCES

Benson, H., Dahl, F., McCubbin, W., & Hunter, E. (1975). Waiting: The dilemma of the MIA wife. In *Family separation and reunion,* Washington, DC: U.S. Government Printing Office.

Hunter, E. (1979). *Combat casualties who remain at home.* Paper delivered to U.S. Naval Post Graduate School, Monterey, CA.

Kautzman, F. (1992). *MIA: WW II.* Delaware, OH: Austin Press.

Knapp, R. (1986). *Beyond endurance.* New York: Shocken Books.

Wolfelt, A. (1990). *Helping children cope with grief.* Muncie, IN: Accelerated Development Inc.

CHAPTER 7

Complicated Grief:
Suicide Among the Canadian Inuit

Antoon A. Leenaars

Across the Arctic, the Inuit have rates of suicide that are three to four times the Canadian average (Royal Commission of Aboriginal Peoples, 1995). This is equally true for Aboriginal people in Alaska and Greenland (Kirmayer, 1994). There are very few people across the world with such staggering rates. My intent here, utilizing both nomothetic and idiographic approaches, is to share my presentation given at the King's College 16th International Conference on Death and Bereavement, entitled "Understanding and Treating Complicated Grief." The chapter served as an opening case illustration of complicated grief, although, of course, other examples could have idiographically demonstrated such grief. The intent was to show the association of complicated grief to suicide, a final action in a grieving person/people.

To begin, I asked the audience to give me some idea of what they meant by complicated grief, a term not often clearly defined. The question was: "What do you mean by complicated grief?"

Here are the audience responses:

- "Sudden, violent, mutilating."
- "What is intent and what lasts longer than what is the norm?"
- "Something that immobilizes."
- "Multiple losses."
- "Suicidal ideation and suicide."
- "Causes are not in the individual but in the culture."
- "Complete denial of grief . . . complete denial of everything, amnesia."
- "They cannot restructure and go on with a new life."
- "Generational."

This will be my working definition. I think that you will see that every one of these definitions will fit with what I am going to share with you about the Arctic, absolutely every one.

EPIDEMIOLOGY AND THE ARCTIC SCENE

The Inuit are a distinct people living in the Arctic; they are distinct from the First Nations people in Canada and the United States. Weyer (1932/1962) was one of the first to suggest that suicide was a cultural trait of the Inuit (although he called them "Eskimos," a Cree word that means eater of blubber). Boas (1964) concurred that suicide was not unusual. These early observers discussed suicide as a way of life, documenting "altruistic" suicide. They noted that suicide, namely in the elderly, disabled, or sick, was undertaken to preserve the group. However, although suicide in the elderly occurred, later more factual observers noted that both Weyer and Boas may have exaggerated the reports from specific cases in specific communities. Even more so, youth suicide was very scarce in the old ways (Kirmayer, 1994; Kirmayer, Fletcher, & Boothroyd, 1997); this, unfortunately, is not the case today. Suicide rates among Inuit in Canada, Alaska, and Greenland are among the highest in the world. The rates have increased dramatically in the last thirty years (Kirmayer, 1994). As an illustration, the Canadian Inuit live in the Northwest Territories (NWT) and that region of Canada has the highest suicide rates in Canada. For example, in 1995 *Statistics Canada* reported a rate of 24.3 per 100,000 (32.1 male; 15.4 female) in the NWT, compared to a total of 13.4 per 100,000 (21.5 male; 5.4 female) in the Canadian population. Table 1 presents the rates of suicide for the North West Territories and Canada from 1980 to 1995. However, the data are probably not accurate. Indeed, in community-based studies, rates of 54.5 to 74.3 per 100,000 have been reported. The highest risk group is young males (Kirmayer, 1994). In 1995, for example, the rate of suicide for fifteen to nineteen year olds was 150.52 per 100,000 in the NWT, and this rate is from the underestimated Canadian rates. There has been, in fact, an increasing rate of suicide for young males, not females. Wotton (1985), in one northern community, reported rates as high as 295 per 100,000 for fifteen- to twenty-five-year-olds. Nowhere in the whole world will you find rates at these levels for young people.

With regard to suicide attempts, there are few studies. Boyer and his colleagues (Boyer, Dufour, Preville, & Beyold-Brown, 1994) reported a life time prevalence of 14 percent. However, in the young people (15 to 24 years), the lifetime prevalence is 27.6 percent for males to 25.3 percent for females. This is interesting because females usually have a higher attempt rate than the males. Yet, this pattern is not occurring in the Arctic. These events are much higher than for the general population of Canada. Domino and Leenaars (1994), for example, found a rate of 3 percent of lifetime prevalence of suicide attempts in the Canadian population. Thus, it is an easy conclusion that suicide and suicide attempts are a serious problem in the Canadian Arctic.

Table 1. Suicide Rates in NWT
and Canada

	Canada	NWT
1980	14.0	20.9
1981	14.0	21.9
1982	14.3	17.0
1983	15.1	43.4
1984	13.7	34.4
1985	12.9	25.5
1986	13.4	28.7
1987	14.0	29.0
1988	13.5	40.2
1989	13.3	58.1
1990	12.7	33.3
1991	13.3	40.3
1992	13.5	28.5
1993	13.1	42.4
1994	12.8	32.4
1995	13.4	24.3

Note: Rates are incidence per
100,000 population.
Source: Statistics Canada, annual.

Why are the rates of suicide so high in the Arctic? One of the people at the conference said that "suicidal ideation and suicide" was an indicator of complicated grief. I agree; and thus, it is easy to conclude, from an epidemiological point of view, that we are truly talking about a tragedy in the Arctic. It is an expression of complicated grief. Yet, we must ask, how can we understand this magnitude of complicated grief, this unbelievable rate of suicides in the Arctic?

A HISTORICAL BACKGROUND

The Inuit people of Canada live primarily in the eastern Arctic, as well as in northern Quebec and Labrador. Approximately 80 percent of the people of the eastern Arctic are Inuit. The present-day Inuit people stem from the Thule whalehunting culture that dates back to about 900 A.D., who overlapped with the Dorset people (approximately 1700 B.C.-1100 A.D.), who in turn overlapped with the pre-Dorset and Denbigh people (approximately 3000 B.C.-500 B.C.) (Houston, 1995; Kral, Arnakaq, Ekho, Kunuk, Ootoova, Papatsie, & Taparti, 1997). Archaeologists have found evidence that people resided in what is now Igloolik four thousand years ago (Punch, 1992). These people have been living on this land and living their life for centuries and centuries. Canadian Aboriginal people, including the Inuit and Dene of the north, have lived in northern Canada well before the Vikings arrived on the shores of Canada around 1008.

The Inuit had foreign visitors or Qallunat (Inuktitut for non-Inuit) notably occurring after 1400 with the arrival of British or European fishing ships, along with colonialism, predominantly by England and France. The Qallunat did not begin to have a major impact in the Arctic, however, until the whaling expeditions and fur trade of the nineteenth century. During those years, hostilities became common with the early, arrivals of the fur traders and whaling expeditions. Great diseases were introduced by the Europeans and took tens of thousands of lives. There were families where everyone in the family died from these diseases. By 1900, only about one-third of the Inuit population was left alive (Leenaars & Kral, 1996). These epidemics continued. There was loss after loss after loss. It has been estimated, for example, that by 1950 one-fifth of the Inuit population had tuberculosis (Kral et al., 1997). The pain, grief, and hostilities increased as the fur trade declined and ultimately collapsed in the 1930s. The Canadian welfare state was introduced in the Arctic and created a human disaster as the significant involvement of the federal government in the lives of the Inuit increased. The presence of missionaries, the government, and large-scale community relocations during the 1940s and 1950s of the Inuit, in the context of attempts at assimilation into Canadian society, changed northern life enormously (Kral et al., 1997; Tester & Kulchyski, 1994). The way of life in the Arctic continued to change. Food and other important resources changed, such that in some communities the Inuit even stopped eating the caribou. These Inuit only ate grocery store foods. Lifestyles, from extended family kinship and nomadic hunting practices, to a modern economy and the establishment of new settlements, resulted in traumatic experiences of grief and aftershocks (Crisjohn & Young, 1996; Royal Commission of Aboriginal Peoples, 1995).

Oil exploration and wells began on Melville Island in 1959, further affecting the pain in the north. Significant increases in social problems and especially suicide have occurred since 1960, primarily among young males (Durst, 1991; Kral et al., 1997; Travis, 1984). Suicide, in fact, increased dramatically with colonialism among Aboriginal peoples in Canada (Anawak, 1994). In the Arctic, during the 1970s and 1980s, epidemic levels of suicide were reported (Kirmayer, Fletcher, & Boothroyd, 1997). The loss of traditional lifestyle has been linked, in fact, to anomie, powerlessness, and grief in not only Aboriginal cultures throughout North America, but also Australia and the world (Berlin, 1987; Leenaars, Anawak, Brown, Hill-Keddie, & Taparti, 1999).

The Inuit continue to experience social disintegration (Durkheim, 1951/1897). They have one of the highest birth rates globally, which is double that of Canada. Fifty-nine percent of its population is under twenty-five years old, compared with 35 percent in all of Canada (The

Globe and Mail, 1997). Infant mortality is 3.5 times higher than it is nationally, and life expectancy is up to fifteen years lower. Their unemployment rate is almost in the 30 percent range (The Globe and Mail, 1997). There is a significant housing shortage (Punch, 1992). Colonial hostilities, thus, continue to impact the people of the Arctic (O'Neil, 1986).

It is now well documented that the Canadian government, beginning particularly in the late nineteenth century, systematically suppressed traditional Aboriginal beliefs and lifestyles through treaties, the Indian Act, residential schools and reservations, and the outlawing of spiritual ceremonies and persecution of those who were caught practicing (Dickason, 1992; Kral et al., 1994; York, 1989). Residential schools were especially endemic (Crisjohn & Young, 1996). The intent of the residential schools was as follows:

> Residential Schools were one of many attempts at the genocide of the Aboriginal Peoples inhabiting the area now commonly called Canada. Initially, the goal of obliterating these peoples was connected with stealing what they owned (the land, the sky, the waters, and their lives, and all that these encompassed); and although this connection persists, present-day acts and policies of genocide are also connected with the hypocritical, legal, and self-delusional need on the part of the perpetrators to conceal what they did and what they continue to do. A variety of rationalizations (social, legal, religious, political, and economic) arose to engage (in one way or another) all segments of Euro-Canadian society in the task of genocide. For example, some were told (and told themselves) that their actions arose out of a Missionary Imperative to bring the benefits of the One True Belief to savage pagans; others considered themselves justified in land theft by declaring that the aboriginal peoples were not putting the land to "proper" use; and so on. The creation of Indian Residential Schools followed a time-tested method of obliterating indigenous cultures, and the psychosocial consequences these schools would have on Aboriginal Peoples were well understood at the time of their formation. Present-day symptomology found in Aboriginal Peoples and societies does not constitute a distinct psychological condition, but is the well known and long-studied response of human beings living under conditions of severe and prolonged oppression. Although there is no doubt that individuals who attended Residential Schools suffered, and continue to suffer, from the effects of their experiences, the tactic of pathologising these individuals, studying their condition, and offering "therapy" to them and their communities must be seen as another rhetorical maneuver designed to obscure (to the world at large, to Aboriginal Peoples, and to Canadians themselves) the moral and financial accountability of Euro-Canadian society in a continuing record of Crimes Against Humanity. (Crisjohn & Young, 1996, p. 2)

The attempts at suppression are, hopefully, no longer in effect and Canada's Inuit are a healing people. A healing has, in fact, recently been started in the Arctic by the Inuit themselves. The lifestyles of Inuit are being restored. A new Inuit territory called Nunavut, first proposed in 1976, came into existence in the eastern Arctic in 1999, promising hope and deliverance to the people.

STORIES FROM THE LAND

Understanding grief and suicide in the Arctic is complex, more complex than Weyer and Boas suggested. They called suicide a trait of the Inuit. These Qallunat merely espoused suicide as a cultural trait in the Inuit, never raising the issue of grief. Yet, it has increasingly been understood that the event is multifarious. Of course, as in all suicides, there is pain, mental constriction, frustration of needs, and so on (Shneidman, 1985). However, it is not simply these psychological factors that explain the tragedy in the Arctic. As our account of the history shows, the Inuit have experienced profound cultural losses and changes in their lives. These people are experiencing complicated grief. As noted in our working definition, complicated grief is not simply within the individual, but within the culture. It is now well established that the rapid changes have had a major impact on the Inuit and all Aboriginal people (Royal Commission on Aboriginal Peoples, 1995).

To understand suicide, we believe that giving voice to the people is a sound avenue to knowledge (Kral et al., 1997; Leenaars, 1995; Leenaars & Kral, 1996). Narrative accounts are increasingly common in the human sciences, including in thanatology. Allport in 1942, in fact, had already argued for such idiographic (the singular, the individual) documentation, showing the importance of personal stories in human science. He argued that letters, logs, memoirs, diaries, autobiographies, personal accounts—and I would add suicide notes—have a place in understanding people. The tabular, statistical, arithmetic, demographic nomothetic approach, such as in our epidemiology section, has a place in understanding the generalizations about suicide among the Inuit. However, the idiographic is equally valuable. The narrative approach, I believe, will in fact give us a better understanding of the complicated grief in the Arctic. Indeed, narrative knowing or story telling is the tradition of the Inuit. No statistics can capture the grief of the people. Thus, we will report some stories from my travels in the Arctic (Leenaars, 1995) followed by a record of the questions from the audience at the London conference about the stories.

To illustrate the land, let me begin with the end of a trip.

My plane was to pick me up at 5:00 P.M. from Pangnirtung ("Pang"; pop. 1,000), a small hamlet near the Arctic Circle on Baffin Island. It's a marvelous little village. My leaving was important because I had to go to Rankin Inlet to meet with my friend, Jack Anawak, Minister of Parliament, and Senator Willie Adams. However, the Arctic controlled my plans. There was a snow storm (on September 23) and the plane could not land. There are few tourist places in Pangnirtung; fortunately, I was able to stay with Rev. Roy Bowkett and his family, who have been friends ever since. Let me tell three little stories about the evening events:

1. I decided to cook supper; so, I went to the "Northern" (previously the Hudson Bay stores) and bought two cans of spaghetti, one-and-a-half lbs. of hamburger, noodles, a bread, and peanut butter. The cost was $44.95. The cost of living is unbelievably high. Indeed, one carver whom I met said, "Groceries are more expensive than carvings."
2. As we were eating, a couple of Inuit children came in to join us. One said, "That smells good." I offered to share, provided they asked their parents. The oldest girl looked at me in a perplexed way and said, "I'm Inuk" (singular for Inuit). From my travels, I knew what this meant. Inuit children make their own decisions and parents respect the decisions, something maybe we all should learn.
3. One of the children—she was eleven—asked me, "Where are you from?" I mentioned Windsor, Ontario and noted the peach trees outside my home. She said, "I've never seen a tree."

To get an idea about the numbers of suicide, let me share with you my favorite trip on the land. I went out for a Kamotiq (sled) ride with two Inuit guides from Apex (pop. 200), a small hamlet near Iqaluit (pop. 3,000) on Baffin Island. We went over the ice of Frobisher Bay and went inland over the small lakes and land, while it was snowing. We traveled and traveled. The caribou were passing us; it was like what one sees on a National Geographic special. The land is not only beautiful, but also healing. On the trip, we stopped at a camp for tea—after all it was 2:00 P.M.—and as we sat, one Inuk told about his sister and brother who had killed themselves and talked about a grandparent. Everywhere there is pain. Everywhere there is grief. Regardless of where you go, one becomes aware of the vast number of suicides. All of the community is experiencing grief. The official statistics of NWT are likely unreliable. Research by Joshie Teemotee, an Inuk, in fact, has shown how unreliable the data are, the statistics under report the actual numbers.

Rankin Inlet is a beautiful community on the very north shore of Hudson Bay (pop. 1,000). One of the most important sites in Rankin is their Inukshuk. Inukshuks are stone figures; they are guideposts for the caribou hunts and for the travelers. They are found across the Arctic.

Once, when I was in "Rankin," the Keewatin Arts & Crafts Festival was being held. Keewatin artists are carrying on the tradition of fine art. There was a Northern Feast, where traditional foods such as arctic char and caribou were served. It was a feast of feasts. It ended with a concert by Susan Aglukark who performed in the native language, Inuktitut. One of her songs, "Arctic Rose" is about a young Keewatin who goes south, leaving the land. She sings about how this man, who comes from a place where it is six months night, did not know darkness until he saw the city lights. He lost himself, turning to alcohol and drugs. The grief grew and in the end, he killed himself, being returned to the land by the spirits after his death. The song is prototypical of the pain of the people.

I was fortunate to meet with young people in the schools on Baffin Island. We talked about suicide. They told me about their friends who had killed themselves. They told me about suicidal people. These young people were quite knowledgeable about the facts about suicide (as much as the young people who I have met in the schools in the south). We talked about helping, the place for peer counselors . . . I could have been speaking in any school in Canada (or the Western world).

The students raised many issues that I have heard before: suicide is just for attention, the complex issue of confidentiality, the lack of services, the need to know what to do, and so on. Some concerns were different, however. The sheer magnitude of the problem is an obvious difference. Most of these young people have not only experienced one suicide but many suicides among their family members and friends. The pain is expansive.

During a visit to Rankin Inlet, after my plane finally left "Pang," I met with Jack Anawak, M.P., and Senator Willie Adams. Both men are federal leaders from the Arctic and deeply concerned about the rate of suicide. I asked what they had learned.

They told about the abuse of the white men. They shared with me about a residential school reunion in Chesterfield, the mayor of the hamlet was also there. During the reunion, tales of abuse and sexual abuse arose. The abuse was namely by the clergy at the schools. Although they also told tales about the rewards of the churches, it was clear that there is an anger toward the predominant churches in the Arctic . . . and equally toward the Canadian government. These children were taken away from their families and put into residential schools. The school staff were supposed to help and foster the children; instead, they were abused and raped. The intent, as quoted earlier, was to obliterate the people.

An Inuk woman shared with me about the abuse by a priest. She said it occurred to everyone. It happened for years; yet, she said, "It never bothered me." Although, at the same time, she tells me of years of grief, asking why she might be that way. This story was shared with me over and over by other people. These people, as noted in our working definition of complicated grief, are in "complete denial of everything, amnesia." The grief is deep, deeper than many are aware.

On one of my trips above the Arctic Circle, I met a young Inuk woman, Sandra Inutiq. She was the 1993 valedictorian at Iqaluit's Inukshuk High School. She also had been on the front page of the *Globe and Mail* (Canada's national newspaper) on August 2, 1993. The article had focused on the story that drugs, suicide, and abuse meant that most Inuit teens never finish high school. Sandra was featured in the article, highlighting that Northern leaders are in short supply to guide the young. The article had caused, understandably, a lot of upset in the north. The article was presented as fact; yet, Sandra herself was very upset at the southern press although she also stated that there are deep problems in the Arctic that cannot be denied. The southern press, however, continue in this approach. For example, a more recent report of the *Globe and Mail* on July 4, 1998, entitled "Inuit find no magic solution on the way," again reports that there are no leaders. Sandra Inutiq's own account is more revealing; she said, "We have witnessed and been deeply touched by so many of the social problems around us." She said that suicide is a major problem "that must be addressed by teachers and parents." Sandra said, "People have to stop saying 'my child doesn't do that.'" The years of denial have to be spoken about. Yet, she equally believes that people are already working to make a successful future for young people. "Elders are available. We do have leaders." Sandra and many others are interested in helping in the Arctic and she concluded, "I think education is the number one priority if Inuit are going to heal."

Young people are now involved in suicide prevention. Yet, the pain/grief continues. One adolescent, on a revisit to his class a year after my first visit, shared with me the pain in his class. Many had left school during the year; school drop-out is a major problem. There had been pregnancy, substance abuse, violence, and suicide. Even in one year, when you listen, you can hear the ongoing losses and pains. As defined, complicated grief is not one loss but continual loss. Even in one year the unbearable pain had gotten deeper in the youth. Suicidal ideations and suicide, fueled by the pain/grief, as defined earlier, becomes a solution, not as an individual reaction but as a cultural reaction. It is not a trait or pathology in these people; it is most often an escape from unimaginable grief.

Jack Anawak has spoken to me many times. He tells me that the pain of the people is "deep in the psyche." He notes how traditional ways had been forgotten. Acculturation is the norm. People do not know who they are, where they came from, and where they are going. Jack Anawak said that the abuse at Chesterfield, for example, is only the surface. He says "How we think . . . how we talk . . . has been affected deep in our psyche." Maybe the best analogy I can offer is the iceberg. What people are beginning to struggle with in the north is likely the tip of the iceberg, and Arctic icebergs are large.

Jack Anawak noted that "only by re-learning the traditional ways with the new is healing possible." Jack Anawak does not believe that people can only heal by going back to the old; he and many leaders in the north see a need for growth and development. To go back to only the old ways, he says, is much too simplistic of a solution.

Jack Anawak admits that there are problems. Substance abuse is a major worry. The alcoholism, the gasoline sniffing, and so on are, of course, also expressions of grief. The alcoholism, for example, is not simply a trait by a "bunch of alcoholics." How would you feel if you came home and your children are taken away? How would you react if you may not speak English (or French or Latino) and you are imprisoned if you do so? The alcohol and drug abuse is a real problem. It is, in fact, a face of suicidal, destructive behavior.

Jack Anawak said many things about how Inuit ways differ. These ways are complex. As an example, he said punishment was less known before the Qallunat. People were rarely punished. They were not told "you're stupid." "When the white people came we were punished and told we were stupid." "We believed that we were stupid." Such cognitions, of course, are central to the suicidal mind. Traditionally, people talked to their children. They would not say one was bad; the children were respected. The elders would guide them. "They would tell us what they had learned."

Thus, it is easy to conclude that there is grief in the Arctic. However, it is deeper than most are aware. There is, in fact, complicated grief and, then, there is *extraordinary complicated grief.* Few griefs, even complicated griefs, should be labeled as extraordinary complicated grief. The surviving of Auschwitz is an example. Suicide in the Arctic is another example, an expression of extraordinary complicated grief. It is a cultural, not only individual, response to generation after generation of multiple losses, death, violence, abuse, diseases, and so on.

Howard Gardner (1997) wrote a fascinating book called *Extraordinary Minds.* There are people who are gifted, who have I.Q.s of 130 or better, and then there are the extraordinary gifted minds such as Sigmund Freud, Wolfgang Mozart, Virginia Woolf, Mahatma Gandhi. These are exceptional thinkers, impacters. They are extraordinary because they are the exception. There are very few people who should be called extraordinary.

I would like to propose here that the same concept can be used when we are talking about complicated grief. What is happening in the Arctic is not simply complicated grief, but extraordinary, unusual. It deserves a more complicated word than complicated grief. Few griefs, even complicated griefs, should be labeled as extraordinary complicated grief. Suicide in the Arctic is an expression of extraordinary complicated grief. It is a response to generation after generation of an intentional cultural genocide, and at times, genocide of the Inuit.

However, there is a healing in the Arctic. Elders are again being respected in the north. In Pangnirtung, I had heard such an elder speak. She told about the old ways, and then the whalers came. People hunted. People cleaned the whale . . . "and then the Qallunat would take the catch, leaving only blubber for us." "In our way," she said, "we share the labour and the catch."

On January 7, 1998, the federal government of Canada unveiled *Gathering Strength—Canada's Aboriginal Action Plan* to renew its relationship to the Inuit and all Aboriginal people. It was a reconciliation and a public apology to the original people of Canada for the atrocities of the Canadian Government. The Government admitted to its abuses, especially the violence in residential schools. The Honourable Jane Stewart, Minister of Indian Affairs and Northern Development stated:

> Sadly, our history with respect to the treatment of Aboriginal people is not something in which we can take pride in. Attitudes of racial and cultural superiority led to a suppression of Aboriginal culture and values. As a country, we are burdened by past actions that resulted in weakening the identity of Aboriginal peoples, suppressing their languages and cultures, and outlawing spiritual practices. We must recognize the impact of these actions on the once self-sustaining nations that were disaggregated, disrupted, limited or even destroyed by dispossession of traditional territory, by the relocation of Aboriginal people and by some provisions of the Indian Act. We must acknowledge that the result of these actions was the erosion of the political, economic and social system of Aboriginal people and nations.

In Canada's apology for its intentional cultural genocide, it makes special note of residential schools. The Canadian document reads:

> One aspect of our relationship with Aboriginal people over this period that requires special attention is the Residential School system. This system separated many children from their families and communities and prevented them from speaking their own languages and from learning about their heritage and cultures. In the worst cases, it left legacies of personal pain and distress that continue to reverberate in Aboriginal communities to this day. Tragically, some children were the victims of physical and sexual abuse.

The Canadian government apologized for the tragedy and the impact, the complicated grief that residential schools and other government actions caused. Yet, many do not believe that the statement is enough. Reconciliation about the extraordinary complicated grief will need to be more and ongoing, otherwise neither the Inuit nor all Canadians can heal.

The Inuit themselves in the north believe healing is possible. The Inuit are again sharing the labor and the catch. People need to speak about the sexual abuse, the alcohol use, suicide, and complicated grief. Suicide needs to be discussed. People need to adjust. Jack Anawak, at the end of one of our conversations, said, "I have no questions about who I am. I'm an Inuk, but I can adapt to other ways."

Many Inuit are now giving voice about the assimilation, the acculturation, being "totally lost"—the deep grief. Accepting acculturation is hard; yet "waking up" is now encouraged. The amnesia is being left behind. Yet, these people will need to understand much. Healing will take a long time because these people have not only lost their way of life, but some, their generational lives. They were stripped of their respect by the white man. There was no dignity. Their children were taken away from them. They were imprisoned for speaking Inuktitut. They were raped. They were abused. They were killed. It was a *cultural genocide* and, at times, *genocide.*

SUMMARY

There is hope for the grief in the Arctic. Lucien Taparti, an Elder and friend from Rankin Inlet, stated that "people have been crying inside for a long time"; however, there is direction. He stated: "It is up to each individual to help. . . . It is up to us to preserve our culture . . . our people." In a Foreword to a book, *Suicide in Canada,* edited by Leenaars, Wenckstern, Sakinofsky, Dyck, Kral, and Bland (1995), he says:

> In the past we hardly used to hear of suicides in our communities and would hear of them every so often only, because there were less people. Once in a blue moon you'd hear of suicides in one of the communities. But nowadays, in one year there would be quite a few suicides. It's hard to grasp the problem. I feel we should look for solutions and start giving this matter more consideration/attention.
>
> So how could we rectify this, working together in our communities, not only in the harsh land, but all of us in Canada? We have to start helping, because we all feel the same way and we live the same way. We all have the same lives. So we need to look for resources that would help in our communities. I wonder how we could start working together on this. . . .
>
> I think we have to start asking ourselves, "Where can we get help with suicidal people?" It is essential that we each have to ask ourselves this. The Inuit must ask themselves. We Canadians will have to ask how we could start to initiate things and how we could rectify problems more so and promote the issue more, so that suicide could decline. It's obvious now, that we will have to really work together on this issue.
>
> We all have different lives, different cultures and we can not say that the Qallunat have a strong culture. All of us came from our ancestors and if we could grasp that back then there were less suicides, perhaps we could start utilizing our culture for prevention. We will have to know more about the cultures of our ancestors, and try to follow them and try to help each other more. We can use many people's cultures, whether they may be Qallunat's, Dene's or even the Inuit's culture. If we can be more aware of people's cultures, then we would be able to come up with something that would be of benefit. (pp. xi-xvii)

QUESTIONS AND ANSWERS

Question #1—Unidentified Female

I would like to ask you to make some comment as a response to this terrible grief and whether it be turned inwards in suicide or outwards in anger. I was in the western Arctic a couple of weeks ago and was involved with the teachers who were discussing two communities that are about thirty miles apart, and on the Mackenzie Delta and about the same cultural composition. In one community, things according to our judgment seem to be going quite nicely. People are cooperating and are friendly. In the other community, there is a great deal of difficulty. The school has been burned down three times, and the day before we flew back we found out that another young person had been arrested by the RCMP because he had burned the Northern store. What would make that difference? You did not mention anger at all and what place does that have in the kind of changes that are happening, and is their terrible problem with suicide and with violence and so forth a kind of a warning to us about rate of change and what we see happening in our cities? Would you please comment on that?

Answer #1—Leenaars

First of all, about anger, I believe that when you talk about suicide, anger is often relevant. Yet, I fundamentally believe that suicide is much more an expression of unbearable pain than anger. Anger is often a secondary feeling or product due to the pain. So, when I talk about suicide, it is unbearable pain that I emphasize and the frustration of needs and mental constriction and so on.

Of course, I believe that anger is relevant in discussing suicide; indeed, there is a great deal of anger in the suicidal person. How would you feel if you came home and your house had just been taken away? Anger would certainly be a reaction to that event. Thus, there is anger and many other feelings in suicide that I did not talk about, like shame, guilt, and anomie, all worthy of discussion.

On the more difficult question that you asked, the one about communities; when I discussed the epidemiology, I mentioned the variation in rates of suicide in communities. Weyer's and Boas' early observations were probably based on specific communities. Indeed, there is great variation in the rates in the Arctic. You will find communities with almost no rates of suicide and then you will find communities with rates of 295 per 100,000 and so on. The question, I believe, should be, why? For example, Igloolik, which is in the eastern Arctic, traditionally had very low rates of suicide and, in the last couple of years, suddenly there is an increase. It is perplexing to the people why this is occurring now.

The variation in suicide rates is not only in the Arctic, but in all Aboriginal communities. You will find in Northern Ontario, for example, certain communities that have low rates and others that have very high rates. What are the explanations? I think, probably, you will need to go into those communities and try to understand the generation after generation impact of what happened to these people. In one of the places in Northern Ontario, for example, people were following a trail of suicide and it appeared to be associated to a specific person who had been in the schools. He had left a series of sexually abused children across the landscape. Thus, I think probably, it is an issue of what happened over time in the various communities that will explain the variation. Each of these communities will also have to understand their own pain. Each will have to heal in their way. Communities have their own ways. There are many different cultures of peoples in the Arctic and Canada as a whole.

The leaders and the elders will be most important in the healing in the community. However, some are not willing to participate, an expression of their grief. As an analogy in terms of schools, I have done a lot of work in suicide postvention in schools and communities. From my front line experience, we learned that certain principals will not let you in the schools after a suicide, whereas others are more than willing to accept postvention in the school. Of course, after a suicide or a trauma, the principal should not be allowed to make the decision about whether you do postvention or not. There should be a standard protocol. It should not be simply because of the principal who believes in "Don't talk about it." In one case, the reason why the principal did not allow the postvention is because his parents had both killed themselves. It had been a homicide-suicide; his own grief, i.e., denial, was stopping the response. The same thing is happening in the Aboriginal communities. There are leaders and elders who have their own dynamics and feelings and emotions; they have their own denial of their complicated grief. They alone should not decide; it should be the community's decision.

Let me give you another analogy to answer your question: The Dakota people in the United States recently had a rash of suicides in one community. What happened after the first suicide of a young person in that community was a big ceremonial traditional celebration. Then, they had another suicide and they had another celebration. Finally, the Chief and his people got together, and they said there shall be no ceremony for the next suicide, and there have been no suicides since. How the people respond to a suicide is so important. The same is true about any aspect of the pain and grief in the peoples. Of course, how all of us respond to survivors of suicide is so important.

Imitation in young people is a real problem. We know that imitation, as a solution, occurs in young people even more than in older people. David Phillips researched this fact. In some communities in the Arctic, you will find imitation. There is a spreading. Once suicide is in the community, it is an issue of how it is addressed and what is being done. One cannot develop amnesia. One of the approaches to imitation, for example, in the Arctic is identifying those communities that have higher rates and the people themselves are going into these communities, introducing a healing.

The truth is that we do not completely understand why some communities have higher rates. Michael Kral has been heading some research into that very question. He and his team are going to various communities and isolating the ones that have high rates and low rates and trying to understand what had happened.

To answer your question, I think that it is historical, what has been happening in those communities. Even if the communities are eighty miles apart, they are not the same. It is like our schools, even if it is down the street, all the schools are not the same in the community. There are different people, approaches, communities. We need to learn what is happening in the communities in the Arctic.

Question #2—Unidentified Person

What do you think about missionary activities that would say unless you accept our god, our all-loving god will burn you in hell now and forever?

Answer #2—Leenaars

There is no question in my mind that the missionaries were in the forefront of the culture genocide that occurred in the land. These people were sent out by the kings and queens to convert and to contaminate the minds and souls of these people. These people had their own beliefs and histories which, from my point of view, are as valuable and as worthy as ours, if not more so. And I think that until we start recognizing that our god is not the only god, that our god is probably with a "g" and that there is probably one, almighty spirit that all people share in various ways and experiences, the cultural genocide will continue. If we can finally start respecting all people in terms of their culture, a healing will occur. I am aggressive on this issue, but going up there and listening to the people, you learn that the people have their own approaches to understanding and healing. This does not mean that the Inuit necessarily alienate Christianity. Some of those people are very strong believers and open-minded to a Christian god. If you, for example, go to Rev. Roy Bowkett's church in Pangnirtung—it is an Anglican church—you will find an interesting mixture in the church of Inuit culture and Christian culture. These cultures mixed together into the services of these people. Other people, however, accept their traditional beliefs. Thus, unless we start recognizing that Christian religion is part of the history in the Arctic, we are not going to be able to address the grief. I am sure that I will offend some people when I say we need to be open-minded about people's spirituality and how they approach spirituality. I have a really hard time when I look back at our churches' histories in terms of their intent, calling the people in the Arctic a bunch of heathens and pagans. I just do not understand that kind of thinking. Of course, I am not from that era and times; yet, if you sit with some of these people in the Arctic, you will learn that many of them are deeply devoted people. They may not share what you or I believe, but they have the same concepts and beliefs of love and healing and spirituality.

The final thing that I will add to my answer is that the residential schools were very much run by the Anglican and Catholic people. Of course, the Canadian government has recently apologized for its role in setting up these residential schools, whose sole intent was to demoralize these people. It was an intent at cultural genocide. Therefore, I think what we need to do in the Arctic is accept our ways and accept their ways. We all need to work together. We all have different cultures. We all have different beliefs. We have our Qallunat culture and our Qallunat religion. They have their Inuit culture and their Inuit spirituality.

Question #3—Lee Thomas from Akenesasne Mohawk Territory

I'm a proud pagan. I guess the history of the Aboriginal peoples of Canada, and we in terms of our own selves refer to the Canada part. It is a long one. One of the main things I would like to state is that "yes" the people know what is good for themselves. If you give them the money and let them run it the way they want to in terms of programs, it should be run and designed by Aboriginal people. I think that one of the struggles, that we have all the time, is when new programming comes forth or designs for dealing with situations that often times these things still come from mainstream and that is part of the acculturation. The assimilation process is when you are programming from a mainstream process. I think that really in terms of balance, because healing is a process but balance is the outcome that we want.

I think there has been a cooperation of the word "healing" here. You are asking why, why, why the suicide rates? Well, back where we are from, we know that the difference is the stronger the community has its traditional ceremonies, the truer it has culture, the lower the stats on child welfare, suicide rates, drinking rates. We know that from our own community where the long house is very strong, it is a community that has both long houses and mainstream churches in it. So really, it is founded in its culture.

I agree with your statement somewhat in terms of the degree of the pain in terms of Auschwitz, but that was three generations. For Aboriginal people. It is 500 years. I think there is a major difference between the two. If anything for those who are mainstream people, they are trying to support I say support, not lead, not go in there to fix because you cannot do it. Encourage them to take their traditional ways back and you can't go there to be a part of that. I think with grace you need to acknowledge that too. So I have a lot of other comments. Overall, I've enjoyed your talk and I have lived many years in the North up in Nunivik and Delta region as well. Thank you.

Answer #3—Leenaars

I can only add one comment, thank you very much.

Question #4—Dr. Ed Pakes, Psychiatrist, Toronto

I was very impressed with the comments this lady just asked because she gave part of the answer to my question. I was going to ask you: If you were given whatever should be provided, what kind of program would you design? I guess part of the answer is to leave it to the people themselves and give them their culture back.

I think your reference to comparison with Auschwitz is that a lot of survivors of Auschwitz, including some of my family, had to deny what went on and had to rebuild their lives first before they could deal with the grief and mourning following that. I do not think it is just a simple answer but I would like to know what you think. What kind of help is needed in the Arctic? What would be the beginning step?

Answer #4—Leenaars

You are asking about programs for healing. Each of these communities have their ways. Lee, could you come up here? I will let Lee Thomas answer the question about programming in her community.

Lee Thomas—What was your question again?

Dr. Pakes—What would you do first, what would be the beginning step? Lee Thomas—In terms of developing a program for suicide prevention? Dr. Pakes—I don't even know if that is the right question because sometimes I think one has to deal with life before you deal with the aftermath of death.

Lee Thomas—Well, you know we look at culture, in traditional means it's a way of life. It is not a religion. One of the places where we really work hard in the community is starting with the youth. It is generational. We have clients who have gone through the residential school. The social learning process that they had was transferred to their children, who are now parents and they lack parenting skills, that are now being transferred to young ones. We like to focus on the young ones. Culture is not like a religion, where there's a place that you go to that you practice. In some means and ways, yes we go by ceremonies; but it is everything from getting back your traditional songs, your dancing, your language, which is the base. The roles and responsibilities of who we are and what we are, as a people, is from the medicine wheel. The elders have a responsibility, the children have a responsibility, the youth, and the adults in terms of. . . . Basically it is getting and empowering those individuals to get back to the philosophical means and ways of the culture. It is not going to be found just in ceremonies. It is not going to be found just in philosophy. It is the whole gamut. If I just talk a little bit about the medicine wheel, you will get the picture, sort of. The medicine wheel has four main colors, and it's because long ago we had a belief that there were four nations that walked on Mother Earth. To the north sat the White nation and their gift to humankind. Because we do not have men and women in our language, it is mostly human beings and the gift was their mental capacity. To the east of the medicine wheel is the color represented by yellow and there sat the Yellow nation and the gift that they gave to human kind was emotion. To the south of the medicine wheel is the color red, and that is where Aboriginal people sat and their gift to human kind was spirituality. To the west sat the Black nation and their gift was their physical endurance to human kind. The reason why it is in a circle is because in a circle all things are in balance, not one governs over another. It is not a hierarchy, but everything comes to the center in one. Now, if we look at it in terms of a people, the Elders sit to the north. They give us wisdom and when you follow the wheel to the east they look over the children and their gift to human kind. They bring us down to earth when we see their true emotions. The children also model from the youth who are to the south and the youth's gift is spirituality. If you have teenagers, like I do, you know they are pretty spirited, they have energy. The gift of the adult, that the youth models from the adult—because it is continual flow, is that they are the individuals that have to go out to look after the community. Again the circle is perpetuated. When you get a system like suicide, through problems you have to go back at government policies as to where the root of most of our issues stem. If you take a component, say the residential school system, they remove the youth and the children from our communities and so the wheel became imbalanced and, therefore, we are dealing with today's children who are acting like adults and adults acting like children. And so, it has been tilted and that is what I mean by our tradition and philosophy and beliefs. It puts us to an understanding of where we are as a people today.

I guess I have some personal comments. When they say we suffer from a cultural identity loss, I guess now that I have gone through academia, I have learned how to analyze in the way that you do. I think we have always known who we are and what we are. The difficulty is when we come into the conflict of the two meeting together. It is the meeting of the two, where one has made us insubordinate to the other. That is where we have become weakened. Even if Aboriginal people have been adopted, I find they still know they are Aboriginal. It is just their process to get there which is the conflict of the two that is what the problem is. So, I guess to make your long story short, empower the traditional culture because many do not have that anymore particularly in urban environments.

Dr. Leenaars—Let me finish our discussions in terms of answering your question with the words from Jack Anawak. He says:

> We need to own this problem. We cannot give it over to the governments, authorities, specialists, professionals, scholars, organizations or consultants. We own this problem. Say it . . . Believe it! We are part of the problem if we do not acknowledge this fact and take both individual and collective action to address it.

We have finally come to realize that:

- WE are the experts of our stories.
- WE know the strengths and weaknesses of our own communities.
- WE have a pretty good idea about how things got this way.
- We have a value system that is worth honoring . . . and WE do have the brains to figure out what to do about it!

The Inuit and all Aboriginal people are now confronting the cultural genocide and genocide toward indigenous people in the Arctic and across the globe. Healing has begun from extraordinary complicated grief. Healing is possible.

ACKNOWLEDGMENT

With thanks to M. Kral, parts of this presentation were presented elsewhere.

REFERENCES

Abbey, S., Hood, F., Young, L., & Malcolmson, S. (1993). Psychiatric consultation in the Eastern Canadian Arctic: III. Mental health issues in Inuit women in the Eastern Arctic. *Canadian Journal of Psychiatry, 38,* 32-35.

Allport, G. (1942). *The use of personal documents in psychological science.* New York: Social Science Research Court.

Anawak, J. (1994). *Suicide and the community.* Keynote address presented at the conference of the Canadian Association for Suicide Prevention, Iqaluit, NT (Nunavut).

Boas, F. (1964). *The central Eskimo.* Lincoln: University of Nebraska Press

Berlin, I. M. (1987). Suicide among American Indian adolescents: An overview. *Suicide and Life-Threatening Behavior, 17,* 218-232.

Boyer, R., Dufour, R., Préville, M., & Beyold-Brown, L. (1994). State of mental health. In M. Jetté (Ed.), *A health profile of the Inuit: Report of Sante Québec health survey among the Inuit of Nunavich. 1992* (Vol. 2, pp. 117-144). Montreal: Ministère de la Sante et des Services Socieux.

Crisjohn, R., & Young, S. (1996). *The circle game: Shadows and substance in the Indian residential school experience in Canada.* A report to the Royal Commission on Aboriginal Peoples, submitted Oct. 1, 1994.

Dickason, O. P. (1992). *Canada's first nations: A history of founding peoples from earliest times.* Toronto: McClelland & Stewart.

Domino, G., & Leenaars, A. (1994). Attitudes toward suicide among English speaking urban Canadians. *Death Studies, 19,* 489-450.

Durkheim, F. (1951). *Suicide.* (J. Spaulding & G. Simpson, Trans.). Glencoe, IL: The Free Press (originally published in 1897).

Durst, D. (1991). Conjugal violence: Changing attitudes in two northern native communities. *Community Mental Health Journal, 27,* 359-373.

Gardner, H. (1997). *Extraordinary minds.* New York: Basic Books.

Houston, J. (1995). *Confessions of an igloo dweller.* Toronto: McClelland & Stewart.

Inuit endorse gender-equal legislature (January 27, 1997). *The Globe and Mail,* p. A6.

Kirmayer, L. J. (1994). Suicide among Canadian Aboriginal peoples. *Transcultural Psychiatric Research Review, 31,* 3-58.

Kirmayer, L., Fletcher, C., & Boothroyd, L. (1997). Suicide among the Inuit of Canada. In A. Leenaars, S. Wenckstern, I. Sakinofsky, R. Dyck, M. Kral, & R. Bland (Eds.)., *Suicide in Canada.* Toronto: University of Toronto Press.

Kral, M., Arnakaq, M., Ekho, N., Kunuk, O., Ootoova, F., Papatsie, M., & Taparti, L. (1997). Stories of distress and healing: Inuit elders on suicide. In A. Leenaars, S. Wenckstern, I. Sakinofsky, R. Dyck, M. Kral, & R. Bland (Eds.), *Suicide in Canada.* Toronto: University of Toronto Press.

Leenaars, A. (1995). Suicide in the Arctic: A few stories. *Archives of Suicide Research, 1,* 131-140.

Leenaars, A., Anawak, J., Brown, C., Hill-Keddie, T., & Taparti, L. (199). Genocide and suicide among indigenous people: The north meets the south. *The Canadian Journal of Native Studies, 19,* 337-363.

Leeraars, A. & Kral, M. (1996). Suizidalität unter Kanadishen Inuit—nomethetishe und idiograpische Perspektivin. *Suizidprophlaxe, 5,* 60-66.

O'Neil, J. (1986). Colonial stress in the Canadian arctic. In C. Janes, R. Stall, & J. Gifford (Eds.), *Anthropology and epidemiology.* Dordrecht: D. Reigel.

Punch, D. (1992). *The Inuit and their land: The story of Nunavut.* Toronto: James Lonimer & Company.

Royal Commission on Aboriginal Peoples (1995). *Choosing life: Special report on suicide among Aboriginal people.* Ottawa: Minister of Supply and Services Canada.

Shneidman, F. (1985). *Definition of suicide.* New York: Wiley.

Taparti, L. (1997). Foreword. In A. Leenaars, S. Wenckstern, I. Sakinofsky, R. Dyck, M. Kral, & R. Bland (Eds.), *Suicide in Canada.* Toronto: University of Toronto Press.

Tester, F. J., & Kulchyski, P. (1994). *Tammarniit (mistakes): Inuit relocation in the eastern Arctic. 1939-1963.* Vancouver: University of British Columbia Press.

Travis, R. (1984). Suicide and economic development among the Inupiat Eskimo. *White Cloud Journal, 3*(3) 14-21.

Weyer, F. (1962). *The Eskimos: Their environment and folkways.* Hamden, CN: Anchan Books (originally published in 1932).

Wotton, K. (1985). Labrador mortality. In R. Fortuine (Ed.), *Circumpolar health 1984* (pp. 139-142). Seattle: University of Washington Press.

York, G. (1989). *The dispossessed: Life and death in Native Canada.* Toronto: Lester & Orpen Dennys.

CHAPTER 8
Grieving in the Context of a Community of Differently-Abled People: The Experience of L'Arche Daybreak*

Jane Powell

At the very beginning of this chapter, I want to take a risk and put forward the proposition that people with a developmental disability, far from experiencing complicated grief, may actually have much to teach the rest of us about grieving in a healthy way. There are, of course, exceptions. But the world of death and bereavement is a world of intuition, symbolism, and ritual, and people with disabilities tend to be much more in touch with these domains than some of the rest of us. I believe that it is precisely because of the lack of cognitive ability that people with developmental disabilities can live more spontaneously from their emotions and, because of this ability, can even give leadership in the work of grieving. But this can happen only if these people are actually enabled to know about terminal illness, to be close to their friends and family members as they approach death, and to participate in the normal expressions and rituals of grieving.

My own learning in this area has taken place in the context of the L'Arche Daybreak community, an intentional faith community where I have lived for many years. Daybreak is a member community of the International Federation of L'Arche Communities, founded by Jean Vanier. In North America, L'Arche communities are predominantly Christian, but other faiths are also welcomed. In L'Arche, people with developmental disabilities share a life together with those who come to assist them. We live together in households, and while some members of the community have employment outside the community, others spend their days together in day and seniors' programs or working in the woodworking shop. Mutuality is a fundamental principle of community life in L'Arche. We believe that each person both gives to and receives from

*This chapter has been developed from a practice report presented at the conference "Understanding and Treating Complicated Grief," hosted by the University of Western Ontario, London, Ontario, Canada, in May 1998.

others in the course of our community life. All that I say in this chapter is based on the experience that "care-giving is not a one-way street," and on the assumption that caregivers have the courage, humility, and insight to receive from those whose care is entrusted to them at some more formal level. Particularly in this most universal realm of death and grief, barriers fall away and we become aware of our common humanity.

Our community of L'Arche Daybreak is rich in diversity of age, intellectual level, religious background, and means of communication. In recent years we have grieved the deaths of several community members, family members, and friends. Because many members of the community have an intellectual disability and some have multiple disabilities, we have needed to find ways to deal with death very concretely and creatively. We have seen the importance of involving each member of our community in the grieving process, whether labeled "disabled" or not. This concrete and shared involvement has greatly facilitated our walking through grief to acceptance and consolation. I share some of our experience here, believing that it can be generalized to other situations.

I will deal with the three stages in the grief process—anticipatory grief, intense grief, and bereavement—describing the steps we have found important to take before the death occurs, the actions we take at the time of death, and the ways in which we facilitate the grieving process after the loss. I give the greatest attention to the first stage because I believe that if it is lived with depth, the actual death and later bereavement is much more likely to be smooth. It will become clear that in each stage, while some steps may be particularly helpful for someone with an intellectual disability, many can be of value to the so-called "normal population" as well.

WHAT CAN WE DO BEFORE A
DEATH OCCURS?

Drawing from our experience at L'Arche Daybreak, I will suggest seven steps that can help the person with a disability prepare for the loss of a loved one. Everything I say here treats as fundamental that honesty will be the rule in communication about illness and impending death and all that ensues. We need to be committed to keeping members informed frankly and clearly of the progression of their own or someone else's illness. In the past, a somewhat patronizing attitude and perhaps fear of unexpected, possibly embarrassingly emotional responses, and also the mistaken assumption that people cannot understand, fed into a tendency to want to shelter people with disabilities from the truth about painful situations. It is now well known that such "sheltering" does much damage that is very difficult to undo later. What I am saying assumes also, of course, the exercise of sensitivity in communication, as would be the case in communicating with any other person about the illness and death of a loved one.

Create a Support Group

At Daybreak, most of the seniors with disabilities belong to the Seniors' Club, which meets Monday to Friday as a social club and peer support group and to engage in various recreational and social service activities. It is the peer support aspect of this group that has proved especially important at times of loss or anticipated loss. This is a group of people who are aging together. They have known one another for some years, and, with good facilitation by a small team who knows the seniors well, they are able to share their fears, sorrows, and frustrations. It is a group where the seniors can gently cope with the variety of losses that accompany aging, and where they can prepare for their own dying and the deaths of others. It is a place to be cared for emotionally and spiritually while becoming more fragile physically. And it is a place to give care to friends and to be respected as a wise elder.

Many in the group have lost parents, siblings, and friends; and with the aid of good facilitation have learned to support others in this situation. George knew that when his sister died too far away for him to attend the funeral, he had a safe group with which to share the story of their relationship and to help him to try to make sense of the loss. He knew others in the group had been through similar experiences and that the moment had come for him to receive the type of support he had offered to them. When she died he brought a photo of his sister and some letters she had written to him, and the others listened sympathetically as he spoke about what she had meant to him and remembered some of the good times of their childhood. At the suggestion of one of the group, he decided to have a memorial prayer service for his sister. All his friends in the Seniors' Club and others who were close to him came to support him at the service.

This group of seniors is able to participate in rituals and to celebrate together. Milestone birthdays and their silver anniversaries of coming to Daybreak are big occasions. It is an environment in which care for others is fostered. When one of the regular recipients on their meals on wheels route died, they sought out the family and sent condolences. The seniors hope for and savor together the many little moments that keep their lives rich and meaningful. For instance, Peggy's being able to go to her family cottage one last time before it was sold, in spite of her increasing problems with mobility, was acknowledged for the significant event that it was in Peggy's life.

A death or approaching death of a significant friend or family member can bring the loss of other activities and contacts very important to an individual's well-being, quite apart from the actual loss of relationship with the loved one who has died. Such loss can be especially pronounced when the individual is already more dependent on these others for support than might be the case among ordinary members of society. And in the senior years this experience of loss and anticipation of further loss can continue to grow over a period of months or years.

One member of the Seniors' Club, Alfred, became depressed when the death of his mother led to his no longer being able to visit the family home for weekends. Over the ensuing years, as his father became less and less able, even visits at home for a meal became impossible. Gradually, Alfred's father began to lose both his hearing and his memory and Alfred's previously consoling phone calls to his father became a source of pain and disappointment. Meanwhile, Alfred himself, who formerly had traveled independently by public transit to visit his parents, became physically disabled and dependent on assistants who were willing to drive him to see his father. Alfred displayed understandable anger, impatience, and frustration during this time. The team in the Seniors' Club facilitated his expressing his feelings to the others and eliciting their understanding, sympathy, tolerance, and forgiveness.

His senior friends helped Alfred not to retreat into sad isolation but to share his sadness and loss with them. Finally, Alfred's father moved to a nursing home and the beloved family home was sold. Alfred continued to be able to visit his father with the aid of assistants, but the loss of the family home was so traumatic that for a time he became quite psychologically disoriented and spent some time in the hospital. Through all this, Alfred's friends in the Seniors' Club remained a constant, kind source of support. Some of the others were experiencing similar diminishment of contact with their families and similar losses of mobility, and as the others spoke about their frustrations, the mutuality of this experience seemed to help Alfred cope. Finally, when his father died, the others rallied around him in friendship and attended the funeral to show him their support. Over the ensuing months some of the seniors joined him when he visited his parents' grave and spent time drawing him out in conversation as he processed the loss and all that his parents had meant to him.

With her friends in the seniors' group, Peggy was able to speak clearly of her hesitations about moving to a new house and to think out loud about the features she would need to help her to maintain as much independence and privacy as possible in the new home. In turn, the group was able to encourage her to ask for what she needed. She can no longer manage stairs, but she wanted, for example, to be able to get to the basement to do her own laundry. After some discussion, she decided to ask that the new house have an elevator and this, in fact, proved possible.

With some team facilitation the group can speak together about Roy's heart being weak, and how this tires him and means he frequently needs to rest or have an easy afternoon—a drive in the country with no clambering in and out of a vehicle, for instance. With this understanding, they are more able when necessary generously to let go of their own plans to accommodate Roy. And the other seniors can help each other understand why Roy is not always in the most cheerful of moods. The Seniors' Club is a place other than Roy's home where he knows he is loved and cared for.

Undertake Life Review and Life Story Work

Life review and the preparation of one's life story is becoming increasingly recognized as important to maintaining good mental health as one ages and as helpful in coming to terms with one's own mortality and preparing for death (Butler, 1963). Life review can be facilitated as people share about their lives and family histories with a close friend or counselor or in a small group with others whom they know and trust and where a safe atmosphere can be established.

The preparation of a life story book can be a therapeutic project during the time of anticipatory grief. It can also be a very good way for a terminally ill person to integrate his or her life experiences and the book itself can be a wonderful legacy for friends and relatives.[1] The therapeutic effect may actually be experienced both by the helper and by the one being helped, as together they examine the many ups and downs of the subject's life journey and the experiences that have shaped who the person has become. And the book itself can be a wonderful legacy for the deceased person to leave behind for family and friends.

Life story work may be particularly important for people who are devalued in our society (Porter, 1998). It provides an opportunity for them to realize how many lives they have touched and been touched by. People with developmental disabilities, of course, are not likely to be able to write down their own memories. An approach that has been used effectively in Daybreak is to assist individuals to write letters to friends and family asking them to send letters with special memories of the person, perhaps humorous little stories or anecdotes, and pictures. We ask that the letters try to highlight the gifts of the person. Tape recordings are also an option if letter writing is difficult. Most recipients are delighted to respond. Often the letters that are sent back to the Daybreak member tell the person of his or her importance in the lives of others. Hearing and discussing these often quite beautiful letters helps the individual to integrate their life history and to see the fruitfulness of their life in their relationships with

---

[1] The Hospice Foundation of America provides a Life Story kit with a video tape and fill-in-the-blank workbooks for the various stages of a person's life. The Foundation's address is 777 - 17th Street, Suite 401, Miami Beach, FL 33139.

others. It is generally a very positive experience for people to work on their life story book with someone they trust. At Daybreak, these books are so sacred that some people have asked to have them blessed.

Find Ways for People with Disabilities to Help Their Dying Friend or Relative

When someone we are close to is living their last months, we can feel very helpless. This can be particularly true for people with disabilities, who may experience even greater powerlessness. They are often assumed to be less able to contribute in difficult situations and may in fact be unnecessarily sheltered or thoughtlessly shut out at such times. We have found that it is important to discover a way for people to be involved directly or indirectly in helping provide care for a dying person. When Helen developed Alzheimer's disease and was having difficulty going upstairs, Gord, a man with a disability who had shared Helen's home with her for a number of years, suggested that he trade rooms with her so that she could have a main-floor bedroom. This was a generous offer on Gord's part and, in fact, one that others in the house quickly saw would benefit Helen. The team in the house ensured that Gord was pointedly credited with making a very real contribution to improving Helen's situation. George, another house member, offered to sit in the living room with Helen on certain afternoons and call for assistance if Helen was about to wander out of the house.

When Adam was being cared for at home, John, a man with Downs Syndrome, was able to help. John was not working at the time and could actually travel to doctor's appointments with Adam and Ann, who was responsible for the home. John was able to lift Adam's wheelchair in and out of the car and to help transfer Adam. Ann speaks very clearly about the great practical and emotional support John gave to her and to Adam. Unfortunately, people with disabilities rarely experience being thanked and feeling deeply appreciated. Such opportunities to give and to be thanked for giving can be very healing when someone is grieving.

The Daybreak members with disabilities are often very generous and quite emotionally mature. The challenge for us is to be creative in involving them in safe ways that they can provide support. Then people can feel they have done what they are able and this can ease the grief when someone dies.

Help Those Who Will be Facing a Loss to Visit the Ill Person in Hospital

Both Helen and Maurice lived their last months on the chronic care floor of our local hospital, much diminished by Alzheimer's disease. We found it very important to convey to the nurses and other staff what we could about Helen's and Maurice's life before they became ill, so that the staff would have some sense of the richness of their lives and their delightful personalities. One way of doing this was to leave their photo albums and life story books by their bedside. Another was to use opportunities to chat with staff about our friendships with their patients when we visited. The Daybreak community set up a roster so as to have someone to give support at mealtimes, since they needed help eating. Friends with disabilities could readily be included in these visits by planning that we visit in pairs. Gord, a fairly independent man who had lived with Helen, usually walked over to the hospital to help her with dinner on Saturdays. The seniors took responsibility for one lunch each week.

A journal was placed by Helen's bedside, with the request that visitors enter a note or draw a picture about their visit. Since eating was difficult for Helen, the note was to include information as to how she had eaten. This book provided a way for visitors to feel a little more connected with Helen's care and was also an additional, more personal and comprehensive means for us at Daybreak to monitor Helen's condition. The Daybreak nurse coordinated Helen's and Maurice's care with the doctors and hospital staff, who, we discovered, were glad to have our support with the patients. Our nurse also helped the rest of us in the community to understand Helen's and Maurice's medical condition and what we could expect would happen to them as the disease progressed. Our nurse's involvement allowed others of us to be free to be present as friends and family rather than primarily as medical liaisons.

All of the Daybreak members with disabilities were encouraged and supported to visit Helen and Maurice if they wished. This meant that all were able to see their decline and when death came, it was with less of a shock. Some of those who visited do not have verbal skills. I believe they were able to grasp intuitively that Helen and Maurice were going to die because they saw them getting sicker, whereas they might not have grasped a merely verbal explanation.

Engage the Person with a Disability in Helping to Plan the Funeral

Early funeral planning, when death is not imminent, helps to ensure that the needs of all parties involved are met as well as possible. Obviously, we include the person who is ill as much as is possible and to the degree they desire. We have found that people with disabilities who are aging or in failing health but mentally able, often want to express their preferences for their funeral and burial, when the subject is introduced gently and by a trusted person at an appropriate time. Some Daybreak members are very clear about their wishes—for example, that they be buried with their parents or in a particular cemetery, or that they be cremated. And they may even want to choose favorite hymns or the leader and readers for their funeral service.

Of course, pre-planning is not always possible. It is helpful to be prepared to include friends or family members with disabilities in arrangements even when such arrangements must be done quickly. When George died suddenly, his family were glad to have his house-mates involved in choosing the casket and contributing to the funeral as readers, ushers, and pall-bearers. This was possible because the family had already become acquainted with George's Daybreak friends and trust had been established.

The need to plan ahead is even greater if the dying person is of an unfamiliar culture or religion and customs and expectations might be very different. Alia, a woman with whom I lived for some time at Daybreak, is of the Moslem faith. In a way, because her needs are great, she is at the center of our community. Doubtless, when she dies everyone in Daybreak will miss her deeply and want to grieve her in some formal way. To prepare ourselves in the event of Alia's death, we asked to meet with her family. We wanted to be aware of and sensitive to their traditions regarding death, and we also wanted to plan ways in which we non-Muslims can join in grieving her. A plan that is acceptable to and that will be consoling for everyone emerged as Alia's family were able to share their wishes concerning Alia's care with us. A "living will" was signed and a copy placed in Alia's file. It is helpful that this discussion took place in a less stressful and emotional way than would have been the case if Alia's life had been in immediate danger. The discussions were precipitated by Alia's needing a feeding tube. Looking back we are grateful that we took the opportunity to have those discussions, as now we can approach the time of Alia's eventual death with clarity and peace of mind, having the assurance that we and her family have the same expectations. The need for this type of dialogue will only increase as our society becomes more diverse.

Encourage Conversation about the Deceased and about Feelings

We intentionally create opportunities to talk about the dying or deceased person. We have found that, particularly for people who have limited verbal skills, it is helpful to have a picture of the person who is ill in a prominent place in the home. We may sit in a circle and perhaps light a candle and pass the picture around, inviting each person to share a memory about the deceased as they hold the photo. The presence of a picture often seems to give people permission to talk. At other times we may notice someone pausing to look at a photo or other object associated with the deceased and take that as a cue to spend time with them. When Lloyd died, his favorite chair at the Seniors' Club looked dramatically empty. Then Francis, Lloyd's closest friend, decided to sit in it. This seemed very appropriate to the others and they affirmed that Francis should have Lloyd's chair and spoke to Francis about the importance of his friendship to Lloyd. This exchange allowed Francis to express his feelings a little more and seemed to be quite consoling for him.

Our experience at Daybreak is that people with disabilities are capable of anticipatory grief, but as caregivers we need to be in touch enough with our own feelings that we do not inhibit this opportunity for those whose grieving we should be facilitating. It is wise to assume that the friends of the dying or dead person understand what is happening, even if they do not seem to be expressing what we would consider to be associated feelings. People who are very limited are also often very sensitive to the feelings of those around them. If nothing else, they will be aware of the concern, anxiety, and tension of their caregivers. It is much easier if the truth of an approaching death is known by all. In the talking together or even in listening to others talk about the person who is dying, their friends may recognize the value of this person and also, perhaps, sense the sacredness of life in general and, by extension, of their own life.

Patrick had a very strong relationship with his mother and found it difficult to make decisions of which he thought she might disapprove. His mother was ailing and Patrick and those around him were concerned about his ability to cope when his mother died. Patrick chose to take part in a special grief-sharing group geared to his needs before his mother died. At the time of his mother's death, Patrick experienced many different feelings but he had a sense that they were not totally abnormal. He was also aware that he needed extra support at this time and was able to seek that out. Our experience with Patrick taught us that someone with a disability such as Patrick's is able to process to some degree what will happen in the future and to develop strategies to use during the difficult period.

Help People to Say Good-by When Death is Imminent

It is important for caregivers to remember that, regardless of the type of service they are helping provide, the people with disabilities who are involved will usually have very long-term relationships with one another. This is true in both residential and work settings. We, as care providers, cannot overestimate the importance of people having a chance to say good-by to their friends when they are actually nearing the point of death. This may mean working closely with people at the hospital or home where the dying person is being cared for.

Certainly, this farewell visit may be an emotional one, but I believe that it provides a healthy way to begin the more intense phase of grieving. Our experience has been, as well, that even for the dying person there is a peacefulness that comes when loved ones come to say good-by. Again, clear communication is very important. Visitors should be prepared as to what to expect. They should know how the dying person will look and be helped to understand that he or she may not be able to respond to them. Mention should be made beforehand of bandages, tubes, machines, or noises that may be alarming. Good preparation will help to make the situation less frightening and the person will be able to focus better on the actual visit. The visitor may choose to make a card to leave behind, or if the visit proves too much at the last minute, to substitute for his or her presence. Visitors can also be helped to think ahead about what they would most like to say to their dying friend—perhaps, a simple sentence like "I love you" or "Thank you for being my friend."

During the actual visit it may be important to help visitors make a connection with the dying person, perhaps by enabling them to stand close to the bed or to hold the person's hand. It may be necessary to work with hospital staff to get permission for people to visit. When Lloyd was dying, many family and friends were able to visit him because he was placed in a separate corner of the ICU. This opportunity to visit was especially important because Lloyd became critically ill quite suddenly and we were not prepared for him to die. Even though he was not able to respond at all, it helped all of us who were his close friends to at least see him, to lay gentle hands on him, and to say a prayer together.

WHAT MIGHT BE HELPFUL AT THE
TIME OF DEATH?

Share the News Fully and Clearly

Again, as with anyone, it is very important to be honest and to use clear language in speaking about a death. Ideally, the language used is language with which people have become familiar over the duration of the illness. If a family member of a person with a disability dies and the person needs to be informed, it is best that this be done in private by someone who is a strong reference for the person. Meanwhile, it may be helpful to see that other people in the bereaved person's house are also informed, so that they can be sensitive and give support to their friend. Some excellent illustrated materials are available for people who have difficulty grasping verbal information.[2]

---

[2] See Sheila Hollings\'92 books, *When Dad Died* (   ) *and When Mom Died* (   ). A third by Hollings, *Feeling Blue* (   ), is helpful in dealing with depression. These books may be ordered from The Department of Psychiatry of Disability, St. George\'92s Hospital Medical School, Cranmer Terrace, London SWLZORE, U.K. at a cost of 12.50 pounds sterling each including postage.

When a member of Daybreak dies, we have discovered that the support of the community leaders (administrators) and the pastor is often helpful. As soon as possible after word of the death is received, these "outside" people visit the houses in which the deceased lived or was most connected. They are present to give security and reassurance and also practical support to both the assistants and the people with disabilities. They can encourage the members of the household to ask questions and ensure that they grasp what has happened.

It is often important to share information about the death a number of times and in different ways, to ensure that each person has fully grasped what has happened. Supplying concrete details is more helpful than it is disturbing. People seem to need to know what happened at the actual time of death. Details such as who was there with the person and whether or not the person was in pain are important. Sometimes, the fact that the information is given seems somehow more important than the details themselves. But generally, people will be less confused and afraid if they know where and when and under what circumstances the person died. It may be helpful to describe how the deceased person looked after he or she died. The bereaved friends will also want to know where their loved one's body is now and what to expect in the ensuing days.

Staff or friends who were very close to the deceased will need extra support. Often many phone calls must be made and practical arrangements undertaken. It may be comforting for those closest to be involved in these arrangements but not to have to make decisions alone. They will also be coping with their ordinary responsibilities and dealing with their own emotions.

Gather Together Soon After a Death

As soon as possible after we have received news of a community member's death, we gather in our chapel. It is important to be together, to hear once again what happened, to ask questions, and to express our feelings. If possible, someone who was with the deceased when they died speaks of what actually took place at the time of death. As we speak about the person, share our memories and perhaps various anecdotes, we may cry, laugh, pray, and feel angry or numb, but the experience of sharing together our sadness about our common loss is a great source of strength in the difficult days to come. I have noticed that people with disabilities are often quite uninhibited about expressing their emotions and in this way may help the rest of us. A gentle embrace can give much comfort. This time together gives all of us permission to grieve and alleviates some of the loneliness and fear that often accompanies the news of death.

Help Those Who are Grieving to be Involved in the Rituals

It is good to encourage people to participate as much as possible in the rituals that are customary at the time someone dies, but also to be very respectful of each person and where they are in the grieving process. We try to provide the necessary accompaniment and support for each one who is grieving so that each may participate as fully as possible. We especially need one another at this time. Linda, a young woman who has suffered many losses, can be quite emotional when someone has died. But her crying and wailing show me that it is all right to be vulnerable. We can cry together. There is a wonderful mutuality because neither of us have any control over the reality that someone we love has died.

At the visitation or wake we find it helpful to call those present to focus together for a time. We gather in a circle to listen to a comforting reading, perhaps to sing, to say a prayer, and allow those present to tell some stories about the deceased. People with disabilities can be helped to prepare, so that they can contribute. This may require asking someone who knows the history of the person's relationship with the deceased to help. At Daybreak, we tell stories about special times we spent with the deceased, about significant moments in the deceased person's life, about turning points in our relationship with the person, and about what we see as the fruitfulness of the person's life.

When it is a family member of a person with a disability who has died, we may need to encourage the family to allow the person to participate as much possible, supplying accompaniment so that he or she can attend the visitation time and the funeral. When Michael's brother, Adam, died, their parents thought, naturally enough, that going to Adam's burial might be too difficult for Michael. They were gently encouraged to allow Michael to join them and others at the graveside. Once there, Michael seemed interested in the priest's sprinkler with which he planned to bless Adam and the casket immediately before the burial. Recognizing this, friends arranged that Michael be allowed to help sprinkle the casket with holy water during this final blessing. For Michael, this proved a wonderful opportunity to express a last gesture of love for his brother. It also helped Michael afterwards to be very clear about what had happened: Adam's body was in the ground; his spirit was with God.

When Henri, our pastor and a much-loved member of our community died, people working in the Daybreak woodworking shop helped build his coffin. Some also drew pictures which were then painted on the coffin lid. At the wake, community members were invited to place a small token in the coffin with Henri. Some people contributed pictures or notes; others, a flower or something that symbolized their relationship with Henri. This was a chance to offer a final farewell gesture and to say thank you to

Henri. Everyone who wanted was able to participate regardless of intellectual or physical abilities.

People who may never have been to a funeral home or a funeral should be helped to know what to expect. If the casket is closed, it may not be evident to the visitor that the body is in the casket. A photo of the deceased placed on top of the casket can be of help in grasping this reality. If the casket will be open for the body to be viewed, the visitors should be told, so that they are less afraid. In either case, they should be helped to approach the casket and make some gesture—to touch it gently or say a prayer, perhaps. If possible, the funeral should be planned with a concern for both accessibility and participation of people with disabilities. At Henri's funeral, the Scripture reading was mimed while it was being read, for instance. Others participated in a reverent dance. And the eulogy was prefaced by one of Henri's close friends with a disability.

When possible, it is usually helpful for people with a disability to be able to go to the cemetery and see the interment. We have found it good to participate together in shoveling the earth down onto the coffin after it is lowered. This may be a painful experience but it gives a sense of completion and makes the reality quite clear. When going to the interment is not an option, we have developed a custom of filing past the casket for a final brief good-by just before the casket is taken out and the service ends. In Daybreak funerals, time is allowed for being sad and serious, but the emphasis is put on giving thanks and celebrating the goodness of the deceased person's life. Usually, there are moments both of laughter and of tears.

Be With One Another

Almost all people wish to have another person whom they trust simply be present with them at a time of intense grief. When Henri died suddenly of a heart attack it was difficult for all of us at Daybreak. He had helped many of us in the community when other members had died, so that we especially missed his comfort when he himself passed away. I had the privilege of sitting at his wake with Tracy, a woman who needs much support because she has profound cerebral palsy. We sat together in silence on some cushions on the floor near the coffin containing Henri's body, with Tracy leaning against me. We had no words to share that would comfort us because Tracy does not speak with words and because my words would not have made our grief any easier. But being there quietly with Tracy was very consoling for me. We needed to be together. It was one of those privileged moments when our common humanity is evident and differences fade away.

We should not assume that someone with a disability has feelings different from our own. People who have a significant loss will be grieving in their own way, even if they are not expressing their grief in identifiable behaviors. We are likely mistaken if we think they do not understand or do not care. The person's feelings need to be acknowledged and attended to for healing to take place. It can be important to ask ourselves who it is whom the person with a disability might be able to talk to at a time of loss. It is good to remember also that a death, for any of us, may trigger memories of other significant losses. For instance, some people with disabilities have been rejected by their families and bereavement may reawaken these feelings of abandonment. Over time, I have noticed that people with disabilities are able to develop skills during a period of struggle or loss that they can then generalize to other experiences of grief. Sitting quietly with a friend over a cup of tea, or with a lit candle, can lead to the gentle sharing of tears. One person I know used relaxation techniques which he had learned for stressful times at work, to help him deal with grief. Others have asked for some warm milk or herbal tea to help with sleep. These are only a few examples of the types of self-care that all of us, disabled or not, can practice when we are coping with intense grief and, perhaps, feel we have little control over a situation.

HOW CAN WE SUPPORT ONE ANOTHER
AFTER SOMEONE HAS DIED?

Visit the Grave and Celebrate Anniversaries

Helping the bereaved person to visit the grave of a loved one periodically can help bring solace and aid in the journey through grief. It is usually helpful for the individual to bring along something to leave at the grave, even if just a single flower or, in the Jewish tradition, a pebble to place on the headstone. We find this is a good time to invite the grieving person to share a few memories of the deceased and perhaps to hold hands and say a prayer together. Expect that some tears may be shed and welcome these.

The seniors at Daybreak have a custom of visiting the graves of friends around the time of the anniversary of the person's death. On some occasions they have invited siblings of the deceased to meet them at the cemetery and have followed the visit to the grave with a lunch or tea outing to renew contact with the family members who have come. This gives opportunity to reminisce further and gives the comforting experience of being together with others who knew and loved the deceased friend. When they visit Lloyd's grave, the seniors invariably recall that Lloyd loved Holsteins, and they recount some of the teasing that they engaged in with Lloyd about his preference for these over Jersey cows. Usually, his sisters will then share about their family life on a Holstein farm before Lloyd moved to Daybreak. Before long, various members of the group have fondly mentioned several favorite stories of Lloyd and the whole experience becomes one of treasuring Lloyd's memory in a way that allows the gift of his life to continue to unfold for each person. I believe this experience also may give the seniors some reassurance that they will be remembered after they die.

The members of the house where Adam had lived decided to mark the first anniversary of Adam's death with a memorial mass and dinner to which they invited Adam's family and a few of his closest friends. The setting was beautiful, with flowers and pictures of Adam arranged around the coffee table altar. It was also a moment for those present to realize they had gotten through the year even though it had been difficult, and to give thanks for Adam's life and all he had meant to them. Adam's parents were grateful to see how much Adam continues to be loved by those with whom he had lived.

Give Permission to Grieve

We have found it helpful to continue displaying pictures and mementoes of the deceased person and to continue telling stories about them for weeks or months after the person has passed away. These items make it clear that those who are bereaved are not expected just to forget about the one who has died and that it is alright to grieve. After some time it may finally feel right to put some of these away and to choose one special photo to display. We find this decision is best made by the members of the household together. A discussion can follow as to how to dispose of the items that will no longer be displayed and perhaps a small ritual created for this changeover, but it is wise not to put a timetable on grieving. People will each grieve in their own way and in their own time. Sometimes the behavior of someone with a disability may change and caregivers may see this as a behavior management issue or merely as attention-seeking. It is important to recognize that the problem behavior may in fact be a way that the person is trying to express grief. We may not be able to see an obvious connection between the behavior and the loss, and the person him or herself may be unable to name this connection, but kindness and patience and the professional help of a grief counselor may be the answer at such times. It may be that unresolved griefs from long ago have been awakened by the more recent loss.

I assist with bathing and personal care for some of the Daybreak members who have profound disabilities. I have discovered that it is important to pay special attention to the body of a person who is grieving. The tension in the person's body may be expressing what they are unable to express in words. People may need to get extra rest and greater care at anniversaries of the death of loved ones. During these difficult periods, often lasting for a few weeks in the vicinity of the anniversary, individuals may be more vulnerable to illness and less resilient. Alia, in my home, expressed what she experienced partly through her appetite or lack of appetite. For a number of years after her mother's death one January and Alia's subsequent placement in an institution, she ate very poorly during the month of January. People can continue to feel the sad effects of losses at anniversary times for the rest of their lives. Probably few of us realize how much the pain we have lived is written in our body. Again, it is important to recognize that individuals may be grieving even if the manifestations of grief are not obvious or typical.

Grief may be especially present at holiday times, when we may expect the opposite. It can help to acknowledge the absence of the people who have died. When Ann said to the others in her house, "It's hard this first Christmas without Adam," everyone seemed to relax a little. They felt they had permission to be sad and the opportunity to express what they may have been feeling. As well, some people recognized that they were no longer feeling quite as sad as they had at Thanksgiving or some of the earlier holidays in the year and this was reassuring. For me, today, nearly three years later, Michael's periodic reminders, "I miss my brother, Adam . . . he is right here in my heart," help me to not forget Adam and to keep him alive in my heart as well.

Name the Gifts and Also the Difficult Realities of the Person Who has Died

When someone has died it is important to ponder the value and meaning of their life, but it is also important to be honest and not to gloss over the pain that may have existed in the relationship. The time spent telling stories is significant in that it helps us to name more clearly the gifts of the deceased person, and also to put in perspective the difficult times. After Maurice died we spoke of his life as being epitomized in his frequently asking friends to "have a cuppa tea," enunciated only as Maurice could enunciate it. Maurice's invitation to a cup of tea very clearly said, "I like you and want to spend some time with you." His invitation was a way of helping the rest of us to slow down, and we loved him for it. But that is not to say that we were not frustrated at times with his attraction to cups of tea and his slowness in partaking of them, especially if it happened to be an occasion when one of us was trying to get Maurice settled for the night. Recognizing this mixture of feelings we sometimes had about Maurice's gifts and his slowness helped us to laugh at ourselves and the situations we recalled and to move realistically toward gratitude.

It is a natural human desire to want to keep the essence of a deceased person's spirit alive. Obviously, naming the gifts of the person helps us to do so. While some of us may think in more general and abstract terms, people with disabilities are likely to recall very concrete moments with the deceased: He liked apple pie. She took me to the exhibition. We remember special qualities of each one who has passed on. As Helen's friends, we want to keep alive Helen's wonderful authenticity and lively energy. We remember Lloyd's gentleness, and Adam's silent gaze that called people together around him. Each of these qualities is tied for us to concrete little stories that we can all share together. This process of sorting out and talking about our special memories of the deceased can also help us to become more conscious of our own gifts and the gifts of those around us, and perhaps to think about the legacy we are leaving.

A memorial book at Daybreak provides a place for community members to memorialize family or friends who have been close to them. Individuals are assisted to prepare a page about their loved one. This activity can allow the grieving person to step back and extract from their many memories the qualities they most want to remember about the one who has died. It can be a wonderful way to move a little further through the grieving process, and it may provide an opportunity gently to hold at a little distance some of the more painful memories concerning the person.

CONCLUSION

I hope that it has become evident that people with development disabilities, given the opportunity and support, can grieve in a healthy and transformative manner. Indeed, because they are often much more in touch with their hearts and sometimes are less inhibited than many so-called normal people, they can call the rest of us to take the time we need to grieve, and to express our feelings in ways that can bring healing. When I give time to someone with a disability to grieve I am more able also to give myself permission to take time. The needs and gifts of people with disabilities in the area of grief and bereavement challenge the attitude of many in society that three days' compassionate leave should be enough and then one should get on with one's life as though nothing has happened.

In some ways, people with disabilities are better prepared to cope with death than are the rest of us. Often they have spent much of their life "being" rather than "doing." When someone is dying, there is usually not much that caregivers can do except to be with the person. People with disabilities may be more at ease in this situation than others. Of course, the dying person does need good care, but mostly he or she may need others to be there and present. The gift of people with a developmental disability often, both explicitly and by their own need for accompaniment, is to call others into relationship around the person who is ill or who has died.

Hospital staff and funeral directors have remarked on the quality of presence Daybreak people bring to the person who is dying and to the visitation and funeral. They have commented that they have never seen the dying person so well "sent off," nor have they seen people, especially people with disabilities, so involved in the rituals and so able both to weep and to talk about the life of their loved one. I believe this is possible because we have touched deeply into one another's common humanity at these times of loss, and from there has grown our sense of mutuality and of honoring the experience of each person.

Wendy, an Anglican priest at Daybreak, tells of being amazed when she arrived in the community at how freely people were able to talk about death and specifically at that time, about the fact that our friend Maurice was not going to get better. This was three weeks before his death. During her time in parish ministry she had found most people less willing to face the reality of a loved one's approaching death. The way that we are able to look at the person's whole life including their suffering and name their gifts while not idealizing the person after their death, seems very healthy to her. The gatherings after a death are times of mourning but also of true, hope-filled celebration. Wendy feels also the "hands on" elements in our celebrations are especially helpful.

It is the people with disabilities who have led us in the community to find ways to be concrete and to use simple rituals. Above all, they point to the centrality of relationship while providing care for someone who is dying or grieving and what we have discovered as a community is our great commonality in the grief process and that the gestures that are very important for a person with a disability in the grieving process are also very helpful for the rest of us. It is a great privilege to walk this journey with people who are differently abled and to experience together the gradual transformation of grief into gratitude and joy and new life.

ACKNOWLEDGMENTS

I thank the members of the L'Arche Daybreak community who allowed me to share their stories. In the original presentation of this material, Ann Pavilonis contributed reflections on Adam and her house. I am grateful to Wendy Lywood, Ann Pavilonis, and Joe Vorstermans for helpful preliminary discussions on this topic. And I thank Beth Porter for her encouragement and editorial assistance.

REFERENCES

Butler, R. N. (1963). The life review: An interpretation of reminiscence in the aged. *Psychiatry, 26*, 65-76.

Porter, E. (1998). Gathering our stories; Claiming our lives: Seniors' life story books facilitate life review, integration, celebration. *Journal on Developmental Disabilities, 6*(1), 44-59.

CHAPTER 9
Minding Mental Illness in the Grief Process

Lynne Martins

UNDERSTANDING AND TREATING
COMPLICATED GRIEF

Mental illness, in and of itself, is a type of loss that is merely whispered about and one that is often wrought with misunderstanding and shame. Even the mention of the term, mental illness, often conjures up images of stereotypical lunacy. Death as a result of mental illness is a type of death rarely mentioned, quietly filed away in the shadows of disenfranchised grief, setting the stage for a complicated grief response. A death by mental illness ushers in a special type of shameful rendering of the thought processes similar to the one experienced when a suicide occurs: it could have been prevented. When this type of relentless torment occurs, there is a strong temptation to find cause, and to appoint blame to such a death.

Discussion about mental illness as a cause of death is as forbidden as its counterpart: coping with mental illness either in the bereaved person or in a surviving family member when a death occurs. Caught in an enormous web of shame, confusion, and blame, the bereaved who is coping with a mental illness may impede and confound the best attempts of professionals to guide them through the grief process. When unchecked, the shame that lurks in the dark secret of mental illness is a cruel, relentless torment to the bereaved. The presence of mental illness in the bereaved profoundly impacts the ability to grieve appropriately and completely.

Through the discussion of case histories, this practice report chapter will assist the professional in assessing grief behaviors apart from mental illness; the use of medications in the treatment of complicated grief; the shame of mental illness; the implications upon the grief process when death triggers unresolved trauma; successes and failures in therapy; and the importance of working in concert with other professionals.

Grief Behaviors or Mental Illness?

Even within a complicated grief response, the ultimate goal of the clinician is to guide the client back to a healthy grief process. It is imperative to be clear about what components constitute a healthy grief response. By understanding how each domain of a person is affected, clinicians can better decipher the emotional responses, physical sensations, cognitions, and behaviors which are within the range of appropriate grief responses (Worden, 1991). The greater our experience of grieving individuals, the greater our appreciation becomes for the range of behaviors which are experienced and *which are expressly not mental illness.*

Still, it is sometimes difficult to clearly identify the line between behaviors which are grief responses and those that mimic a mental illness in the grief process. If there is a lack of understanding about what constitutes a healthy grief response, then it will be difficult to ascertain the line between complicated grief and the presence of mental illness (Rando, 1993). For example, when does the obsessive nature of pining and yearning for the deceased become a concern? How do we determine when a sense of depersonalization is actually a pattern of dissociative episodes? When does a repetition of rituals cause alarm? If we have not stopped to ask ourselves these questions, it is my opinion that we are at risk, as professionals, to do harm to our clients.

Assessing for differences between grief responses and mental illness has a starting point by examining three primary areas: 1) the display of the disturbance, 2) the duration of the disturbance, and 3) the disruption to the level of functioning. An outline of questions pertaining to these areas can be found in Appendix A. While this does not promise an exhaustive or conclusive outcome, it can begin to help the professional and client to more clearly define whether the disturbance is a grief response or whether it is a symptom of mental illness. Likewise, it can serve to alert the helping professional to the limits of their expertise and assist in determining if a referral is appropriate.

It is critical to understand that an accurate assessment involves a cluster of elements—and the clinician must not rely upon one single component. If a disturbance is present, it is not necessarily an indication that mental illness is present. Rather the goal of the assessment is to provide a broader landscape of the client's functioning and distress as a backdrop against clear criteria for mental illness described in the *Diagnostic and Statistical Manual of Mental Disorders IV.*

Medication: Does It Help or Harm the Grief Process?

The temptation among the bereaved is often to alleviate the sadness, depression, and anxiety of the grief process in the quickest manner possible. Equally as often, there is a helping professional ready to prescribe a medication. I am convinced that this action is well-intended but often it is based on misinformation about the intensity or duration of the grief process. For individuals not experiencing complicated grief, I have assisted dozens of people and their physicians to discontinue a prescribed medication in exchange for a undistracted, clear journey through the grief process with much success. Likewise, I have worked in concert with many physicians to create the best treatment plan possible for individuals whose grief may not be complicated, but nonetheless extremely disruptive to their functioning. To believe that medication is only appropriate for someone experiencing a complicated grief response would be a mistaken assumption. I believe there are many factors to consider in how a person moves through their grief process and that every case must be assessed according to the strengths of the individual.

The presence of mental illness in the grief process renders it complex, complicated, and challenging to the client and the clinician. While the question of medications remains a heated debate among professionals working with grieving persons, the context of this discussion is neither intended to convince or dissuade the use. Instead, the intent is to pause to examine the use of the medications in the cases presented. The treatment of mental illness with the use of psychotropic medications will continue to provoke a great deal of controversy among mental health professionals, physicians, the clients, and their families. The advantages, disadvantages, and challenges that the use of medications present to the helping professional is most poignantly clear in the following pages of Sarah's case.

The Shame of Mental Illness

The presence of guilt is usually considered a normal part of the grief process. When shame overshadows the guilt, the result can be grief that stays stuck. Mental illness as a cause of death evokes deep feelings of shame and blame among many of the bereaved and often the legacy of mental illness in the deceased is ignored or minimized. As with suicide, there is an enormous stigma attached to mental illness either as a cause of death or as a part of life to be dealt with throughout the grief process (Allen, Calhoun, Cann, & Tedeschi, 1993-1994); (Dunn & Morris-Vidners, 1987-1988; Ranger & Calhoun, 1990). As will be seen in the case of Marla, the acknowledgment of mental illness both induced and relieved the guilt and shame which she experienced. In Nancy's story, we will see a clear example of how coping with mental illness in a surviving family member rendered life extremely difficult.

When Death Triggers Unresolved Trauma

Often at the very heart of unresolved and complicated grief is a traumatic event or a series of traumatic events suffered within a short period of time. Sometimes the trauma has been inflicted at the hands of another; sometimes it has been witnessed; and sometimes the trauma has been due to an act of nature. Regardless of the etiology of the trauma, one of the responses which can occur is an anxiety response known as Post Traumatic Stress Disorder (PTSD). It is critical for the professional to understand the nature of post traumatic stress, the behaviors which present obstacles to the grief process and how the grief process and tasks can actually facilitate the healing of PTSD symptoms. Sarah's relief from relentless nightmares was due, in part, to her courage to grieve the death of her sister.

SARAH'S STORY

Sarah, a forty-two-year-old European-American veteran, has been clean and sober for five years following a twenty-year-plus history of poly-substance abuse and alcohol abuse. She is happily married to her third husband of eight years, who is ten years her senior. Over the past three years, Sarah has become increasingly withdrawn, paranoid, and depressed. She is unable to work due to the internal distress she experiences and lacks any significant social supports. She quit attending spiritual services with her husband a few months ago and struggles with continued contact with her five siblings, mother, and stepfather, who continue to abuse drugs and alcohol.

Sarah described her main problem as "I can't keep the memories back anymore." She exhibited symptoms of PTSD in our initial meeting. Due to recurring nightmares, she had not slept through the night for more than two years. Currently, she could not sleep for more than two hours at a time. Her husband accompanied her into every session as she was terrified to meet with me alone in my office.

In the first few sessions, Sarah was unable to sit in a chair, paced frantically across the floor and became nauseous at the sight of a child's chair with a stuffed animal on it. During one session, all doors and windows in the office had to remain open; and she was unable to face me for much of the session. She was extremely depressed and displayed a moderate risk for suicide. She refused psychotropic medications due to her mother's history of bi-polar disorder (which had remained untreated) and was adamantly opposed to voluntary hospitalization.

Within the first eight sessions, she revealed fragments of a recurring nightmare which eventually told a horrifying tale. At the age of two, she had witnessed the murder of her younger sister at the hands of her mother. Her mother had taken a pillow from her crib and suffocated her sister. A maternal aunt had helped the mother dispose of the body by wrapping it in newspaper and placing it in the trash can.

Within two weeks of remembering this murder, Sarah's mother died unexpectedly. Although she had a known history of multiple health problems, there was no warning that she was in immediate danger of dying. The death of Sarah's mother had a profound effect. It was as though the death unleashed memories of a lifetime of extremely sadistic psychological abuse, physical abuse, and sexual abuse. Sarah was extremely relieved that her mother was dead and for a short period believed that "she was safe for the first time in her life."

Sarah felt enormous anxiety and terror about attending her mother's funeral and having contact with other family members. A month after the funeral, she (at the urging of her husband) confessed that she spent a considerable portion of her day performing rituals that she could not control (up to 4 hours a day checking the locks on the doors, windows, basement, and attic of her home and relentless washing of her forehead to the point of severe chaffing). To cope with the anxiety of the events that had unfolded in her life, Sarah's Obsessive-Compulsive Disorder (OCD) surfaced. She did have insight into her OCD, but felt a great deal of shame about her inability to control it. She adamantly refused hospitalization and simply did not meet the criteria for involuntary commitment.

Following this, Sarah reluctantly agreed to an evaluation for medications. Due to her long history of substance abuse, it was difficult to find medications which would prove effective. Sarah would continue to be extremely unstable for the next three to four months until she began to realize the benefits of serizone (antidepressant), ambien (sleeping aid), and ativan (for agitation). She remained a moderate to high risk for suicide.

As Sarah continued to report relentless physical abuse and psychological torment at the hands of her mother and stepfather, some of her nightmares dissolved. During this slight reprieve, she agreed to attend a trauma survivor's group at the Veteran's Hospital and to remain in individual therapy with me. Each step was significant as Sarah confronted her profound mistrust and fear of adult females.

As therapy progressed, Sarah was able to appropriately grieve the death of her sister and began to address the unspeakable amount of loss she had suffered in her lifetime. She remained a substantial risk for suicide. However, as the issue of sexual abuse surfaced, Sarah began to deny that she could have endured such a thing, even though she had previously admitted its occurrence. The memories became increasingly intrusive for Sarah and her sleeplessness ravaged her. She sought to convince herself that it "really didn't happen." She demanded that I remove the child's chair from my office prior to each appointment. In an attempt to provide a safe environment, I complied with her request. Soon after, she quit the survivor's group. Months later, Sarah admitted that if "that *sexual abuse* had really happened, it would have meant that I never existed as a person."

Following the first anniversary date of the death of her mother, Sarah experienced increased anxiety, agitation, and despair. She began to skip appointments, and she began to self-medicate with alcohol. She began acting out in the community (confronted a gang member, terrorized a young boy who had broken flowers in her yard). She became increasingly hostile and agitated. She began to use marijuana; and in one instance, nearly over-dosed on prescribed medications and illegal drugs. It had not been an intended suicide attempt, but rather an attempt to stop the painful memories.

In the final two months, Sarah continued to avoid and deny the issues of sexual abuse, which circumvented her ability to grieve the death of her mother and incredible loss of self sustained through years of sexual abuse. She continued her high-risk behavior with self-medication and finally her prescriptions were terminated. Her transference of rage became threatening phone calls to me and out of control behavior in my office. She continued to refuse to voluntarily commit herself to a hospital.

Therapy was eventually terminated due to Sarah's non-compliance with the use of medications, her refusal to seek treatment/discontinue substance abuse, her refusal to return to any type of support group, and her insistence that I conduct therapy solely in the home.

It is helpful to summarize Sarah's story by examining the factors which complicated the grief process and to examine how the presence of mental illness impacted the grief process.

Factors that Complicated the Grief Process

- History of unresolved trauma, history of multiple losses in every domain: physical, emotional, psychological, sexual, spiritual, by multiple individuals: mother, step father, foster father, previous husbands, military.
- Psychic numbing and dissociative episodes inside and outside of therapy sessions.
- Long-term history of poor coping skills: chronic substance abuse (teens to mid-thirties).
- Unresolved trauma over witnessing murder of sister and keeper of the "family secret."
- Highly conflicted relationship with deceased mother.
- Isolation, poor social skills.
- Presence of Post Traumatic Stress Disorder, Obsessive-Compulsive Disorder, and Major Depression.
- Sudden, unexpected death of mother.
- Honest recollections of mother were not tolerated or supported by other family members.
- Debilitating, dangerous, and dysfunctional family system prior to death(s) and following death of mother.
- Break in sobriety to resume use of drug/alcohol to extinguish pain of intrusive memories.

How Mental Illness Impacted Grief Process

- Obsessive-Compulsive Disorder (OCD) surfaced in order to cope with mother's death.

- PTSD/OCD exacerbated (intensified) grief responses.
- PTSD/major depressive symptoms were sometimes impossible to separate from the grief surrounding the death of Sarah's mother.
- Mother's history of refusing treatment for bipolar disorder remained a major factor which negatively influenced Sarah from considering hospitalization.
- Shame internalized, unrelenting guilt over inability to cope with life.
- High risk of suicide.

Sarah's story is one that causes the term complicated grief to turn pale in definition. Despite the backdrop of pervasive neglect, abuse, and trauma in Sarah's life, she had been grieving losses throughout her entire life. Albeit, her coping mechanisms through the use of drugs and alcohol was extremely destructive. Although the death of her mother was her most current loss, it was the trauma of witnessing her sister's murder, forty years earlier, that Sarah had to begin with. It is my contention that in order for Sarah to find some completion point in grieving the death of her mother, she would have to complete her grieving for the life with her mother and the torment she endured at the hands of her mother.

NANCY'S STORY

Nancy, a fourteen-year-old European-American, is in her first year of high school. Nancy was adopted and the only child in this family. She was referred to me for her escalating depression over the sudden death of her father.

The previous Christmas, Nancy found her mother unconscious as they were leaving for a party. Her mother had suffered an aneurysm. Having called 911, Nancy was told by many that she had been *responsible for saving her mother's life*. Tragically, ten days later, during her mother's recovery in the hospital, Nancy came home to find her father in the kitchen suffering a massive heart attack. Again, she called 911. Ushered off to a relative's house, she never saw her father again. He died upon arrival to the hospital. Nancy was very close to her father and was devastated that her "best friend" had died. She recalled little about the funeral she attended.

Nancy's primary support was her paternal grandmother who lived on the same road. Her grandmother had arranged therapy but was unable to provide further support due to family conflicts. Nancy's maternal aunt lived about seventy miles way. She visited frequently, but the visits were very stressful. Nancy was very involved in her church's youth group and enjoyed a variety of sports at school.

After four months of therapy, Nancy had made significant movement in mourning the death of her father, but had become more withdrawn, anxious, and depressed, despite the fact that she had been on Prozac (antidepressant) for nearly one year. She was unable to get a complete night's sleep and was constantly exhausted. During this period, Nancy's somatic complaints increased: multiple colds, headaches, bouts of bronchitis, and a proneness toward accidents (sprained wrist, ankle). When she attempted to run track, she complained of shortness of breath and feared she was having a heart attack.

Through collaborative efforts, it was discovered that Nancy's mother was non-compliant with therapies following the aneurysm. Her recovery was compounded by a twenty-year history of major depression and histrionic personality disorder. Asleep during the day, awake throughout the night, she demanded that Nancy sit up and keep her company. She refused to accept that Nancy had homework, needed her sleep, or had her own issues.

Nancy felt conflicted toward her mother as she was terrified that her mother would actually die. At the same time, she became increasingly resentful at her mother's admonition that it was "now Nancy's responsibility to keep her mother alive." It was during this difficult time that Nancy quit taking antidepressants for fear that she would "end up like her mother." Instead, she became sexually active and bounced from one boyfriend to the next.

After a family session (mother and aunt), it was discovered that Nancy's mother had insisted on keeping a monitor that ran between the two bedrooms so that Nancy could "listen for her mother at night in case of an emergency." Nancy also revealed that her mother often pressured her to sleep with her because she was "so lonely and Nancy was her companion now that daddy was gone." When confronted with the inappropriateness of her requests, the mother became highly dramatic and sobbed uncontrollably for the remainder of the session. On many occasions, Nancy's mother would continue to dominate conversations with the central focus on herself with little regard for Nancy's losses or her progress.

Over the next twelve months, the maternal aunt became an extremely disruptive and domineering influence. She abruptly moved Nancy and her mother seventy miles away. Nancy was very distraught and angry about the move. She could not imagine how she would survive living with her mother in an even more isolated, remote area without her support system. She was told that "she had to make sacrifices for her mother." Despite repeated attempts to work with the family, the aunt continued to ignore the impact of the situation upon Nancy.

After the move, Nancy's therapy was abruptly terminated by her aunt. However, Nancy contacted me on four occasions, one in which she had run away (now age 16). She had run back to her hometown, her friends, and her church. Her aunt was furious and threatened to have Nancy arrested on several occasions. Nancy's belongings and social security benefits were withheld in an effort to punish Nancy for her "incredibly selfish behavior." Nancy received extremely hostile letters in which she was blamed for her mother's unhappiness and health problems. In one such letter, she was told, "If your mother dies, it will be your fault. You're killing her!" Shortly after, in an exceptionally disturbing visit, Nancy's mother attempted to engage her in making a suicide pact.

At Nancy's request, I resumed therapy with her. She was extremely anxious, experienced dissociative episodes, and was very depressed. In the next eighteen months, she would have to move five more times before finding a stable place to live. Despite the incredible obstacles, she remained in school, in therapy, rejoined the youth group, choir, and found a full-time job. As Nancy was able to separate herself from her mother and recognize her mother's behavior as mental illness, she was able to release the burden of responsibility and guilt that she felt and grieve the loss of her ideal mother as well as the death of her father. At eighteen, she terminated therapy and relocated to another part of the country.

Factors that Complicated the Grief Process

- Sudden, unexpected, multiple losses.
- Nature of father's death: sudden, unexpected.
- Nature of mother's recovery: uncertain.
- Loss of primary caregivers simultaneously.
- Central question abandoned: Who will care for me? Replaced with: How will I take care of mother?
- Premature death of father, a death out of life sequence.
- Disruption/termination of developmental phase of adolescence.
- Truncated grief response: buried/delayed.
- Role reversal: primary caregiver to mother.
- Lack of debriefing for Nancy by adults following trauma of finding parents in distress.
- Lack of information/understanding about mother's premorbid state.
- Highly dysfunctional family system prior to the traumas.
- Multiple major life changes (multiple moves, change in status, financial strains, legal problems).

Impact of Mental Illness on Grief Process

- Premorbid state of mother: twenty-year history of major depression and histrionic personality disorder. Disabled family system fueled personality disorder and ignored non-compliance with treatment for major depression.
- Conflict/ambivalence to adjusting to death of father meant forgiving him for dying first and abandoning her to cope with her mother.
- Conflict/confusion toward father in recognizing that he had served as a buffer between Nancy and her mother prior to his death.

- Grieving was done in isolation: did not share grief in public due to her mother's inappropriate histrionic behavior.
- Preoccupation with mother's behavior rendered Nancy's grieving for her father sporadic, disrupted, and incomplete.
- Repeated retraumatization of client by mother and aunt.
- Mental illness induced a type of mourning for "what could never be" with her mother and essentially the loss of both parents.
- Unauthentic guilt for missing her father, interpreted as lack of loyalty to mother.
- Confusion over mother's behavior: recognition of manipulation created cycle of anger followed by guilt.

MARLA'S STORY

Marla, was a thirty-year-old European-American grieving the death of her only husband by suicide. She began therapy with me approximately eighteen months after the death. Together, they had one son, aged three. Marla's husband had committed suicide by jumping from a highly populated public place at the age thirty-three. The suicide had been videotaped by witnesses, including his delusional remarks and was repeatedly dramatized by the media.

Her husband had previously held a very prestigious position with the government as an engineer. By the age of thirty he was highly successful and described as: "an extremely driven, high achiever who was adored and admired." Six months prior to the suicide, he had been fired from his job due to erratic behavior, mood swings, and suspected alcohol and marijuana abuse. During this period, he had been diagnosed with diabetes and bi-polar disorder. He had experienced many manic episodes within the six-month period, one in which he charged $70,000 on their joint credit cards. Marla was completely unaware of the long history of bi-polar disorder and suicide in her husband's family as he had remained estranged from them.

One month prior to his death, he had reluctantly begun taking lithium for the treatment of the bi-polar disorder. Unfortunately, he had not yet begun to realize the benefit of lithium to gain relief from these episodes. Marla was haunted by the fact that her husband remained more hypomanic than depressed. In this way, there were no warnings, indications, or threats of suicide. The day Marla's husband committed suicide, she had been at home waiting for him to return from a shopping errand to enjoy a evening out on the town.

Following the death of her husband, Marla was unable to sleep and displayed immobilizing levels of anxiety. She had been advised by her physician to use ativan to control her anxiety and agitation. She continued to use ativan for the first six months following the death, but voluntarily discontinued its use due to unpleasant side effects.

Approximately fourteen months after her husband's death, Marla became involved in another relationship which resulted in a relocation to Washington state. Her primary support included her boyfriend and her housekeeper.

Prior to her initial visit with me, another physician had prescribed zoloft (antidepressant), which she taken for six weeks but disliked and abruptly discontinued. Marla had done a great deal of education on her own about bi-polar disorder, but had little understanding of the grief process and the complications of a death by suicide. Marla continued therapy with me for approximately ten months during which time she was able to unravel the pain and guilt induced by suicide and come to a greater acceptance of her husband's mental illness as the cause for his suicide.

As Marla was able to accept mental illness as a cause for death, she relinquished the need to blame herself as her husband had chosen to hide his illness and the history of the illness in his family. She had believed that his erratic behavior and disappearing episodes had been her fault. This remained a focus of therapy as she initially described her husband as "faultless, perfect." It was a painful, but crucial step of growth for her to allow a more accurate, realistic picture of her deceased husband. As she came to understand the nature of the illness through collaborative communication and education, she could further resolve the notion that "she should have seen it coming."

Factors that Complicated the Grief Process

• Sudden, unexpected death.
• Death by suicide—complication: delusional state due to bi-polar disorder.
• Highly publicized death, witnesses captured delusional statements on film which were broadcast on radio, television, newspapers, and tabloids.
• Major life changes: relocation, financial, legal.
• Lack of support systems.
• Developmental stage disrupted.
• Denial/shame at recognizing mental illness as cause of death. It was easier to admit to depression than to accept mania and delusions.
• Distraction from grief by prematurely entering new relationship.
• Difficulty accepting the deceased's mental illness caused idealistic recollections.

Impact of Mental Illness on Grief Process

• Lack of knowledge about mental illness (family history) caused extraordinary anguish in grief process.

- Ambivalence toward mania behavior in deceased: high energy, funny, outgoing person laced with confusion and guilt: "how could I miss the part of him which caused him to be so ill and ultimately caused his death?"
- Shame: overwhelming stigma of mental illness combined with suicide.
- Relief: by understanding the nature of the mental illness, Marla was assisted in resolution of guilt she felt over the suicide. She was able to absolve self from the guilt of "I should have known."
- Anguish over knowledge of mental illness: With such a strong family history of bipolar disorder (3 of husband's siblings), will her son develop the disorder?

SUCCESSES AND FAILURES IN THERAPY

Some of the best kept secrets among professionals are our successes. If we have difficulty sharing our strategies which succeed, it is not difficult to understand why we would keep our failures to ourselves. However, neither secret harbored is a service to ourselves, our colleagues, or our clients. By sharing what has worked and what has not, it is hopeful that we can learn from each other's experiences.

In Sarah's case, I regret that I allowed the removal of the small chair and stuffed animal from my office. In this way, I may have contributed to her inability to come to terms with the trauma of sexual abuse which needed to be resolved before she could grieve the actual death of her mother. However, despite a rather tumultuous ending with this case, I believe there were many instances of success.

Success, in Sarah's case was not found in the traditional approaches to therapy. One of the first strategies attempted was to find a meeting place which did not invoke such intense post-traumatic responses. Until a therapeutic alliance was formed, we met in the yard of my office, under a tree and sipped tea. I read stories to her and allowed her husband to attend sessions until she felt safe in my presence. I often used phone check-in appointments with her in between our scheduled appointments to monitor her suicidal risk. The months following the death of her mother, I agreed to go to her home for therapy appointments. I also accompanied her on her initial visit with a psychiatrist and on her initial interview with the trauma survivor's group leader.

Sarah's shame and mistrust prevented her from allowing me to attend her mother's funeral with her. She was able to incorporate some strategies we developed together to survive her attendance without becoming further disabled by the experience. One such strategy was to purchase a gardenia to wear to be assured that her family was unable to render her invisible (she enjoyed the idea that the gardenia's fragrance was so potent, it could not be ignored). She was able to allow her husband to attend with her and speak/act on her behalf, if necessary. The accomplishment of participation in the funeral on her terms remained a solid part of Sarah's healing, and she referred to it often with a great deal of pride.

Although Sarah's journey was not as complete as I would have preferred and resulted in a return to substance abuse, I did not render her case as a failure. I was her first experience with therapy and given the extreme nature of her case, believe that our work together resulted in resolving the nightmares surrounding the violent death of her sister. She was able to properly grieve the death of her sister. At times, I was utterly amazed at her ability to continue therapy for nearly eighteen months and not commit suicide. Admittedly, those are not the usual measures of success, but Sarah's case was far from usual.

In the case of Nancy, it was sometimes difficult not to become over-involved. She often did not have another adult who would elect to become involved due to the volatile nature of her family system. Nancy's case did not qualify as child-abuse and due to her age, she would not have been a candidate for foster care in our state. Given the extraordinary challenges of her living situations and lack of family support, it was difficult to remain in a strict therapist role with her. When she was unable to obtain transportation to our sessions, I would often meet her in places which were safe: her school or her church. Twice, I attended a choir performance. Did I cross a therapeutic line? I struggled to find the harm in supporting her positive choices and believe that an occasional attendance throughout the duration of our work together was more therapeutic than not. Nancy faced many obstacles in the grief over the death of her father and the mental illnesses of her mother. It would be my contention that Nancy moved through her grief to the best of her ability given her developmental stage in life.

In comparison, Marla's case was relatively simple, although her grief was complicated. Success in Marla's case was realized in her ability to remove the unauthentic guilt she harbored due to the mode of her husband's death. As she was able to understand her husband's mental illness, she was able to relinquish blame and detach from the stigma of both mental illness and suicide.

WORKING IN CONCERT WITH OTHER PROFESSIONALS

When cases are extraordinarily challenging, collaboration with other professionals, family members, and other trusted individuals is essential not only to provide the best treatment available, but to preserve the professional from burnout. Issues of confidentiality, obtaining permission to collect or release information, collaboration, and the value of educating professionals and family members about the grief process were paramount to the success of cases presented.

A routine part of my practice incorporates the use of collaborative communication with the family physician. I have come to deeply appreciate the depth and history that the family physician may have with the patient. In turn, I have been able to educate many professionals about the grief process and use of medications. I have also come to rely upon this relationship to partnership with others and avoid isolation as a clinician.

In each case presented, I obtained numerous consents to collaborate with family members, psychiatrists, family physicians, support group leaders, school counselors, teachers, pastors, and any other significant person whom I or the client believed would be helpful in the therapeutic process. I also consulted with other professionals and continue to do so on a regular basis as much of the work I do is with extraordinarily complex cases.

APPENDIX A
Assessing for Differences between Grief Responses and Mental Illness

Display of Disturbance

- What type of disturbance is being reported or observed? (Is it physical, emotional, cognitive, psychological, spiritual, sexual, or developmental)?
- If the disturbance is only reported by the client (and not observed by the professional), is collaborative report possible? (Such as physicians, other family members, friends, school counselors, spiritual guide, mentors, etc.)
- Is there a previous history of disturbance in the individual or another family member?

Duration of Disturbance

- How long has the disturbance been occurring?
- What time of the day or night does it occur? How long does it last?
- What is the intensity level of the disturbance?
- Can the disturbance be disrupted? Can it be controlled?
- Is the person aware that the disturbance is occurring?
- What feelings are present during or after the disturbance?
- Is there a rapid shift in the individual's personality?

Disruption to Level of Functioning

- How does the disturbance interfere with the individual's overall level of functioning? (At home, school, work, social settings?)

• Does the disturbance interfere with activities of daily living and/or occupation?
• Does the disturbance cause significant disruption to areas of social life and/or personal relationships?
• Does the disturbance cause involvement with the legal system?

REFERENCES

Allen, B. G., Calhoun, L. G., Cann, A., & Tedeschi, R. G. (1993-94). The effect of cause of death response to the bereaved: Suicide compared to accidental and natural causes. *Omega: Journal of Death & Dying. 28*(1), 39-48.

Dunn, R.G., & Morris-Vidners, D. (1987-88). The psychological and social experience of suicide survivors. *Omega: Journal of Death & Dying, 18*(3), 175-215.

Ranger, L. M., & Calhoun, L. G. (1990). Responses following suicide and other types of death: The perspective of the bereaved. *Omega: Journal of Death & Dying, 21*(4), 311-320.

Rando, T. A. (1993). *Treatment of complicated mourning.* Champaign, IL: Research Press.

Worden, J. W. (1991). *Grief counseling and grief therapy: A handbook for the mental health practitioner* (2nd ed.). New York: Springer.

CHAPTER 10
Dementia: A Cause of Complicated Grieving

Catherine Anne Quinn

Using the author's experience as a social worker specializing in dementia care with a community aged care team in the north-western suburbs of Sydney, Australia, the chapter explores some reasons for the complexity of the grief caused by Alzheimer's disease and other dementing illnesses for carers, especially spouse-carers, but also for those sufferers whose insight remains. Using the constructs of the *psychological, sociological,* and *mythological "planes"* wherein grieving must take place, the chapter shows that it is the absence of one or more of these in mourning the numerous losses occasioned by dementing illnesses that may explain the complicated nature of this grief. Carers and sufferers are "disenfranchised" and disempowered by the nature of the illness, the lack of social awareness and understanding of this, and the apparent meaninglessness of the process of the illness and its destruction of the uniqueness and individuality of the sufferer. The author offers practical suggestions for ways in which some of these problems can be addressed on each of these "planes."

A woman was recounting her breakfast-time experience. Her husband of fifty-eight years of marriage has Alzheimer's disease. He stood beside her in the kitchen that morning and said "Let me get this straight. Are you my wife?" When asked what she had done, she said "I hugged him tightly and said 'yes dear, I am' then I went to the bedroom and cried."

Dementia is not a disease in itself but a broad term used to describe the loss of mental function caused by a number of different diseases which have a physical affect on the brain. This interferes with the person's daily life and relationships by affecting the memory, especially for recent events. It may also produce other problems such as word-finding difficulties, recognizing spatial relationships, having difficulties with daily tasks like dressing (*apraxia*), loss of social skills, and sometimes normal emotional reactions. In Alzheimer's disease especially, the sufferer's frequent absence of insight into his/her own difficulties as well as the feeling and needs of the carer is a painful and isolating experience for the carer as it becomes a change in personality.

Someone has described the process of caring for a person with dementia as "the funeral that never ends." Certainly it falls into Dr. Kenneth Doka's categories of "disenfranchised grief." Disenfranchised grief is the experience of suffering a loss which one is not permitted, in various ways, to grieve. The loss may not be recognized for what it really is either by the person or by their social group. Examples include such losses as having an abortion or surrendering a baby for adoption, the death of a friend or perhaps a companion animal, and many others. Alternatively, there are some people who are not acknowledged as having the right to mourn, for instance the family of a criminal, homosexual partners, children, the disabled, the very elderly.

This chapter will attempt to explore how the concept of complicated grieving/disenfranchised grieving applies to dementia sufferers and their carers. Some suggestions will be made about practical responses to the problem. The discussion will mainly focus on the issues for carers, in particular spouses, of people with Alzheimer's disease, the most common cause of dementing illnesses and one of the most complex. However, it is applicable to the other dementing illnesses and also to people with acquired brain injury, especially that involving the frontal lobe.

THE GRIEF OF DEMENTIA

The dementia sufferer, as well as the carer, often faces a complex grieving, made harder by the isolation and loneliness imposed by factors like the carer's grief, misinformation, misunderstanding of the sufferer's feelings, and the carer and sufferer being "out of step" with each other's emotional "pace." One sufferer confided to her husband "I cannot tell you how afraid I am." Her husband said that until that moment he had not understood that she was even aware of her illness, and he felt chastened and humbled by her remark. For many sufferers, this misunderstanding of their experience is part of their grief and isolation which they cannot bridge. A very real existential loneliness pervades the progress of this illness which can cause its victims to awake in the night not knowing who it is who stands beside them but also who they are themselves. Their sense of continuity as a human person is shaken to its very core and torn apart by their brain's failure to hold these connections together. It is somehow reminiscent of beads which lose their connection to each other and their form and pattern when the string that threads them is broken. Many sufferers report nightmares. Fears for the future are very real for the sufferer.

Like many "bereavements" which are not caused by the final loss of death, Alzheimer's disease and the other dementing illnesses bear a complex range of losses. To many people dementia seems like a psychological death, preceding the person's physical death by perhaps ten or fifteen years, which is in itself a complicating factor.

Among the most obvious losses for spouses are the loneliness resulting from loss of companionship within the marriage and the sad but inevitable falling away of friendships and other social contacts. Carers and sufferers often make the wry but telling comment that dementia really shows who one's real friends are. Even family members can be among those who avoid contact with a dementia sufferer and, by default, the carer. This sometimes conceals the family member's fears that the illness may somehow be passed on to them. It may also cloak their uneasiness in dealing with their own feelings of loss and grief.

Another aspect of this loss is the radical and deteriorating change in the balance of the couple's relationship as the spouse moves increasingly into the role of parent to their partner: thinking for them, making decisions for them, and as the illness progresses, having to take up humiliating personal tasks such as toileting and physical care. Issues regarding sexuality such as disinhibition or, alternatively, loss of libido on the sufferer's part are often not discussed but add to the pain and loneliness experienced by the carer. Carers speak of experiencing difficulties with sexuality because they are doing the intimate and sometimes unpleasant personal tasks such as dealing with bowel and bladder incontinence, something more readily associated with infancy. Both partners may then find themselves becoming very "touch hungry" where the physical contact born of affection and love is no longer present. Spouses are not the only ones for whom these personal tasks of caring bring an element of grief. The adult son or daughter caring for a parent with dementia finds the role reversal from "child" to "parent" uneasy and disquieting, and sometimes distasteful. In some situations the adult child is watching not only one parent's declining cognitive abilities but the other parent's failing health or their inability to withstand the distress of the demands inherent in their partner's deterioration, and, for example, taking refuge in alcohol abuse or outright denial of the problem.

The endless grind of hard work, both physical and emotional, and the erosion of freedom and independence can contribute to a carer's sense of having lost command of their own life and becoming disempowered by factors beyond their understanding and control. Sometimes a carer has to abandon employment and career, sometimes a move from the family home becomes a necessity. Financial burdens may accumulate; the insecurity caused by fears for the future may also go with the abandonment of plans and dreams. This latter is often a major grieving for men. One support group for men caring for wives with dementia frequently described their forced abandonment of plans for retirement relationships and activities, along with the loss of their wives' companionship, as the most painful losses they were experiencing.

The history of the marital and family relationship may itself uncover issues from the past which will impact upon the loss. This will affect adult children as well as spouse carers. Sometimes there are rifts or divisions within the family. Long-standing dysfunctional patterns or unhealed disputes may interfere. Sadness and anger may surface if the marital relationship has been unsatisfactory, and the spouse resents the expectations that he/she will be the devoted carer. Once dementia is established it is almost impossible to set relationship problems to right. In some instances a carer's long-suppressed anger and frustration can surface as abuse or neglect. Carers can be locked into the role by family expectations. Emotional blackmail and other forms of control such as manipulation and guilt can impose caring on spouses or family members. Conflict may arise, not only about who should be the carer and how they should undertake this, but also about the use of family resources such as savings or other inheritable assets. This may cause enormous distress to the older person even to the person with the dementing illness.

People who develop "early onset" dementia, while aged in their thirties, forties, or fifties, may still have dependent children in their care. This places another range of stresses on the marital and family relationships, especially as the dementing illnesses in this group appear to be more strongly hereditary.

Finally, for many the end result may be placement of the sufferer in residential or institutional care. The decision to take this step is one of the hardest that anyone can face. Studies indicate that carers may approach the final step as many as seven times before actually taking it. Many carers experience profound feelings of guilt when making this decision, and a sense of having betrayed a trust or failed in their role as carer. They fear that they are abandoning the person to whom they are committed. This can be mixed with feelings of relief, about which they may also feel guilty. Their sense of loss may well be misunderstood by family and friends. Family members may complicate the experience by their differing expectations of what is appropriate care for a parent or sibling and be critical or unsupportive of the carer's need to take this choice. Carers and sufferers alike face the problems associated with transferring or sharing the caring tasks and role. There is often implicit or even explicit dispute about who "owns" the patient and the family carer can feel pushed aside by the institution staff.

GRIEVING AND DEMENTIA

Grieving is that complex emotional process involving shock, confusion, anger, guilt, longing, and sadness which follows loss experienced by individuals or groups. Its purpose is to allow disengagement from that which is lost so that those who suffer the loss can re-engage with their own future. This disengagement inexorably changes the nature of the relationship. This is something that can be seen, for example, where people grieve the loss of someone "missing, presumed dead." If the person is restored to them, the relationship cannot be resumed as it was because the disengagement process has already begun, however subtly.

One of the reasons why the grieving for dementia carers is so difficult is that the disengagement process must remain incomplete because the person with dementia is still a part of the carer's future. However, there is a danger that beginning this disengagement process may result in an emotional distancing that reduces the sufferer to an "object" or a patient, someone to whom things are done. There may be additional factors such as previous ungrieved losses, "unfinished business." These are often present in complex or unsatisfactory relationships.

The eventual death of the sufferer can itself lead to a grief that the carer and others can find hard to understand, as it may include feelings of relief and liberation about which the carer may feel guilty.

Another important reason for the complication is the fact that all grieving must take place on three "planes," the *psychological*, the *sociological*, and the *mythological*, in order to be complete. If any of these are omitted the process is compromised, sometimes severely. This is in part an explanation of the concept of "disenfranchised grief." In disenfranchised grief at least one of these elements is absent.

Psychological

The significance of this is evident when the loss caused by dementing illnesses is examined. The *psychological* "plane" is recognized by most people when grief is discussed and applies largely to the individual inner life of the grieving person. Most people understand, at least where a death has occurred, the need to allow the experience and expression of some or all of those emotions associated with grief: the shock and disbelief, the anger, the confusion and chaos, the guilt and the "if onlys," the longing and yearning for the restoration of what has been lost, the despair and desperation, and the drifting feeling of having nowhere to go and no connection with anything meaningful any more. Grieving people need to be able to articulate these in some way, openly and fully. However, many carers and their families believe that even owning such feelings, let alone giving them expression, is inappropriate and callous. They will say "I shouldn't feel this way. After all it's not his fault that he has dementia." Family members or friends will sometimes imply that grieving should be reserved for death alone. If carers have a poor understanding of the causes and process of dementia, they find the anger and frustration they feel even more inexplicable. This is also frightening, isolating, and confusing for the sufferer. For example, one carer persisted, in spite of attendance at carer information sessions, to insist that her husband was "mad" and to treat him with exasperation, impatience, and some contempt. People with dementing illnesses retain their capacity for feeling hurt and humiliation until very late in the progression of the illness and perhaps to the end.

Sociological

Grieving people also need to know that their loss is understood and appreciated by the group or society to which they belong. They need to know that their feelings are acknowledged and to some extent shared, and that they will still have a place within their own social context even though they have been changed by the loss-experience and are no longer exactly the same as they were prior to the loss. They must know that they are still accepted and can return to the group when they are ready. This is where the concept of *mourning* as a function of grieving is important as this describes the social, visible, or conventional expression of grief, such as the wearing of black arm bands or clothing or the observance of silence. For the carer of someone with dementia, there is no such possibility of mourning in this sense since there are no social conventions for expressing an invisible loss. The "object" of the loss, the person with the dementing illness, is still present. The losses are largely unseen by the external observer.

For sufferers of dementing illnesses and their carers the passage of time is of great importance as this process can last many years. The carer may find himself/herself in a very solitary space by the time the sufferer has died. Younger carers may have disrupted careers; family life may have become very fragmented; the older carer may be in poor health. Carers and sufferers alike will also comment on the fact that the friends are rare who remain in contact once the diagnosis is known or the behavioral problems become obvious.

Mythological

The mythological plane addresses the need to be able to confront or be confronted by those great human questions: What is the meaning of this? What is the meaning of life? the "why me?" or "why him?" questions. For spouses there may also be the re-examination of what was meant in the marriage vows which stated: "In sickness and in health until death do us part." What indeed is meant by death? For some people these questions may also have a theological component: "Why did God let this happen?" "Who is God for me now?" Most human beings have a strong need to assign meaning to or make sense of any loss, and it is through the "myths" or core beliefs of our culture and, for many, through religion that this need is addressed. This is why adequate and appropriate funeral rites are so important. They not only give expression to the emotions, they are a social recognition of a loss, and they articulate the founding myths of the culture or the social group regarding the meaning of life and death for those who are bereaved. Some of these myths are expressed in the sentiments in sympathy cards. In religious funerals the prayers state the beliefs: "For the life of your faithful people, Lord, is changed, not ended. . . ."[1] The person with dementia and the carer stand at a serious disadvantage here. In part this is because so little is currently known about the causes of illnesses such as Alzheimer's disease. It is easily misunderstood, the pain and distress ignored or trivialized, and the whole process experienced as meaningless, destructive, wasteful, and even punitive.

The principal way in which we can appropriately approach and integrate these three "planes" of the process is through ritual. Good ritual, culturally appropriate and rightly done, gives us access to the various dimensions of our humanity because it deals in the currency of both the spirit and the body, the symbolic and the tactile. Gerald Arbuckle, in *Grieving for Change* (1991), quotes Bocock (1974): "Ritual is the stylised or repetitive, symbolic use of bodily movements and gesture within a social context to express and articulate meaning." Examining this definition, it can be seen that ritual involves our whole being, our bodies through movement and gesture, our mind and spirit through symbols and through expressions such as music. Because we are social beings, when we perform rituals, we act in conjunction with our fellow human beings even if we act privately. Thus ritual is stylized, simplified, and able to be repeated. Rituals give voice to those complex layers of feelings and experiences which reside within us at the conscious and the unconscious levels of our being and for which words alone are often inadequate. Ritual, through the use of movement, gesture, and especially symbols, will often unite our experience to those of others where words might only serve to confuse or alienate.

Ritual does not have to be derived from religious or any other formal or institutional context. Some of the rituals with which we are most familiar are in fact the simple stuff of everyday life, the story we read each night to a small child to reassure him that the darkness is not permanent and that life has continuity, the way we celebrate family events like birthdays, the gestures and words we use in greetings and farewells.

Rituals are needed to express such issues as closure, continuity, transition, healing, reconciliation, forgiveness. In so doing they enable us to deal satisfactorily with endings and move on to new beginnings without carrying too much "unfinished business" (divorce is a major loss and transition requiring ritualization). Thus, for a ritual to be effective and to give voice to the psychological, sociological, and mythological issues that

---

[1] *The Roman Missal*, English Translation, 1973, Preface of Christian Death I for the Mass for the Dead.

concern the person, it must arise from the story of that person's experience. It is particularly important to mention that any effective ritual for addressing the grief associated with dementia must emerge from the lived experience of the people involved. The telling of their story is a major part of the process of developing any ritual. There is no "one size fits all" answer since everyone's story is unique while still containing elements of similarity which serve to bind us together as members of the same human family. Grief is one human experience which transcends all manner of boundaries and can unite rather than isolate if people are given the opportunity to express to one another what they know and are learning. Grieving is more complicated where this process is not available. Isolation and alienation from oneself and one's place in the human family are the outcome if this is the case.

One problem with a disease like Alzheimer's is that its insidious onset and gradual progression may also be a factor in delaying the grieving process. There is rarely a single event or point in the story which marks a place at which a ritual of closure or transition could be effectively employed. Another problem for many carers is the characteristic denial of the problem by many Alzheimer's sufferers and their lack of insight into the needs of their carer. This means that some rituals may not be able to involve the sufferer directly.

SOME POSSIBLE RESPONSES

Let us return to the three planes of grieving. First are the *psychological* needs to be addressed. Family carers in particular need to be informed and reassured that they are entitled to their feelings of loss and all that goes with that. The fact that they are grieving may need to be named so that they may recognize and understand what they are experiencing. They need opportunities both private and public to express these feelings. Groups which meet for the education and support of carers have an important role in facilitating this process. Similarly, such things as the practical task of putting together a "This Is Your Life" or "Book of Memories" by a carer for their person with dementia can be more than simply assembling an album of old photographs. It is an opportunity for retelling and reflecting on their life story. It is, therefore, both preparation for and ritualization of a major life transition. It can be equally important to both the carer and the sufferer, and the book can be used repeatedly if necessary. Family gatherings of all kinds, but especially those concerned with the problem, can use this opportunity to tell the story as it touches each of them and share their different feelings.

From the *sociological* level, public awareness needs to be raised, not only about the dementing illnesses but of their impact on sufferers and carers alike. Events such as National Alzheimer's Week could include some form of public ceremony which not only affirms and applauds the carers for the job they are doing but also acknowledges more definitely the grieving that goes with the task. At the more informal and intimate level, carers and sufferers should be supported more through the process of diagnosis, and later on of residential placement, should that become necessary. The importance of not abandoning the sufferer and their carers when the diagnosis is made should be stressed. Carers often express their dismay and distress at being told that the person about whom they are concerned has a dementing illness and then not being offered any support, follow-up, or opportunity to express their anguish. One younger wife recalled driving her fifty-eight-year-old husband home after days of clinical testing and sobbing to herself, "I want my mother."

Other landmarks along the journey could also be noted, for example the sufferer's first admission for institutional respite care or loss of driver's license. Carer Support Groups can be encouraged to find sensitive ways to mark these events with one another. Opportunities for lobbying for research funds and other forms of recognition of the illnesses may also be means by which some people can articulate and channel their anger and concern.

At the *mythological* level, it can be helpful to situate an illness such as Alzheimer's disease in its proper context in the process of raising public awareness. More information about research can be an effective way of clarifying some issues. Disabusing people of the idea that dementia is a mental illness and means "going crazy" or "losing your marbles," "getting senile" or "childish" can be a start. These notions have a randomness and meaninglessness about them that further isolates the sufferer and the carer. Public education about illnesses like epilepsy has already changed attitudes. Religious organizations such as parishes and church groups can be more helpful and supportive by devoting some time and thought to carers and to those sufferers whose awareness of their disability causes them distress and raises questions about the future and issues of meaning. People need the opportunity to explore the theological issues for themselves individually as well as hearing them preached for the community as a whole. These issues of the spirit need to be addressed at the institutional and formal level as well as at the personal and informal level. Calling together those people in a parish or church community who are affected by these illnesses and eliciting their opinions can be a very effective way to give them access to the importance of their stories. In itself this is an empowering step to take, but it will be even more valuable if it flows out into the wider group as education and practical support.

The place of support groups in dealing with such a complicated grieving experience cannot be overstated. There is also a need for individual counseling for carers and some sufferers, especially those who face the problem already burdened by any of the unresolved issues alluded to earlier in this discussion.

CONCLUSION

The dementing illnesses are involving a greater proportion of the population of Western societies where people now live longer in better health than a generation or more ago. These illnesses affect not only the very elderly and their spouses and families, they are now being recognized and diagnosed in middle-aged people as well. Besides representing a challenge to the community in terms of services and support, this development demands that we broaden our understanding of the implications of loss and grief. This is a silent hidden grief, already complicated by that very fact and rendered more complex by a host of other factors, some of which have been discussed here. The ultimate outcome of grieving should be healing of the loss and the hurt, so that the surviving person may embrace their future with more rather than less than they were before: more courage, more wisdom, more peace and wholeness. This cannot be the case if the grieving person's loss goes unrecognized and is devalued, their inner resources compromised by the absence of affirmation of their sorrow and their need for compassion.

REFERENCES

Arbuckle, G. (1991). *Grieving for change.* Homebush, Australia: St. Paul Publications.
Babcock, R. (1974). *Ritual in industrial society, a sociological analysis of ritualism in modern England* (pp. 35-39). London: Allen & Unwin.

CHAPTER 11

Grief Complicated by Spiritual Abuse

Boyd C. Purcell

THE ROLE OF RELIGIOUS FAITH

The potential for a person's religious faith to help or hurt the believer was wisely articulated by Dr. Kenneth Doka (1998) who said, "Sometimes these belief systems will provide comforting answers. But sometimes they will not." He explained, "In other cases, the belief system itself may be a source of spiritual pain. For example, religious beliefs that see suicide as an unforgivable sin offer scant comfort to survivors." Doka concluded, "A person's perspective of God as gracious will have far different implications than a perspective of a punishing God." To the question "What are the most prominent fears that a dying person experiences?" Carroll (1991) listed four categories, the first of which was "Religious fear: fear of damnation, retribution, punishment in the afterlife." When asked the question "What are the particular fears experienced by a dying person?" he listed more than a page of questions asked by those who are dying, one of which was "Will I be punished for my sins after I die?" He also listed among specific fears "fear of the devil."

The author of the chapter "Christians in Grief," McConnell, a Christian pastor, correctly contended, "The Christian faith offers both great comforts and great challenges to the person in grief" (in Doka & Davidson, 1998). McConnell addressed the implications of one's understanding of who God is, God's perceived part in causing or allowing the loved one to die, belief in life after death, and the role of the church in the grief process. "What one believes may complicate or facilitate grief and loss."

Stuart (1998), the Medical Director for VNA and Hospice of Northern California, reported that patients' religion appears to be helpful 50 percent of the time, while in the other 50 percent it appears to be hurtful. Kübler-Ross (1973) observed that most religious patients experienced fear of judgment and punishment in the afterlife. It appears that the degree to which a person's religious faith is helpful or harmful is proportional to the degree to which one has been exposed to what this author refers to as "spiritual abuse."

McConnell did an excellent job of addressing potential problems in the Christian faith, such as a griever feeling guilty or selfish that one is not experiencing the joy of believing that his/her loved one is enjoying the glory of heaven. In such a case, the Christian community may be a source of pain for the griever. For example, "All too often within the Christian community bereaved individuals are not given permission to feel and express the deep pain that may remain in spite of the assurance of eternal life for their loved one. Sadly, there are even those who are likely to cast doubt upon the faith of a griever who continues to traverse the valley of the shadow of death longer than expected, or who wonders aloud why God would allow such a death to occur" (in Doka & Davidson, 1998).

Lastly and briefly, McConnell dealt with the issues of heaven and hell. He declared, "A discussion of Christian beliefs regarding death and response to it is incomplete without touching on the issue of salvation and judgment. Many Christians believe that heaven is not necessarily a guaranteed destination. Thus, grief can be complicated by a bereaved person's doubts about the salvation of the deceased and the possibility that, due to God's judgment, he/she is, in fact, not in heaven but in hell" (in Doka & Davidson, 1998, p. 44). It is this author's belief that the doctrine of eternal damnation is at the heart of spiritual abuse which greatly complicates grief for Christians and others with this particular religious belief.

DEFINITION OF SPIRITUAL ABUSE

Spiritual abuse can complicate the process of grief for both dying patients and their families. Spiritual abuse can be defined as the fear, stated or implied, that a person is going to be punished in this life and/or tormented in hell-fire forever for failure to live a good enough life to earn admission to heaven. The most extreme form of spiritual abuse is labeled "spiritual terrorism." Purcell (1998), in "Spiritual Terrorism," stated, "Thus, spiritual terrorism, depending on the age of onset, intensity, and duration, may be as harmful to people's emotional, mental, and spiritual well-being as any other form of abuse and perhaps even more injurious than all other forms of abuse put together!" With other forms of abuse, victims have the possibility of getting away from or defending themselves against the abuser. With God who has all knowledge, all power, and is everywhere present, victims do not even have freedom of thought. They have no defense, and no place to hide! Perhaps motivation by fear is why U.S. News & World Report (March 1991) reported that hell is every believer's worst nightmare.

A great deal has been written about various forms of abuse: physical, mental, emotional, verbal, and sexual. Spiritual abuse is a form of abuse about which very little has been written. In fact, it is only now, in the decade of the 1990s, beginning to be recognized as a serious problem by mental health professionals (Booth, 1991).

Spiritual abuse is definitely at the heart of the fear and emotional pain this writer, as a Board Certified Chaplain, has encountered with hospice patients and, as a Licensed Professional Counselor, with clients in private counseling practice. In order to understand and to effectively deal with this problem, one must consider the nature, the scope of, and the solution to this mental health menace.

THE NATURE OF SPIRITUAL ABUSE

The inherently abusive nature of spiritual abuse, though he does not actually call it that, is portrayed by Swindoll (1990) in his excellent book, *The Grace Awakening*. He explained:

> There are killers on the loose today. The problem is that you can't tell by looking. They don't wear little buttons that give away their identity, nor do they carry signs warning everybody to stay away. On the contrary, a lot of them carry Bibles and appear to be clean-living, nice-looking, law-abiding citizens. Most of them spend a lot of time in churches, some in places of religious leadership. Many are so respected in the community, their neighbors would never guess they are living next door to killers. They kill freedom, spontaneity, and creativity; they kill joy as well as productivity. . . . This day—this very moment—millions are living their lives in shame, fear, and intimidation who should be free, productive individuals. The tragedy is that they think it is the way they should be. They have never known the truth that could set them free. (p. 4)

Swindoll concluded that these unfortunate persons are victimized, existing as if they are living on "death row!" George (1991) observed that victims of spiritual abuse are living in "abject fear of God." As victims of spiritual terrorism, they are, therefore, experiencing a living death.

The principal symptoms of spiritual abuse are: anger, anxiety, fear of God/eternal torment, guilt, low self-esteem, panic, a feeling of never being good enough, hopelessness, and shame. Richard Anderson, in an unpublished paper, listed an entire page of symptoms of spiritual abuse. In its worst form, spiritual terrorism, has been called "The Spiritual Walking-Zombie Syndrome" by Elliott (1991), a licensed social worker in private practice.

THE SCOPE OF THE PROBLEM

Addressing the nature of spiritual abuse leads logically to a consideration of the scope of the problem. While the incidence of spiritual abuse appears to be most prevalent in the lower socioeconomic level of society, it can be found at all levels.

Is the belief of some Christians in punishment in hell, literally in eternal fire, spiritual abuse . . . even terrorism? According to the Bible, persons who fear are not perfected in love because fear involves torment; perfect love casts out fear (I John 4:18). How can people ever be perfected in God's unconditional love while they are motivated by fear?

Some readers of this chapter may conclude that the harmful effect of eternal hell-fire and brimstone theology is here overstated. It is this author's belief that, if anything, the widespread harm is understated. Tasker (1979) refers to Matthew 25:46 in which Jesus is supposed to tell the unrighteous to depart into eternal (aeonian) punishment, Tasker contended that the Greek word "aeonian" should be translated "indefinite" rather than as "eternal." He concluded, "It would certainly be difficult to exaggerate the harmful effect of this unfortunate mistranslation, particularly when fire is understood in a literal rather than a metaphorical sense."

The Chaplain of Kanawha Hospice Care, in the state of West Virginia (in the Bible Belt), sees dying patients every day. The typical patient tells him that he or she is seventy to eighty years of age and has been "trying" to be a Christian for sixty to seventy years but is afraid to die for fear of not being good enough for God to accept into heaven. Spiritual abuse, however, is not confined to any one region of the country. According to a Gallup survey, 56 percent of Americans worry about dying without having been forgiven by God. (*NHO Newsline,* January, 1998).

If we accept the existence of spiritual abuse, we must next look for a solution to this problem. In order to prevent or effectively treat victims, they must be presented with a theology with no mixed messages, that characterizes God as both loving and just. God must not be seen as the cosmic tyrant who can never be pleased and who threatens divine wrath and inflicts eternal punishment. It is essential, for effective treatment, that victims of spiritual abuse develop a positive conception of God.

Alan Anderson (1995) contended that, for the abused, God is not a problem among various problems; but, since this problem is so all-pervasive, God is the problem! Until this problem is resolved nothing else really matters. The famous theologian and writer George MacDonald (1990), the mentor of an even more famous writer, C. S. Lewis, said that unless people perceive God to be as tender as the most tender-hearted person they have ever known and an infinitude better, they can never trust themselves to God. Neither can they trust their loved ones to God, whom they perceive to be the cosmic tyrant.

It does not help victims of spiritual abuse to attack God or try to discredit the Bible. People can best be helped to develop a positive conception of God by helping them understand the meaning of Biblical symbolism. Spiritual abuse is not confined to Christians alone and non-Christians need to be helped in other ways. However, in the Bible Belt almost all patients identify themselves as Christian or say that they are trying to be one. Therefore, for them, addressing Biblical issues is essential. Questions most frequently asked are about how to be saved, the necessity and mode of baptism, the security of the believer, divorce and remarriage, and "the unpardonable sin," but the issue which, by far, strikes the most fear in the minds of spiritually abused patients is the doctrine of eternal punishment in literal hell-fire—the lake of fire and brimstone!

Prominent among the reasons given by Russell (1957) for rejecting Christianity as his faith was the doctrine of eternal punishment in the fire of hell. He believed that teaching this doctrine was a character flaw in Jesus since many people have lived in fear that they may be forever damned in hell-fire. Russell contended that a person with much compassion would not have taught something which would cause so much fear and terror in so many people.

He, though a gifted writer, was not a theologian. He was only responding to the version of Christianity to which he had been exposed and to what he had observed in people's lives. Russell's position is a good example of what MacDonald (1990) meant when he stated that some things the Bible teaches and Jesus taught, on the surface, appear to be harsh and even cruel but, underneath the surface, they show the extent of God's love in action.

How can one see God's unconditional love in action in a teaching that superficially appears to some to be absolutely sadistic? In Mark 9:49 Jesus taught about sinners being "salted with fire" in hell. Interpreted literally, people being "salted with fire" is spiritual terrorism. Underneath the surface, this is beautiful, timeless, cross-cultural symbolism for purification. *The Good News Bible* (1976) translated this symbolic language as, "Everyone will be purified by fire. . . ." In the context of Holy Scripture, fire is consistently used to symbolize cleansing. The fire of hell is the same Greek word for "fire" used elsewhere with a beneficent connotation. This is the same word from which comes the word "purgatory" meaning to purify. The authors of *Good Goats Healing our Image of God* insightfully address the problem of spiritual abuse from a Roman Catholic perspective (Linn, 1994). They do a good job of explaining Biblical symbolism.

Jesus, according to Gerstner (1990), was a "scare theologian" per Jesus' use of the word "fire" in order to try to scare people into being good. If Gerstner's belief were correct, then Jesus was not only a "scare theologian," he was a spiritual terrorist. As in-depth study of Biblical symbolism reveals, Jesus was neither a "scare theologian" nor a spiritual terrorist.

What about the "lake of fire and brimstone?" Even below the surface, is there anything positive here? *The New International Version* (1978) of the Bible translated fire and brimstone as "burning sulfur" (Rev. 20:10). Webster (1961) defined "brimstone" as an outdated word for sulfur. Sulfur was known widely, throughout the ancient world at the time the Bible was being written, for its medicinal value and fumigation properties (Douglas, 1973). The ancients used sulfur daily to cure body sores and heal infections. They burned it in homes to disinfect them after people had died of an infectious disease and to disinfest them of insects, mice, and vermin. People used sulfur to preserve produce such as apples. Sulfur was also burned as incense in religious observances to symbolize prayers of purification. God does things on a grand scale, not just an incense pot but a whole lake of burning sulfur!

A positive conception of God, based on this symbolism, would be that the God of love, grace, and justice spiritually heals or "fumigates" sinners of their sins. God reconciles and restores all of creation! This understanding is in accord with the best in Biblical scholarship and the latest in medical and scientific research on death and dying.

People who have had near-death and out-of-body experiences have reported that there is perfect justice with God. God is always encountered as The Being of Light who gives each person a review of one's life with loving commentary about how one could do better. There is, however, no condemnation. In the life review, each person sees and feels the effect one's life has had on others. In fact, each person feels like one is the other person—feeling the pain one has inflicted on that other person. This process is total freedom with total accountability! The common transformative experience is meeting The Light (Morse & Perry, 1992). Ultimately, all are reconciled and restored to The Light in love, peace, and universal harmony.

This therapeutic approach, using Biblical symbolism in cognitive therapy, is used with patients who are victims of spiritual abuse and who ask pertinent questions. In actual practice, this is not a quick-fix, one-shot deal. It is a process which may take a few or many sessions, giving patients only as much information as they are able to understand and internalize. A few patients, who are eminently dying, may need a massive dose of grace to counteract the toxicity of their past spiritual terrorist exposure. With other patients a different modality is employed in helping them explore their spirituality and find peace with God, other people, and themselves. A non-religious approach is used with patients who are agnostics or atheists.

Therapeutically, a broad brush is used to paint a picture of God who is the essence of justice, love, hope, and forgiveness. An unpublished poem, "Better Than God???" has proven effective in bringing comfort, hope, and peace to people who have been spiritually abused. It may also be helpful for those who have lost loved ones and have been told that they will be tormented in hell forever because they failed to believe and/or live right. This poem has been especially beneficial for parents whose child was gay and who died of AIDS, spouses whose husband or wife died without having made a verbal confession of faith in Christ, and those who have lost loved ones to suicide. Patients can trust themselves and beloved family members to this God who is total forgiveness, unlimited hope, amazing grace, unconditional love, and perfect justice personified:

BETTER THAN GOD???
By Peggy Kociscin

The day you died, my mind, my heart
Became obsessed by fear.
Where are you? Did a hell now claim
The son I hold so dear?

For I recalled the "thou shalt nots"
instilled within my brain;
Will judgment for the failure mean
An everlasting pain?

Addiction gained control of you
(A rebel through and through);
Appalled and hurt, my heart would break
At things you'd say and do.

But through my fear, God came to me
And touched me tenderly.
He smiled, and with a loving voice
He kindly spoke to me.

"Did you love your son no matter what?"
"Certainly," I said.
"Did you forgive him for the pain
For all the things he did?"

"Of course," I said, "He is my son,
How could I not forgive him?
An unconditional mother's love
Was all I had to give him."

I thought I heard God chuckle then
As He whispered His reply,
"Why would you think that you can love
More perfectly than I?"

Chastised, ashamed, I understood,
All fear and doubt now ceased;
My son is in the hands of God
In glory and at peace.

I find that I can let him go
And the pain is now abating;
For I know that when I meet my God
My John will be there . . . waiting.

This is a totally, positive conception of God. Such a loving characterization of God does not give people false hope as some contend.

Conversely, it portrays The Supreme Being, in words and symbols, as the God who is the giver of life, the forgiver of sins, and the restorer of creation! Even victims of spiritual abuse can trust this kind of God to restore their spiritual balance and empower them to be survivors who experience freedom from fear, peace of mind, and joy of living! Grievers are able to progress through normal grieving without that process being complicated, or made more painful, by spiritual abuse.

Spiritual terrorism can be seen as blatant abuse, but most people who have been spiritually abused have not experienced it this blatantly. Spiritual abuse comes in various forms, some of which may be very subtle. Consequently, victims of spiritual abuse, in its more sophisticated forms, may not realize that their feelings of anger, anxiety, depression, stress, etc. are caused and/or exacerbated by spiritual abuse. Physical illness is common for persons in complicated grief. According to the principles of psychopathology, there is an integral connection between the body and the mind. Therefore, stress caused by spiritual abuse, or any other stressor, has the potential to depress a person's immune system making it more likely one will become physically ill (Barlow & Durand, 1995).

EXAMPLES OF GRIEF COMPLICATED
BY SPIRITUAL ABUSE

Anticipatory grief is the process people go through as they contemplate a death, even their own. A terrible case of anticipatory grief, due to spiritual abuse, involved a seventy-six-year-old great grandmother who was a patient of hospice. The nurse who made the referral for the chaplain to see her stated, "This lady is really afraid to die!"

When the chaplain arrived for the home visit, the patient had only talked for a few minutes when she burst into tears crying, "I don't want to go to hell!" Asked why she was so afraid of going to hell, she related that she had been trying to be a Christian since age twelve but she was afraid that she had not lived a good enough life to gain admission to heaven. The chaplain asked the patient to tell him about her life in order to ascertain whether there was some deep, dark sin which she had committed and of which she had never confessed to God and asked for forgiveness or for which she might believe was unforgivable. She stated that she had worked hard to rear her family, to be a good person, good wife, and mother. She had accepted Christ at age twelve, been baptized, gone to church regularly, and had never committed any sin which she had not confessed and asked God to forgive.

This woman had been taught in her church that in order for a person to get into heaven one had to accept Christ, be baptized, and live "right." In spite of having accepted Christ, being baptized, and trying to live "right," she was never sure whether her life was good enough to gain admission to heaven. Based on the preaching to which she had been exposed, in a fundamentalist church, not just deeds but sinful thoughts and sins of omission would send a person to hell. Hell, in her understanding, was conscious existence forever in literal fire.

The chaplain explained to this patient one of the most basic doctrines of the Christian Faith . . . salvation by grace rather than by good deeds. She responded that this sounded wonderful but too good to be true. She said that she would think about it.

On the second visit, she was more hopeful but still expressed doubt about going to heaven. On the third visit, the chaplain asked her if she believed that God would lie. She immediately replied that the Bible says that God cannot lie. The chaplain responded, "That means that you cannot go to hell because the Bible also says, 'If we confess our sins God is faithful and just to forgive us our sins and to cleanse us from all unrighteousness' " (I John 1:9,10). This approach apparently scored a home run with her because the light appeared to come on and she smiled and nodded understandingly. This is cognitive restructuring. Truth can set one free from morbid fear. This patient died a few days later, before the next scheduled visit. When the chaplain called to follow up with the family, they reported that she died in peace. Without fear of going to hell, she had been able to complete the work of anticipatory grief and die peacefully.

Sometimes spiritual abuse delays grief and further complicates the grieving process. Depending on the time lag and circumstances, the complications may be diagnosed as Post-Traumatic Stress Disorder. This situation is illustrated by Jane, an elderly woman, who was a hospice patient.

On the first home visit, Jane stated that she had been a Christian for more than seventy years and was confident that she would go to heaven after death. The chaplain asked Jane to tell him more about her life and her family. She reported having several children all of whom had become Christians except one son. When she mentioned his name she burst into tears and cried uncontrollably for a few minutes. Through her tears, she apologized for crying and for being so out of control. The chaplain assured her that it was okay to cry and that there was no need to apologize nor to hurry or to stop crying.

After she had regained her composure, he asked her if she would like to talk with him about this son. She informed him that her son had died about forty years ago and that it broke her heart to know that she would never see him again because he was an alcoholic who died a suicide. Jane explained that she had always heard it preached that alcoholics went to hell, as did all people who committed suicide, even if they had been persons of good moral character.

The chaplain talked with Jane, on this and subsequent visits, about a person being saved by grace not by lifestyle. Therefore, heaven is a gift and a gift is not earned. He assured her that God's grace, which is unconditional love in action, supersedes alcoholism and even suicide. He tried to comfort her, in her dying days, by telling her that he was confident that when she gets to heaven she will find her son there waiting for her arrival.

Jane took heart and said that she would take what she had heard preached as a grain of salt and trust God to do the right thing. Since she loved her son, who was an alcoholic, in spite of the fact he committed suicide, she came to believe that God, who claims to be our heavenly Father, will not do less. By restructuring her conception of God, Jane was able to effectively work through thoughts which were so frightful that she had repressed (pushed them from conscious memory) for forty years. The mind is better than a "ziploc" bag at keeping things preserved and fresh including sights, sounds, smells, thoughts, and feelings. Unless such painful feelings are effectively dealt with, it is probably impossible for the griever, regardless of how many years have elapsed since the death, to work through one's grief and find peace of mind. Dealing with spiritual abuse as the root cause of her repressed memories enabled Jane to find peace with God, in regard to her son, and to die with peace of mind.

A multidimensional case of complicated grief is illustrated by Martha. The chaplain met Martha when her boyfriend, Sam, was a hospice patient. On the first and only visit, Sam informed the chaplain that he had never had God in his life up until now so he was not going to start at this late date. He died a couple of days later.

Two weeks after Sam's death, the chaplain called to follow up with Martha in order to provide spiritual care for bereavement. Martha tearfully poured out her heart's overwhelming pain. She presented the most complex case of complicated grief with which the chaplain had ever dealt in over a quarter century of pastoral, mental health, and chaplaincy counseling.

Martha was not just experiencing the usual painful feelings of loss, loneliness, anger, depression, and guilt from not having been able to have done enough to prevent Sam's death. She was also feeling overwhelmed by catastrophic bereavement issues.

Martha "knew" that Sam had gone to hell! She related that Sam had been a good man even though he had been an alcoholic. She stated that she had always heard it preached that a person went to hell for drinking alcohol or for being an alcoholic. Even if God would somehow overlook Sam's alcoholism, he still went to hell because all of the thirty years they had been together, including giving birth to their two children, they had, according to her church's doctrine, been "living in sin" due to not being married. Actually, even if they had gotten married, they would have still been "living in sin" since, according to Martha's church, there are no grounds for divorce and both had been divorced. This was literally a case of being damned if they did and damned if they did not.

The largest Christian denomination, which represents the vast majority of Christians, holds that even if there are valid grounds for divorce, remarriage is not permitted. The only basis for a valid Christian marriage is for a person who has been divorced in a civil court to go through the long, and sometimes expensive, process of obtaining an annulment which states that the first marriage never existed. Many persons who are divorced and remarry outside the church live in fear of judgment and eternal damnation due to this practice which some see as a form of spiritual abuse.

In addition to their two children, Martha had a son from her previous marriage to whom Sam had been a good stepfather and with whom he had been very close. In less than two weeks after Sam's death, her son felt so overwhelmed with grief that he committed suicide.

The pain of losing her beloved son and her common-law husband within two weeks of each other was almost more than Martha could bear. She stated that the only thing which kept her from taking her own life was that she felt that she had to keep living in order to care for her youngest son who was in junior high school. The pain of two deaths in such a short time is beyond the emotional coping ability of many people. Almost any person in this situation could be a good candidate for hospitalization.

Martha's emotional pain was made immeasurably worse by her belief that her son went to hell for taking his own life. She would, therefore, never again see her son, or Sam, unless she too ended up in hell which she thought she would likely do.

Martha was a recovering alcoholic. She had not had a drink in many years but she had been unable to break her smoking habit. She had also been taught that people go to hell for smoking! This is a common belief in fundamentalist, Christian churches and is another manifestation of spiritual abuse. Taken as a whole, in her frame of reference, Martha was spiritually terrorized!

On each visit, the chaplain assured and reassured Martha of God's love which is unconditional and everlasting. The chaplain talked with her about God's grace which is truly amazing, since she liked the hymn, "Amazing Grace." He shared with her that God's grace is so amazing that it is greater than alcoholism, nicotine addiction, sexual sin, suicide, or any other sin.

They discussed God's understanding of why Sam had rejected religion. Sam had come from an abusive home. As a child he had prayed and asked God to help him, but as far as Sam could tell, God never helped him. As an adult, therefore, Sam felt he no longer needed God. Martha and the chaplain talked about God's acceptance and forgiveness of Sam. They, of course, spent much time talking about God's acceptance and forgiveness of her son.

Poetry is a powerful medium of communication. The thing which helped Martha the most seemed to be the poem, "Better than God???" As soon as the chaplain had recited this poem to her, Martha exclaimed, "That is beautiful! I want a copy to share with my family and all my friends." He provided a copy and share it she did! Apparently, each time she shared it with someone, she became more convinced of its validity. On each visit Martha became more and more hopeful of going to heaven and finding her loved ones there waiting for her arrival. Martha was very quiet and not well-educated but, as she got better, she wanted to help others who were victims of spiritual abuse.

At that time the chaplain was teaching a class on spiritual abuse to students who were working on their Master's Degrees in counseling. Martha came to the graduate college to serve on a panel of persons who had suffered spiritual abuse. The graduate students expressed their appreciation for the insights they gained from Martha and the other panelists who had the courage to share their painful experiences, especially in regard to complicated grief.

This writer has taught a graduate course on grief counseling and has incorporated instruction on spiritual abuse into the content of that course. An assignment given in that class was for the students to write an integration paper on their understanding of the grief process, personal insights, and professional applications. One student wrote about growing up in a dysfunctional home with her father, an alcoholic, who abused her, her mother, and her siblings.

The student "knew" her mother was finally at peace in the presence of God when she died because she had been such a loving, godly mother. This was not the case with her father, who died seven years later, after a year and a half of terminal illness during which time this student and her siblings had cared for him. She concluded, "During these months my father refused to discuss his death and gave no clue to his spiritual beliefs. He died without ever saying, 'I love you,' to any of his children. However, more important, we shared (unspoken) among us the fear of an alcoholic ever entering heaven's gate. The poem, 'Better Than God???,' has brought peace to my heart and now I am ready to emotionally relocate my father into the arms of God and move on with my life."

Hopefully, graduate students are being educated who will be able to effectively deal with their own bereavement issues and then be able to counsel others experiencing both uncomplicated and complicated grief. They will, thus, also be better able to recognize grief complicated by spiritual abuse and to professionally treat it or make a helpful referral to a therapist who has theological expertise dealing with spiritual abuse in regard to complicated grief.

The hospice philosophy is that the patient and family are one unit of care. The mission is to meet the needs of both. At times these needs may appear to be, and in fact are, mutually exclusive. The case of the patient, John, and his wife, Sue, illustrates this dilemma in relation to complicated grief.

John was bedfast and very weak. He told the chaplain that he knew he was going to die and that he was okay with that, except for one thing. He was concerned about whether he had had a valid, Christian baptism. He explained that he had been baptized as an infant by sprinkling. At age twelve he had confessed the Christian faith and had joined his current church. He had no doubts about his baptism until after he had gotten cancer and the doctor had told him and his wife that he was going to die in a few months. At that time, Sue and some friends had expressed their fear that he might go to hell due to not having been baptized in the "right way." For them the "right way" was being immersed as an adult.

John asked the chaplain who was right. The chaplain did not answer that kind of controversial question because the answer is sure to alienate one or the other, so he asked John what he thought about it. John replied that he thought that God looks at the intention of the person rather than the external details. In this case, God would look at his confession of the Christian faith and the fact of his baptism, so his age and the mode of baptism would not matter. Since the chaplain was not disagreeing with his rationale, he could see that John's wife was getting upset with him.

The chaplain addressed Sue, "I get the impression that you are afraid that by my not disagreeing with John that I am giving him false hope about going to heaven." She replied, "I hate to say that but, based on what I have heard all my life, that is true." She said, "Well, I probably should not say anything about his baptism because I have been baptized by immersion as an adult, after accepting Christ, and I am still not sure that I am going to heaven." She bent her knees and leaned forward, in a cowering posture, and wrapped her arms around herself. Then, in a whining voice, she cried, "I don't want to burn." She was terrorized by the thought of being tortured in literal hell-fire.

The chaplain responded, "I assume you mean burn in the lake of fire and brimstone according to the Book of Revelation in the Bible." She exclaimed, "Yes, exactly." He told her that he was not trying to sound superior, because he had to look it up himself, but he wondered whether she was aware of the dictionary definition of the word, "brimstone." She replied that she had no idea. He informed her of the Webster (1961) definition of "brimstone" as an outdated word for sulfur. The chaplain then asked Sue if she knew what sulfur was widely known for in the ancient world at the time the Bible was being written. Again, she had no clue.

After the chaplain had explained to her the medicinal and fumigation uses of sulfur in Biblical times, he asked her what she thought a "lake of burning sulfur" (which is how the New International Version of the Bible translated "fire and brimstone") would symbolize. She immediately responded, "That would symbolize spiritual healing or purification!" He then said to her, "If that is true and you were to believe it, what would that understanding do for you?" She thought for about a minute while he silently waited. A smile replaced the scowl on her face and she exclaimed, "I could stop being afraid!"

It was not immediate, but Sue did stop being afraid for John's and her own salvation. When John died, she was able to grieve his death without the catastrophic complication of fearing that he was burning in literal hell-fire. It is hard enough to deal with the loss of a person's loved one without the bereavement process being complicated by spiritual abuse. No one should also have to deal with the fear of that loved one being tortured in hell forever.

When people, of whatever religious faith, come to the end of life, hopefully, their faith will be a source of comfort rather than distress. A positive, loving conception of God can facilitate this process both for patients and their loved ones. Their grief will not be complicated by spiritual abuse. Not just during bereavement, but in life in general, a positive conception of God promotes optimal emotional, mental, spiritual, and physical health.

REFERENCES

Anderson, C. (1995). *The problem is God.* Walpole, NH: Stillpoint.

Arterburn, S., & Felton, J. (1991). *Toxic faith: Understanding and overcoming religious addiction.* Nashville: Oliver Nelson.

Barlow, D., & Durand, V. (1995). *Abnormal physchology.* Pacific Grove, CA: Brooks/Roe.

Booth, L. (1991). *When God becomes a drug: Breaking the chains of religious addiction & abuse.* New York: Jeremy P. Tarcher/Perigee.

Carroll, D. (1991). *Living with dying: A loving guide for family and close friends.* New York: Paragon House.

Doka, K., & Davidson, J. (1998). *Living with grief: Who we are how we grieve.* Philadelphia: Brunner/Mazel.

Douglas, J. (Ed.) (1973). *The New Bible Dictionary.* Grand Rapids, MI: WM. B. Eerdmans.

Elliott, R. (1991). *Wide awake, clear-headed, & refreshed.* Winfield, IL: Relaxed Books.

Enroth, R. (1994). *Recovering from churches that abuse.* Grand Rapids, MI: Zondervan.

George, B. (1991). *Growing in grace.* Eugene: Harvest House.

Gerstner, J. (1990). *Repent or perish.* Ligonier: Soli Deo Gloria Publication.

Good New Bible (1976). New York: American Bible Society.

Kübler-Ross, E. (1973). *On death and dying.* New York: Harper & Row.

Linn, D. (1994). *Good goats: Healing our image of God.* Mahwah, NJ: Paulist Press.

MacDonald, G. (1990). *Knowing the heart of God.* Minneapolis: Bethany House.

Morse, M., & Perry, P. (1992). *Transformed by the light.* New York: Villard Books.

NHO Newsline (1998 January). Gallup releases survey findings on spirituality and dying.

Purcell, B. (1998, May/June). Spiritual terrorism. *The American Journal of Hospice & Palliative Care,* 167-172.

Purcell, B. (1998, July/August). Spiritual abuse. *The American Journal of Hospice & Palliative Care,* 227-231.

Russell, B. (1957). *Why I am not a Christian.* New York: Simon & Schuster.

Stuart, B. (1998, April). Annual hospice teleconference.

Swindoll, C. (1990). *The grace awakening*. Dallas: Word.

Tasker, R. (Ed.) (1979). *Tyndale new Testament Commentaries: The gospel according to St. Matthew*. Grand Rapids, MI: WM. B. Eerdmans.

The Holy Bible: New International Version (1978). Grand Rapids: Zondervan.

U.S. News & World Report (1991, March). The rekindling of hell.

Webster's New Collegiate Dictionary (1961). Springfield: G & C Merrian Co.

CHAPTER 12
Spirituality and Religion: Risks for Complicated Mourning

Richard B. Gilbert

> Spiritual crisis can come to any of us no matter how many preventive or protective filters or barriers we may have in place. (McBride, 1998, p. 4)

> Many honest seekers have turned away from the church and formal religion or, at least, have been puzzled by how their spiritual lives have not fit into the neat pattern so often presented of the faith journey. (McBride, 1998, p. 4)

> Trauma occurs when one loses the sense of having a safe place to retreat within or outside oneself to deal with frightening emotions and experiences . . . Trauma made them feel cut off from God, from others and even from themselves . . . How can a viable spiritual life exist in the midst of all this? How can a connection with God be established in the midst of radical separation? (McBride, 1998, pp. 12-13)

> Soul appears, then, to be a concept of the self that speaks of the whole person integrated in his or her unique way. Trauma disrupts or destroys this integration of the total person. (McBride, 1998, p. 13)

My baby died. Don't talk to me about a loving God.[1]

In the monumental work which has become the authority on complicated mourning, Dr. Therese Rando provides the setting and assessment tools for affirming the practical reality of complicated mourning in the journeys of the bereaved (Rando, 1993). Rando identifies the losses that typically come wrapped in risk factors (natural, accidental, suicide, homicide) (Rando, 1993, p. xiii), the seven high-risk variables for complicated mourning (suddenness and lack of anticipation, overly lengthy duration of demise, loss of a child, preventability, existence of concurrent losses and stresses and elements of disenfranchised grief) (p. xiii), the needs of those experiencing complications in their mourning for additional and

---

[1]A personal note from a bereaved parent.

intentional assistance ("individuals experiencing such complications require more extensive, more intensive, or different interventions") (p. 3) and, quoting a study by Raphael from 1983, documents the severity of the problem ("one in three bereavements result in 'morbid outcome or pathological patterns of grief") (p. 5).

THESIS STATEMENT

While spirituality and religion are typically identified as sources of meaning and comfort for the bereaved (including Rando's work) we often find it difficult or otherwise uncomfortable to highlight (and respond to) examples of spirituality and religion that compromise our grieving and thus are themselves complicating factors.

Many studies are emerging on the subject of abusive spirituality and religion, and several of them are cited in the Bibliographic Notations at the close of this article. Spirituality and religion are still subjects that are frequently taboo subjects for many healthcare professionals, therapists, counselors, and bereavement caregivers. Typical arguments for moving away from the sensitive subjects of religion and spirituality are that spiritual/religious matters do not fit conveniently into the medical/therapeutic models. They take time, and time is a rare commodity for many professionals. We feel uncomfortable intruding into the beliefs and practices of another person, we lack training, and, probably the issue most crucial, the spiritual and religious questions and longings of others get too close to our own journey or to the issues within us that we otherwise would choose to ignore.

Workable and measurable definitions of spirituality, religion, spiritual and pastoral care provide assessment tools that bring us closer to the stories and experiences of the bereaved, and offer recognizable dimensions of faith (as determined by the individual) that are more likely to present themselves as risks rather than sources of comfort are the focus of this chapter.

FILTERS . . .

Filters generally represent flow, purification, and, on some occasions, compromise. A filter is something that another, whether it be fluids in an automobile, various bodily functions, what we bring to grief experiences, grief, itself, that flow. The filters are there and must be recognized.

Filters are essentially neutral until the individual gives meaning to them. If our meaning makes the filter problematic, then the purifying process is supplanted by the compromising or complicating factors. Filters can either facilitate the flow or dam up the entire process.

It is important to remember that it is our privilege to walk with the bereaved as they are willing to "let us in." That does not give us permission to negate or criticize the filter. I regularly meet people whose beliefs and practices are, at a minimum, not suitable to *my* beliefs, and thus subject to scrutiny. I question, I join in the assessment struggle to help the person come to a point of meaning which is the spiritual connection. The filters, even the clogged ones, are still my filters and I have a right to them until I choose to do something with them or about them. This becomes particularly sensitive and cumbersome when related to a person's beliefs.

GRIEF AS A FILTER . . .

Grief is itself a filter. For a time, and that time varies from person to person, everything about us is filtered by or otherwise influenced by grief. We say that grief is physical, emotional, social, and spiritual. We measure its effects through our personal experiences and our observations of others. Figure 1 demonstrates the role of grief as a filter.

GRIEF IS FILTERED . . .

There are many factors that influence how we do or do not grieve. Many studies are available that highlight these factors. Just to list a few . . . gender, cumulative effects of loss, ethnic or cultural, health of the griever, relationship with the deceased, *and* spirituality or religion. Figure 2 illustrates the process of filtering that our grief journey can experience.

DEFINITIONS . . .

Despite extensive research and study, as well as the familiarity of these words in conversation and professional practice, seldom have we found a subject where the operative words are subject to so many definitions and subtle nuances based on personal preferences, prejudices, beliefs, and practices. For example, while many of us would suggest that, even on a generic level, all people are spiritual, and that the bereaved demonstrate the common thread of a search for meaning that speaks of their spirituality, there are many who suggest that you cannot be spiritual without God. There are many who express no particular belief system and therefore want to substitute other words (psychology, philosophy, ethical standards) for "spirituality" since they do not believe in God. It is my observation that you cannot begin to understand the uniqueness of each journey, and each set of beliefs, unless you provide a common definition or foundation point on which to build. So we offer some definitions.

Spirituality

"Our spirituality has to do with the way we conceive of and express our relationships to the creator. Spirituality has been called the

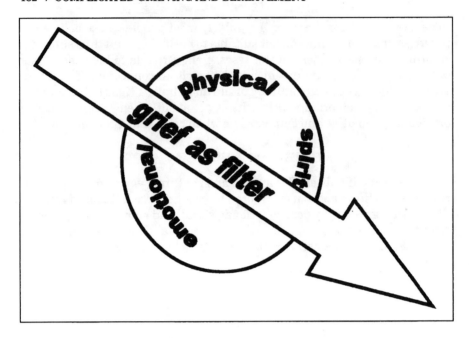

Figure 1.

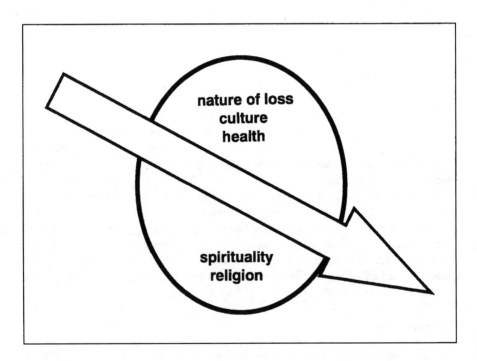

Figure 2.

psychological or experiential counterpart of dogma" (Steere, 1997, p. 44). Spirituality is the connection to meaning, hope, and inner strength, and a sense of purpose that becomes challenged through many of life's experiences, especially loss. Spirituality is a powerful filter for our grief experiences, powerful enough to determine even whether we do or do not grieve, and a filter strong enough to redirect our lives and our desire to live. "The spiritual beliefs shape the way individuals view the world around them" (Cox & Fundis, 1991, p. 82). Leo Booth, who specializes in addiction and abuse, especially providing care and intervention for those at risk because of spirituality or religion, reminds us, "Each of us contains a spark of the divinity, and that spark enables us to connect with each other and with God . . . I have come to believe that spirituality is the 'soul' of religion" (p. 36). While there is a contemporary trend of drawing lines in the sand and demanding absolutes as we define them (expecting others to conform to our definitions and standards), John Fortunato would remind us, "Spiritual growth is more of the nature of proceeding from hunch to hunch rather than from conclusion to conclusion" (1997, p. 14).

In a conference worksheet, Dr. John Morgan offered these statements about spirituality:

1. Each person has a spiritual dimension.
2. The spiritual orientation influences mental, physical, and emotional dimensions.
3. Adversity can be an opportunity for spiritual growth.
4. Spiritual beliefs and practices are exhibited in widely different ways.
5. Spiritual needs can arise at any time or place.
6. Joy and humor are essential parts of human spirituality.

Religion

While it is often so intertwined to be indistinguishable from spirituality, spirituality and religion are different. They serve different purposes or functions. It is not unusual for one to yield to another, at least modestly in order for them to mesh. It is important to remember that they are different (that is not a value judgment; we did not say better or worse, just different) and, for spirituality (which is central to the individual) it is essential to remember that the function of religion is to build a person spiritually. When the reverse flow is emphasized from beyond the person, there is a tremendous risk for complications, damage, or abuse.

The word "religion" comes from the Latin root *religio* which signifies a bond between humanity and some greater-than-human power. Scholars identify at least three historical designations of the term as follows: 1) a supernatural power to which individuals must respond; 2) a feeling present in the individual who conceives such a power; and 3) the ritual acts carried out in respect of that power. Religion has been transformed from an abstract process to fixed objective entity expressed through a definable system . . . the pivotal role of religion . . . is to facilitate personal sensitivity to ultimate questions, while urging the individual to continue his or her search for answers to those questions. (Larson, 1998, p. 15)

Religion is the "we" that balances the "I" of spirituality, and gives us places to find tradition, continuity, community, and support.

The longings produced by grief are often most painfully explored in our spiritual centeredness. Many of the complicating filters that seem to emerge in our spiritual quest through sorrow and loss are really invitations to dig deeper into our inner strength and resources. Many of the religious filters can be compromising, controlling, or place expectations upon us that become blocking filters. A common example, "Your minister tells you, 'The Bible says that anger is a sin,' " and you will probably have difficulty with anger, a natural partner in our grief journey. As a result of loss and how religion has or has not influenced the grief journey, McBride notes, "Many honest seekers have turned away from the church and formal religion or, at least, have been puzzled by how their spiritual lives have not fit into the neat pattern so often presented of the faith journey" (1998, p. 4). A comparison of the two is noted in Figure 3.

	Spirituality		Religion
I AM . . .		WE ARE . . .	
	Loved		loved/loving
	Nurtured		nurtured/nurturing
	Valuable		valuable/valuing
	Valued		valued/valuing
	Forgiven		forgiven/forgiving
	Journeying		journeying/facilitating
	Hopeful		hopeful/hope-bearing
	Respected		respected/respectful
	Productive		productive/enabling
	Eternal		eternal
	Nourished		nourished/nourishing
	Safe		safe

Figure 3.

Spiritual Care

Spiritual care is the work of all of us, empathetically devoted presence in the life and journey of those in our care. To be spiritually present is to be open to their longings, quests, struggles, doubts, and tough questions, as we willingly set aside those same dynamics within us. It also means that empathetic listening leads to emptiness; we must commit to our spiritual connections so that we might be replenished.

While in the context of hospice or palliative care, Wilcock (1997) offers this definition,

> To comfort God's people (and that is *all* people, not just a select few) and make straight the road along which God may come to them is the work of spiritual care. It is team work, because the obstacles on the road are many, and need different disciplines to dislodge them. (p. 18).

Spiritual care asks the following questions:

1. What is spiritual assessment? Religious assessment?
2. What do they mean for *this* person/client?
3. What is my relationship, on these issues, to the larger team?
4. What does faith/belief mean to this person?
5. What beliefs are operative for the person at this time?
6. What rituals or practices are helpful for this person?
7. What does "religious leader" mean to this person?
8. Would you like to pray?

To be involved in spiritual care is also to monitor the spirituality within ourselves. It was once suggested why doctors avoid dealing with bad news with their patients. It offers some wise counsel in exploring our spiritual connectedness with our patients.

1. Fear of the unknown and the untaught.
2. Fear of unleashing a reaction.
3. Fear of expressing emotion.
4. Fear of not knowing the answers.
5. Fear of illness and death (or what, for this discussion, we would call the wilderness experience of struggle).

To be involved in spiritual matters with the bereaved is also to flag dynamics that might appear abusive or unhealthy. Of course it serves well to remind us of a point mentioned earlier that, unless the client is quite literally "in danger," we must move cautiously if we are thinking of "removing" what is abusive. It may be the only thing the individual has to hold on to. It may appear abusive to us, but it may be sanctuary for that person. We do not pull out the props, but rather walk with and through them so that the client can give meaning to these props or filters and then determine whether or not they are still useful.

In a very thorough and troubling review of abusive religion in various expressions of religion within the Christian fold, dynamics which the authors suggest crush the voice of the individual's own spirit, Ritter and O'Neill (1996, p. 5) identify specific feelings often associated with unsafe religious experiences (see Figure 4).

Pastoral Care

Pastoral care is the work of those who specialize in spiritual care, bringing the special gifts associated with call, office, training, and how the person is envisioned and trusted by the individual receiving that care. It is important that we remember that the work of spiritual care, that special invitation afforded to us as we glimpse the inner stories of our clients, is the work of all of us. Pastoral care is a specialized care and deserves its rightful place on the bereavement team.

This is what pastoral care brings to bereavement care and the team . . .

✓- helps caregivers explore deeper spiritual issues
✓- symbolic presence of another "word" or perspective
✓- linkage to religious communities, traditions, values
✓- administers sacraments and rituals requested by patient
✓- represents sanctuary or a safe place
✓- represents spiritual matters to the team and treatment plans
✓- advocacy

Feelings Associated with Unsafe Religious Experiences

1. UNSAFE . . . no longer responsive to my needs.
2. INVALIDATED . . . my goodness is refuted.
3. ABANDONED . . . I am cast aside when I don't fit in because of my diverse needs.
4. APPREHENSIVE . . .increased fear.
5. GUILTY . . . we can't meet someone else's expectations.
6. SHAMEFUL . . . I have failed God; I am a bad person.
7. UNWORTHY . . . I must again "qualify."
8. DEVALUED . . . group over the individual.
9. FRUSTRATED . . . no one listens.
10. THWARTED . . . no room for negotiation.
11. STIFLED . . . creativity crushed.
12. SHUNNED . . . I am cast aside.
13. DISEMPOWERED . . . I am powerless.

Figure 4.

✓- provides for the spiritual needs of the caregivers
✓- "keeps track" of the extended circle of family and friends
✓- keeps the focus holistic
✓- represents institution/team to the religious community

Within pastoral care we also have specialists. Chaplains are the "specialists" in pastoral care (in a particular setting or around a special need).

A considerable amount of a chaplain's time is spent in simply hanging loose with patients and staff, talking and laughing over inconsequential things, and time spent like this is not wasted. It is thus that ground is established so that when a patient or family member or member of staff needs to talk, a friendship has been established, a foundation for trust. Also, as faculties diminish with illness, and maybe speech goes, the chaplain will know the idiosyncrasies and personal characteristics which enable this person to continue as a complete individual, living, not dying, to the very end. (Wilcock, 1997, p. 18)

This anecdotal note from a very early book on chaplaincy summarizes this well:

A chaplain is one with a foot in two worlds: the world of faith and the world of modern medicine,
Not a doctor, but often asked to "explain" an operation.
Not a priest, but sometimes a baptizer of Catholic babies.
Not a social worker, but often a family counselor.
Not a professor, but on and off a teacher of young doctors.
Not a parish pastor, but usually a pastoral counselor.
In a society where medicine is more and more complex and impersonal, one who sometimes can make the hospital seem more human. (Mitchell, 1972, p. 16)

ASSESSMENT . . . HISTORY

If we are to walk with people in the valleys of their sorrow, we must understand what the individuals are trying to "understand," namely, what of my past understandings of spirituality and/or religion are present in this current valley or struggle and how do they help or hinder me in my search for meaning and healing?

For many people (especially adults) the struggle may appear less complicated. It is usually the struggle (and it *is* a struggle) to bring the simplicities of what we call "The Sunday School faith" or the spiritual truths we learned "at our mother's knee." For others there are some very specific (though often hard to identify) "tapes" of past experiences and understandings that will put us at risk in the wilderness. For these people (and it can be any person at any time) it becomes not only the struggle of loss that has created this valley, but also the buried valleys of past issues, abuses, misunderstandings, and wounds that now become magnified and become concurrent valleys.

Here is a useful assessment tool that has served me well in helping patients and clients sort out feelings, issues, doubts, and areas of strength. It offers an essential truth. Our toughest (and often most meaningful) struggles are in the valley. We cannot move to tomorrow's healing without exploring the valleys of today and the experiences of yesterday that influence (and occasionally corrupt) our current struggles (see Figure 5).

In the classroom setting I often use cartoons to capture the penetrating insights that are otherwise untouchable when exploring the deep truths and even deeper wounds that are part of our spiritual stories. They still serve here. The cartoons help us understand (column 1) what the person is bringing into the present valley (column 2) and now serving as filters in the struggle to find hope and meeting.

Illustration #1. A little girl passes a radio that is blaring out the song, "God is watching over you, God is watching over you." The little girl replies, horrified, "Oh, no! Not God AND Santa Claus." What do we remember from our childhood or in our parenting about Santa Claus? How often has it been said, "If you aren't good Santa Claus will not bring you any presents." Therefore, "if something is wrong (the death of a loved one or my own dying) I must have done something wrong." What does that do to disrupt the journey and heighten expressions of guilt and shame?

Illustration #2. "The Lord is my shepherd, I have everything I need." In this paraphrase of Psalm 23 we have a sense of certainty or guarantee of God's providential care. A drunk driver runs a stop sign and kills your son. What happened to the shepherd?

Illustration #3. Rev. Will B. Dunn, a cartoon character, has an automatic teller machine at his church. On observing it one notes that it takes deposits only. Many view their religious practices (attendance at

	"back when . . ."	in the valley . . .	moving toward . . .
spirituality			
religion			

Figure 5.

Presentation	"In the valley"	assessment
"Christian Science was discovered by a woman who had been in ill health and pain much of her life and for whom illness was a metaphor for learned female helplessness" (Wilson, 1997, p. 90).	"It doesn't seem likely that she would have told her grandmother about the lump . . . I know that my mother didn't tell her closest friend in the church . . . what did she fear from telling them? That they would see her as a failure— someone who said she wanted to become a healer and instead developed cancer. For my mother, schooled in Christian Science, which had told her since childhood that disease was unreal and a lie, hiding must have been second nature" (Wilson, 1997, p. 168).	
A cartoon, "Do you believe in heaven or hell?" "It depends on what I did the night before."	"Am I 'saved.'" "Will I go to heaven?" "What is heaven like?" "There is no heaven."	
"You should look upon suffering as an opportunity from God. Give the suffering over to God in humble service and God will lift your burden."	"Why did God take my baby?" "See cancer as a gift." "If that is what God is all about, I want nothing to do with God."	
"In our humanity, many of us act as if we enjoy a certain inalienable right to answers to all of our questions" (Davis, 1996, p. 69).	"I had to accept the fact that the God I had always believed I could rely on had moved out of my life and left no forwarding address" (Davis, 1996, p. 61).	
"God answers all of our prayers."	"With the darkest hours of my life bearing down on me like a freight train in the night, I knocked desperately on God's door . . . and heard only the sound of it being locked and double locked from within" (Davis, 1996, p. 49).	
"Part of the problem lies in the way sin doctrines have been used judgmentally to affix blame or culpability apart from the presence of understanding and forgiveness" (Steere, 1997, p. 105).	"It's all my fault!"	
"My minister won't come to see me."	"Some priests, ministers and rabbis compound the situation by setting themselves above grief and tears, either as an example of fortitude or self protection. A greater problem is that most members of the clergy receive little training in bereavement during their formal education" (Moe, 1997, p. 8).	

Figure 6.

worship, financial contributions, service on various committees, ethical processes, and decision making) as a form of "making a deposit." What happens when we find that we are unable to make withdrawals, or the panicked fear when we cannot remember our PIN number?

Illustration #4. A parishioner shares with her minister the deep sorrow she is feeling in her grief. The minister replies, "You mean you have been carrying all of these feelings all of this time and you haven't come to talk with me? Shame on you!"

Illustration #5. (Reported to me by a neighbor who went to her minister to share her struggles about doubt and sorrow after the death of her husband). "You are a Christian, you believe in Easter, Jesus has taken care of everything for you. Grief is contrary to Easter. If you believe in Easter, you will no longer grieve. Get on with your life. It is what Jesus would want you to do."

ASSESSMENT . . . STORIES

Figure 6 is a series of quotes from books, statements, or cartoons that make a statement. The second column translates them into experiential remarks "in the valley." The concluding column is the assessment track. It is imperative that we remember that assessment is not what we do, but the meaning that comes when the client and caregiver come to this meaning together. The worksheet is left incomplete so that you can use it as a worksheet while you develop a format that you can then use as you listen to the stories of others.

REFERENCES

Booth, L. (1994). *The God game: It's your move.* Walpole, NH: Stillpoint.

Cox, G., & Fundis, R. (1991). *Spiritual, ethical and pastoral aspects of death and bereavement.* Amityville, NY: Baywood.

Davis, J. M. (1996). *In the shadow of evil: Where is God in a violent world?* Dubuque, IA: Kendall/Hunt.

Fortunato, J. (1987). *AIDS: The spiritual dilemma.* San Francisco: Harper & Row.

Larson, D. (1998). *Scientific research on spirituality and health: A consensus report.* Rockville, MD: NIHR.

McBride, J. L. (1998). *Spiritual crisis; Surviving trauma to the soul.*Binghamton, NY: Haworth.

Mitchell, K. R. (1972). *Hospital chaplain.* Philadelphia: Westminster.

Moe, T. (1997). *Pastoral care in pregnancy loss: A ministry long needed.* Binghamton: Haworth.

Rando, T. (1993). *Treatment of complicated mourning.* Champaign, IL: Research Press.

Ritter, K., & O'Neill, C. (1996). *Righteous religion; Unmasking the illusions of fundamentalism and authoritarian Catholicism.* Binghamton: Haworth Pastoral Press.

Steere, D. (1997). *Spiritual presence in psychotherapy: A guide for caregivers.* New York: Brunner/Mazel.

Wilcock, P. (1997). *Spiritual care of dying and bereaved people.* Harrisburg: Morehouse.

Wilson, B. (1997). *Blue windows: A Christian science childhood.* New York: Picador.

BIBLIOGRAPHIC NOTATIONS

Anderson, R. S. (1997). *The soul of ministry: Forming leaders for God's people.* Louisville: Westminster John Knox Press.

Bowman, G. W., III (1998). *Dying, grieving, faith and family: A pastoral care approach.* Binghamton: Haworth Pastoral Press.

Dayringer, R. (1998). *The heart of pastoral counseling: Healing through worship.* Binghamton: Haworth.

Denshimer, R. (1990). *Counseling the bereaved.* New York: Pergamon Press.

Doka, K., & Morgan, J. D. (1993). *Death and spirituality.* Amityville: Baywood.

Enroth, R. (1992). *Churches that abuse: Help for those hurt by legalism, authoritarian leadership, spiritual intimidation,* Grand Rapids: Zondervan.

Fitchett, G. (1993). *Assessing spiritual needs: A guide for caregivers.* Minneapolis: Augsburg.

Fitzgerald, H. (1994). *The mourning handbook.* New York: Simon & Schuster.

Gilbert, R. (1996). *HeartPeace: Healing help for grieving folks,* St. Meinrad, IN: Abbey Press.

Gilbert, R. (1997). *Responding to grief: A complete resource guide.* Point Richmond, CA: Spirit of Health!

Grollman, E. (1995). *Bereaved children and teens.* Boston: Beacon.

Guntzelman, J. (1995). *124 prayers for caregivers.* Winona, MN: Saint Mary's Press.

Hagley, N. (1985). *Comfort us, Lord—Our baby died.* Omaha: Centering.

Irish, D. et al. (1993). *Ethnic variations in dying, death and grief: Diversity in universality.* Bristol: Taylor & Francis.

Koenig, H. G. (1997). *Is religion good for your health?* Binghamton: Haworth Press.

Magida, A. (1996). *How to be a perfect stranger.* Woodstock: Jewish Lights.

Miller, J. (1995). *A pilgrimage through grief: Healing the soul's hurt after loss.* St. Meinrad: Abbey Press.

Meyer, C. (1998). *A good death: Challenges, choices and care options.* Mystic, CT: Twenty-Third Publications.

O'Brien, M. (1997). *Healing prayer services for those who mourn.* Notre Dame: Ave Maria Press.

Sims, D. (1994). *If I could just see hope.* Wenatchee, WA: Big A & Co.

Zurheide, J. (1997). *When faith is tested: Pastoral responses to suffering and tragic death.* Minneapolis: Augsburg Fortress.

CHAPTER 13

Can We Predict Complicated Grief Before the Bereavement? A Report on Bereavement Risk Assessment in a Palliative Care Setting

Christine Hodgson, Lynda Weaver, and Pippa Hall

Many authors have offered specific definitions of grief and mourning that distinguish one from the other. There seems to be no real consensus. In this chapter the two terms will be used interchangeably to refer to the process that a bereaved person experiences as a result of the bereavement.

Bereavement support for the family, both before and after a patient's death, is generally considered to be an integral part of a palliative care program. In a sense, these families are fortunate since this support is not usually available to those whose relative has died at home or in an acute care hospital. Even in palliative care, however, as the number of patients increases and human resources are depleted, it becomes ever more difficult to decide when to offer more intensive counseling and to whom. Who needs the help most and who will be most able to use it? There is a tendency in North American society to label the expression of intense grief reaction as pathological, implying a need for some form of "treatment" (Wolfelt, 1992). Can grief not be seen as a natural process, albeit one that results in irreversible changes for the person who is bereaved? Can it not be assumed that this grief will evolve to some point of reconciliation unless there are complicating factors present? This being the case, interventions should be focused on those individuals and families where such complicating factors are present. Not only does this imply a service more focused on prevention, it also suggests a more efficient deployment of resources.

Of critical significance in a palliative care setting is the fact that a person's risks can be identified and facilitation of the mourning process can begin before the death occurs. With a more precise method of identification of those at highest risk, the incidence of complicated mourning may be lowered, thus preventing the occurrence of the distressing symptoms that arise. With this in mind, the Ottawa Regional Palliative Care Centre embarked on a research project, the goal of which is to identify and quantify the circumstances, both external and internal, that predispose people to cope or not cope well with the death of someone significant to them. Not surprisingly, this is proving to be a major undertaking and one that is very much still in process.

Risk factors put one's well-being in jeopardy by confounding the situation, making it much harder to work through the grief toward reconciliation. Outcome measures refer to the magnitude of the person's grief, indicating the extent to which the person is experiencing normal or complicated mourning. We would assess the person's risk before the death of the loved one and use an outcome measure to see whether or not the person does indeed display the characteristics of complicated mourning one year after the death.

A major part of this research is still pending. In the meantime, as the result of an extensive literature search, a tentative list of risk factors has been drawn up; and this list is being used, informally, as part of the psycho-social assessment conducted routinely with all patients and families admitted to the Centre. Equally informally, the "outcome" for certain family members has been monitored over a period of a year and compared with the initial risk assessment. The results are sometimes surprising, and in the case study that will be described it becomes clear that there are factors that cannot be assessed, measured or quantified, but which may be critical in determining how someone copes.

TOOL DEVELOPMENT

For a full review of both risk indicators and outcome measures as found in the literature search, see Appendix (Tables 1, 2, and 3). After a list of risk factors was identified from the literature, a group of local professionals working in the field of bereavement was brought together to form an "expert panel." This panel was asked to review the list and to rate the individual factors according to their significance in predicting complicated mourning. This final list of significant risk factors is currently being used at the Centre. A similar rating process was attempted with outcome measures; but this proved to be more difficult, particularly in reaching any consensus in the expert panel. Outcome assessment, therefore, has been more intuitive, looking at characteristics such as depression, staying active, and adjusting to a life without the deceased.

The following indicators are those that have been identified as the most likely predictors for a person to have difficulty in the process of grief or mourning:

- Other dependents/commitments
- Work stresses
- Financial problems

- Other losses
- Physical illness/disability
- Mental illness, particularly depression
- History of abuse (physical, sexual, psychological)
- Conflicted relationship
- High level of dependency on the deceased
- High level of anxiety
- High level of anger
- High level of guilt
- Perceived lack of support from family, friends, community
- Lack of spiritual resources
- Circumstances of the death

CASE STUDY: LAURA'S STORY

The following case study describes the situation of a particular young woman whose husband died at the Centre and who is referred to as "Laura." In presenting Laura's life history and psychological situation, it will become apparent that she was considered to be at high risk for having serious problems after the death of her husband. These risks will be discussed, followed by an account of how her situation has evolved during the past year. Her husband, Bill, died in October 1997, from cancer of the bowel. He was forty-seven years old and had been diagnosed in 1994. At the time of his death, he and Laura had been married for five years.

Laura had experienced a very unhappy and deprived childhood. She had been physically and emotionally abused by her mother and sexually abused by her father. Not surprisingly, Laura found it extremely difficult to talk about this pain in her past. She chose instead to share with the palliative care team poems that she had written referring to the abuse—poems written to both her mother and her sister. One of these poems, written in 1996, is entitled "Motherly Love."*

"You left us with no self-esteem
You left us with nothing,
Not even a dream
You said you loved us all so much
But all we needed was your loving touch.

Whatever happened to you?
You never did any of the things a mother should do
Year after year,
We lived in constant fear.

Now we all look up above
and wonder
Whatever happened to Motherly love?"
*©LH

And in 1995 Laura had written to her sister:

> "I'd change it, if I could:
> The pain within our childhood,
> But reality tells me
> That this is not to be.
>
> The pain is the past,
> To be put behind us at last,
> Because dear sister of mine
> Somehow we keep each other in line."
> *©LH

Through her poetry writings Laura had been able to express her suffering; and she felt that this had contributed significantly to her ability to achieve some healing.

Laura had been married twice. Her first marriage had lasted for seventeen years but had not been a good relationship. She described her first husband as someone who "never grew up," and from the time that the first of their two children was born he could not tolerate sharing her with them. From that time he was either out, or unavailable to her or abusive when home. Laura had a daughter and a son. It was only when her daughter reached the age of sixteen that Laura was finally able, with this daughter's strong support, to leave her husband. These young people are now twenty-five and twenty-three respectively.

Laura's second husband, Bill, had also been married before; and his ex-wife introduced him to Laura. His divorce had been more amicable than Laura's. He had remained on relatively good terms with his ex-wife and had regular contact with his sixteen-year-old daughter. He and Laura knew each other for a few months before moving in to live together, and they were married about a year after that.

At the time of their meeting both Laura and Bill had a history of drug and alcohol abuse, but other family members were able to confirm that they found some real stability and security together. Laura felt that Bill was the first person in her life on whom she could depend. Laura had a history of depression going back to at least her first marriage and including several suicide attempts. For many years her daughter had clearly been trying to "parent the parent"; but both her children, while supportive to her and available in real crises, had had to distance themselves somewhat from their mother in order to survive. The siblings were living together, with the daughter's boyfriend, both working and doing well.

As well as having major psychiatric problems, Laura also had several physical health problems which were chronic in nature and rather vague in diagnosis. She reported that she had been diagnosed with hepatitis; and she also seemed to have some ongoing bowel and bladder complaints, for which she said that she was supposed to have surgery. She had become so dependent on benzodiazepines that she had been hospitalized for four weeks in January 1997 for addiction treatment.

Bill was admitted to the Palliative Care Centre from acute care in June 1997. This admission was difficult for both him and for Laura because he had very much wanted to return home. After admission, his condition initially improved; and he was, in fact, able to go home for a period of about a month. He was readmitted as his condition continued to deteriorate; and eventually he became increasingly confused, agitated, and weak. He died in October 1997. During Bill's time at the Centre, Laura talked on several occasions of feeling suicidal again. She felt at times that she simply could not face the prospect of watching Bill die and this was compounded by her ongoing guilt that she could not take him home to die. She vacillated between wanting to escape all the pain and responsibility and reaffirming her commitment to be with Bill to the end. During the last week or two before he died, Bill, in his confusion, talked constantly about going home and accused Laura of not being with him enough. He had never been able to acknowledge the fact that he was dying, and his extreme fear was now paramount. Eventually this situation proved to be more than Laura could handle and her own suicide intent resurfaced. Through this period she was in regular contact with her family physician who had been treating her for her depression and had known her for many years. She was persuaded to admit herself to psychiatric care, and she was actually an in-patient at the time of Bill's death. Laura was allowed out on a leave-of-absence, in the company of her sister-in-law, and was at Bill's bedside, with many members of his family, when he died. His death was peaceful and although Laura appeared to be heavily medicated and showed little reaction at the time, she was able to recall events afterwards. Laura returned to the psychiatric hospital but discharged herself within a few days.

From the time of the initial psycho-social assessment after Bill's admission, Laura was identified as someone at high bereavement risk for many reasons. At the end of June she agreed to an interview in which she and the social worker reviewed her perception of her ability to cope. The results confirmed she was positive for many of the factors on the list of risks. In terms of commitments, Laura felt overwhelmed with the demands of housework and daily tasks. Her financial situation was very precarious, and it seemed inevitable that she would have to move out of the apartment they had shared because she could not afford the rent on her own. Her physical illnesses were an ongoing problem and she reported being in frequent pain as well as being unable to sleep or eat normally. Her depression was also ongoing, treated with various medications, and she had, as has already been pointed out, a considerable history of abuse.

As has been mentioned, she felt that she had been able to depend on Bill for her emotional support. Her level of anxiety, particularly at the prospect of being alone again, was very high; and she felt an extreme guilt at having, in some way, failed Bill. Although very proud of her children, she felt that they had their own lives to live and she could not burden them with her troubles. She did not feel that there was anyone that she could really count on within her family other than a sister of her first husband, who happened to live in the same apartment building. When asked with whom she had been most able to share her feelings about Bill's illness and pending death, Laura identified her family physician.

About three weeks after Bill's death, Laura agreed to complete another "coping checklist" similar to the first one and this time some of the difficulties that she had noted before had clearly intensified. Her concern about the commitments of daily tasks had lessened, simply because she was too tired to care, but her financial problems were worse, as predicted, without Bill's disability pension. Her depression felt worse; her eating and sleeping difficulties had increased; and she felt that her anxiety had also increased. When asked about her sense of self-esteem, Laura's response both before and after Bill's death, was that she "liked herself somewhat." In answer to the question of how she would see herself coping in a year's time, her answer was the same both times, "I don't know." Given so many risk factors, the predictions for Laura's mourning process were not optimistic. The team admitted to having serious doubts as to her survival, and if suicide following the death of a loved one can be seen as the ultimate inability to cope with loss, then it was felt that Laura was very vulnerable.

Laura had always said, before Bill's death, that afterwards she would want to isolate herself. It soon became apparent that she was doing this, seeing very little of friends or family. On the other hand, she quickly set up a network of professional support with whom she was in regular contact, consisting of her family physician, the staff on the psychiatric unit, her psychiatrist, and the social worker at the Palliative Care Centre. She seemed reassured that both her doctor and her psychiatrist were now agreed that her major problem was an anxiety disorder, and she was on a new medication for this. She also asked her doctor to limit the amount of medication that she could get at any one time.

In January 1998, Laura went to visit her mother's sister for a week. This was important because this aunt was aware of all the abuse that Laura had suffered as a child and enabled Laura to talk about it, something that she had not done before. During this same time period, Laura was reliving Bill's death a great deal, remembering it as a peaceful release for him; but she was still tormented by her guilt of not keeping him at home. She reported dreaming that Bill was reaching out to her but not touching her. She had also been writing more poetry, about Bill and also about herself "as if I had already died." There were new health problems and she was falling for no apparent reason. Panic attacks were increasing and she had developed a real fear of going out other than to see her doctor. Through all this, however, Laura felt that she was "coming to terms" with Bill's death, and she also maintained an ongoing faith in God, a God whom she felt had never deserted her in the past and would not do so now.

At the beginning of April, Laura again admitted herself to the hospital for depression and suicidal thoughts. She discharged herself after three days. Still on medications for anxiety, she was off anti-depressants, and summed up her general well-being as, "some days I'm great, some days I'm not." Her guilt seemed to have modified, giving way to more simple regret at Bill's last weeks, without blaming herself. If anything, she felt she had been let down at the end by the promises that he would be "comfortable" and have a "good quality of life." She would not admit to anger, preferring to use the word "disappointment."

Since January she had not been able to use her car following a minor accident, and could not afford the repairs. (In fact, soon after Bill's death, her psychiatrist had told her that she should not drive.) By May, Laura was still without the use of her car and feeling very lonely because of the imposed isolation. She had decided she was not depressed any more and that she should put an end to the pattern of admitting herself to the hospital on, more or less, a monthly basis. At this point, her professional supports had been cut down to her contacts with the social worker at the Centre about once a month, and visits to her family physician, usually every few weeks.

In June, Laura was feeling much better emotionally, although still physically unwell. She had her car back and was going out more. She had also started writing poetry again. In July, she reported, in great excitement, that she had been accepted for a course to train as a Personal Support Worker and was talking, somewhat unrealistically, about working in a palliative care setting. She had written more poems, one of which had been accepted for publication. She was sleeping better and had spent a great weekend with her sister-in-law at a cottage. It all sounded too good to be true, and so it proved to be.

Laura's doctor had, not surprisingly, advised her that a full-time course would be more than she could handle. In early September, Laura got herself a job delivering newspapers, which lasted only a few days. She then reported that her TB (tuberculosis) test was positive, which meant she could not take the Personal Support Worker course. Laura seemed determined, however, that she would not give up her search for a job; and she had been able to move into a smaller apartment in the same building to ease her financial situation. At the end of September, she acknowledged that she was in something of a "bad patch" and had returned to using tranquilizers again. She insisted, however, that she was not feeling suicidal. She admitted to "reliving" much of the previous year as the anniversary of Bill's death approached.

DISCUSSION

What can we learn from Laura and her coping during the first year of bereavement? The team's first and honest reaction is to marvel at the very fact that she *has* survived it; and yet, on reflection, this clearly shows how much we underestimated her. From the very beginning, Laura herself said she was a survivor. When asked what kept her going, she would usually find this difficult to define, sometimes referring to God, but more often simply saying that she had overcome so much in her past that she knew she could do it again. The poem quoted earlier, written to her sister is entitled "Survival" and it is probably in Laura's following words that the key to her coping ability lies:

> So we'll forge ahead
> and live life, instead,
> Though memories lie within
> We will survive again and again.*
>   *©LH

In the original meeting of the "expert panel," it was stressed by several social workers and counselors that any risk assessment must take into great account the importance of self-perception. It is not enough simply to identify factors that may be associated with a poor bereavement outcome, because for every individual the degree of stress that is associated with each factor will be different. What may be a comparatively minor issue for one person may be totally overwhelming for another because that is how it *feels* to them. If they feel they cannot cope, then chances are that they will not; and if they feel that somehow, whatever the odds, they can cope, then, as Laura has shown us, they probably will.

The critical significance of perception was brought home again in the situation of another woman whose husband also died at the Centre not long before Laura's husband. In palliative care, we are used to witnessing patients' deaths and, regrettably, sometimes fail to recognize the impact this may have on the family or friends who are present. This particular woman was an emotionally strong and capable person who had had a particularly positive relationship with her husband, both as his wife and also as a professional partner. Although we recognized that she would grieve his death very much, we had no doubt that she would cope well with her bereavement. Her husband's death was, in our terms, "peaceful"; but that was certainly not the way that she saw it. It had been preceded by a considerable period of intense and uncontrolled pain, during which time she had felt helpless, angry, and frustrated, wishing only for an end to that pain even if this meant euthanasia. For many months after her husband's death, these feelings persisted and, despite the fact that in all other respects she would have been considered as "low risk," she nevertheless had a very difficult time in her mourning process.

CONCLUSION

In his keynote address at the 1998 ADEC Conference in Chicago, Alan Wolfelt talked of "companioning" rather than "treating" those with whom we are in a counseling relationship. He further explained "companioning" as "honoring the spirit" and "learning from others rather than teaching them." He warned against the dangers of the medical model that seeks to assess, diagnose, and treat grief as an illness that demands a cure. Finally, he cautioned that we should be wary of joining in and supporting the "managed care" approach to what is really a soul-based journey. It is all too easy for us, as trained professionals, to overlook the journey into grief as being "soul-based": but we must never forget the "mysterious, spiritual dimension of grief that harbors the capacity to go on living until we, too, die." Dr. Wolfelt advocates strongly for a new model of bereavement counseling that is more life-giving and hope-filled, one that will incorporate "not only the mind and body, but the soul and spirit."

There are some things that we cannot measure, some indefinable qualities that defy all attempts at classification. While we would never deny that in our work with the bereaved it is important to be aware of risk factors that have been well studied and documented, we also recognize that no assessment tool can ever be foolproof. While individual strength and courage continue to be a factor and while the human spirit continues to surprise us with its refusal to be conquered, there will always be those individuals who defy all statistics and assessments. We believe that Laura is one of those, and we thank her for reminding us.

REFERENCES

Beckwith, B. E., Beckwith, S.K., Gray, Th., Micsko, M.M., Holin, J.E., Plumber, V., & Flaa, S.L. (1990). Identification of spouses at high risk during bereavement: A preliminary assessment of Parkes and Weiss' Risk Index. *The Hospice Journal, 6*(3), 35-46.

Byrne, G. A., & Raphael, B. (1994). A longitudinal study of bereavement phenomena in recently widowed elderly men. *Psychological Medicine, 24*, 411-421.

Cowan, M. E., & Murphy, S. A. (1985). Identification of postdisaster bereavement risk predictors. *Nursing Research, 43*(2) 71-75.

Farnsworth, J., Pett, M. A., & Lund, D. A. (1989). Predictors of loss management and well-being in later life widowhood and divorce. *Journal of Family Issues, 10*(1), 102-121.

Gabriel, R. M., & Kirschling, J. M. (1989). Assessing grief among the bereaved elderly: A review of existing measures. *Bereavement Care: Hospice and Community Based Services*, 29-54.

Gilewski, M. J., Farberow, N. L., Gallagher, D. E., & Thompson, L. W. (1991). Interaction of depression and bereavement on mental health in the elderly. *Psychology and Aging, 6*(1), 67-75.

Jacobs, S., Hansen, F., Kasl, S., Ostfeld, A., Berkman, L., & Kim, K. (1990). Anxiety disorders during acute bereavement: Risk and risk factors. *Journal of Clinical Psychiatary, 51*(7), 269-274.

Kissane, D. W., Bloch, S., & McKenzie, D. P. (1997). Family coping and bereavement outcome. *Palliative Medicine, 11*, 191-201.

Kurtz, M. E., Kurtz, J. C., Given, C. W., & Given, B. (1997). Predictors of postbreavement depressive symptomatology among family caregivers of cancer patients. *Support Care Cancer, 5*, 53-60.

Levy, L. H. (1991). Anticipatory grief: Its measurement and proposed reconceptualization. *The Hospice Journal, 7*(4), 1-28.

Levy, L. H., Derby, J. F., & Martinkowski, K. S. (1992). The question of who participates in bereavement research and the Bereavement Risk Index. *Omega, 25*(3): 225-238.

Parkes, C. M. (1990). Risk factors in bereavement: Implications for the prevention and treatment of pathologic grief. *Psychiatric Annals, 20*(6), 308-313.

Parkes, C. M., & Weiss, R. S. (1983). *Recovery from bereavement.* New York: Basic Books.

Prigerson, H. G., Maciejewski, C. F., Reynolds, C. F., Bierhals, A. J., Newsom, J. T., Fasiczka, A., Frank, E., Doman, J., & Miller, M. (1995). Inventory of complicated grief: A scale to measure maladaptive symptoms of loss. *Psychiatry Research, 59,* 65-79.

Ransford, H. E., & Smith, M. L. (1991). Grief resolution among the bereaved in hospice and hospital wards. *Social Science & Medicine, 32*(3), 295-304.

Robinson, L. A., Nuamah, I. F., Lev, E., McCorkle, R. (1995). A prospective longitudinal investigation of spousal bereavement examining Parkes and Weiss' Bereavement Risk Index. *Journal of Palliative Care, 11*(4), 5-13.

Sanders, C. M. (1988). Risk factors in bereavement outcome. *Journal of Social Issues, 44*(3), 97-111.

Shanfield, S. B. (1987). Chapter 6: The prediction of outcome in bereavement. In S. Zisook (Ed.), *Biopsychosocial Aspects of Bereavement.* Washington, DC: American Psychiatric Press.

Sheldon, A. R., Cochrane, J., Vachon, M. L. S., Lyall, A. L., Rogers, J., & Freeman, J. J. (1981). A psychosocial analysis of risk of psychological impairment following bereavement. *Journal of Nervous and Mental Disease, 169*(4), 253-255.

Steeve, L. (1992). Risk factor profile for bereaved spouses. *Death Studies, 16,* 387-399.

Vachon, M. L. S., & Stylianos, S. K. (1988). The role of social support in bereavement. *Journal of Social Issues, 44*(3): 175-190.

Windholz, M. J., Marmar, C. R., & Horowitz, M. J. (1985). A review of the research on conjugal bereavement: Impact on health and efficacy of intervention. *Comprehensive Psychiatry, 26*(5), 433-447.

Wolfelt, A. D. (1991, March/April). Toward an understanding of complicated grief: A comprehensive overview. *American Journal of Hospice and Palliative Care,* March/April: 28-30.

Wolfelt, A. D. (1992). *Understanding grief helping yourself heal.* Muncie, IN: Accelerated Development Inc.

Wujcik, D. (1984, Fall). Grief response of the primary caregiver receiving bereavement follow-up care at home. *American Journal of Hospice Care,* Fall: 15-22.

APPENDIX: Table 1. Summary of Risk Factors from Literature

Domain	Risk Factor	Author	Findings
Demographics	Age & Gender	Beckwith et al., 1990; Farnsworth et al., 1989; Kurtz et al., 1997; Levy, 1991; Parkes, 1990; Sanders, 1988; Shanfield, 1987; Sheldon et al., 1981; Steele, 1992; Windholz et al., 1985; Wujcik, 1984	Conflicting findings. May not be age but other factors affected by being older/younger and bereaved. Older age seems to exacerbate existing health problems. Younger bereaved are coping with young families, financial issues, etc. Studies can be found to say young age, old age are significantly worse for differing outcomes. Gender is not directly found to be associated with complicated grief, though at certain ages, one gender may do worse than the other.
	Socio-economic status	Sheldon et al., 1981; Steele, 1992; Beckwith et al., 1990; Sanders, 1988; Windholz et al., 1985; Farnsworth et al., 1989; Byrne & Raphael, 1994	Low socioeconomic status increased problems. Low socioeconomic status increased problems. Low socioeconomic status increased problems. Lack of income, changes in financial situation led to poor outcomes. Poverty led to poor outcomes. Education and income not predictive. Income and education were negatively associated with bereavement phenomena.
Commitments	Number of children at home	Parkes & Weiss, 1983; Windholz et al., 1985; Beckwith et al., 1990	Having more children at home led to poor adjustment. Having more children at home led to poor adjustment. Having more children at home led to poor adjustment.
	Work Retirement Unemployment	Beckwith et al., 1990	Lower levels of employment resulted in a high bereavement score.
Concurrent Stresses	Concurrent stresses	Sanders, 1988; Windholz et al., 1985; Cowan & Murphy, 1985	Concurrent crises led to additional debilitation; caused situation to be overwhelming. Multiple stressful events led to poor outcomes. Higher score on Life Experience Survey (measure of concurrent life stresses) resulted in higher depression.

APPENDIX: Table 1. (Cont'd.)

Domain	Risk Factor	Author	Findings
Major Losses	Death of someone else close	Parkes, 1990 Windholz et al., 1985	Dealing with multiple deaths was a risk factor. Experience with previous losses led to better outcomes.
Social Support	Availability	Sheldon et al., 1981	Isolation led to problems; more social contacts did not.
		Sanders, 1988	Isolation occurred consistently with loss.
		Windholz et al., 1985	Survivors' perception of social support mitigates response to spouse's death.
		Cowan & Murphy, 1985	Lower support predicted higher depression.
		Wujcik, 1984	Higher number of bereavement visits from a counselor resulted in lower (better) Grief Experience Inventory scores (Sanders, 1979).
		Vachon & Stylianos, 1988	Inadequate social network was associated with high distress during bereavement.
		Ransford & Smith, 1991	Those whose loved one died at a hospice (with good social support) did better in bereavement than those in hospital (poor social support).
Physical Health	Poor Health or Disability	Farnsworth et al., 1989 Sanders, 1988	Poorer health before bereavement led to poorer outcomes. Poorer health before bereavement led to poorer outcomes.
Psychological Health	Depression, mental illness	Parkes, 1990	Existing problems were exacerbated.
		Sanders, 1988 and Kurtz et al., 1997	Poor premorbid adjustment strategies were exacerbated by bereavement.
		Jacobs et al., 1990	Past history of panic disorder resulted in higher panic scores.
		Gilewski et al., 1991	Depressed elderly were at risk for complications.
	Self-esteem	Parkes, 1990 Farnsworth et al., 1989	Low "self-trust" led to intense grief. Greater self-esteem led to less depression.
	Optimism	Kurtz et al., 1997	High optimism on Life Orientation Test (Scheier & Carver, 1987) resulted in less depression symptoms.
	Suicide	Parkes, personal correspondence, 1993	Previous history of suicide is important to capture as it may be associated with poor outcomes.
	Drug or Alcohol	Kissane et al., 1997	Spouse using psychotropic drugs had poor outcomes.

Category	Subcategory	Reference	Description
Relationship with Deceased	Closeness	Steele, 1992	Extreme closeness resulted in higher (worse) subscores on Grief Experience Inventory (Sanders, 1979).
		Kissane et al., 1997	Higher level of spousal contentment resulted in better bereavement outcomes.
	Conflict	Parkes, 1990	Conflict between spouses led to anger, guilt, complicating mourning process.
		Farnsworth et al., 1989	Greater marital happiness led to better outcomes.
	Emotional dependency	Parkes, 1990	Reliance on patient for reassurance and strength was associated with chronic grief.
		Sanders, 1988	May be associated with poor outcome.
		Beckwith et al., 1990	Greater clinging resulted in high bereavement score.
Dealing with Death	Acceptance	Prigerson et al., 1995	Disbelief, not accepting death led to impairments in functioning.
	Ability to cope	Kissane et al., 1997	Perception of poor family coping resulted in greater psychological morbidity.
Circumstances of Death	Length of time on ward	Beckwith et al., 1990	No significant difference between high and low risk scores.

Table 2. Summary of Grief Symptom Indicators Found in Literature

Domain	Outcome	Test	Used By:
Coping Styles	Social withdrawal, hyperactivity	• UCLA Hospice Evaluation Study (probably not available or validated) • Reorganization Activity (developed by authors to measure constructive social activity, p. 298)	Ransford & Smith, 1991
	Avoidance	• Impact Event Scale (Horowitz, 1979)	Levy, 1991
	Substances (drugs, alcohol, smoking)	Questions created by authors	Parkes & Weiss, 1983 Ransford & Smith, 1991
	Management of Loss	• Glick, Weiss, & Parkes, 1974 (self-rated perceptions of ability to cope, stress, feelings of self-worth)	Farnsworth et al., 1989
Psychological Distress	Clinical depression	• Beck Depression Inventory (Beck, 1967) • Self-Rating Depression Scale (Zung, 1965) • Center for Epidemiologic Studies—Depression (CES-D) (Radloff, 1977) • Profile of Mood States—Depression (POMS-D) (McNair et al., 1981)	Levy, 1991 Jacobs et al., 1990 Ransford & Smith, 1991 Kurtz et al., 1997 Levy et al., 1992
	Anger	• Profile of Mood States—Anger (POMS-A) (McNair et al., 1981)	Levy et al., 1992
	Anxiety	• Psychiatric Epidemiology Research Interview Anxiety Scale (PERI)	Jacobs et al., 1990
	Personality Factors	• Cattell 16 factors—e.g., emotional instability, conservatism (Cattell, 1970)	Sheldon et al., 1981

	Psychological distress	• Brief Symptom Inventory (BSI): 9 dimensions, 3 global questions: somatization, obsessive/compulsive, interpersonal sensitivity, depression, anxiety, hostility, phobic anxiety, paranoid ideation, psychotocism.	Robinson et al., 1995
	Subjective stress	• Impact of Events Scale	Ransford & Smith, 1991
Physical Health	General health	• General Health Questionnaire (GHQ) (Goldberg, 1979)	Sheldon et al., 1981
	Mortality	Vital statistics	Windholz et al., 1985
Overall Health	Overall health	• Medical Outcomes Shortform (MOS) (Stewart & Ware, 1988): general health, mental health, physical health, social functioning, role performance and bodily pain.	Prigerson et al., 1995
	Subjective well-being	• Ware General Well-Being Scale (Ware, 1976) • Life Satisfaction Scale, LSI-A (Neugarten, 1961)	Ransford & Smith, 1991 Farnsworth et al., 1989

Table 3. Grief Measurement Tools Found in Literature

Test	Author and Year
*Adjustment Scale	Carey, 1977
*Bereavement Items/CES-D	Jacobs, Kasl, Ostfeld, Berkman, & Charpentier, 1986
*Boulder County Hospice Bereavement Assessment Referral	Lattanzi & Coffelt, 1979
*Grief Experience Inventory	Sanders, 1980-81
*Grief Resolution Index	Remondet & Hannson, 1987
*Impact of Event Scale	Horowitz, Wilner, & Alvarez, 1979
*Present Feelings about Loss	Singh & Raphael, 1981
*Texas Inventory of Grief	Faschingbauer, DeVaul, & Zisook, 1977
*Texas Revised Inventory of Grief	Faschingbauer, 1981
Anticipatory Grief Scale	Levy, 1991
Bereavement Phenomenology Questionnaire	Byrne & Raphael, 1994
Inventory of Complication Grief 1995	Prigerson, Maciejewski, Reynolds, Bierhals, Newsom, Fasiczka, Frank, Doman, & Miller, 1995

*Reviewed in Gabriel & Kirschling (1989).

CHAPTER 14

Personality as a Variable in Grief Response

Susan K. Parker

Personality is a variable seldom considered in the adult grief process. Using the constructs of the Myers-Briggs Type Indicator, four questions are considered when assessing complications in the adult grief process. What style of rejuvenation is preferred? What type of information is gathered and processed? How are decisions made? What level of closure is needed? A discussion of the questions is held in the context of the adult grief process. This forum creates potential personality profiles for grief response.

We grieve uniquely. We grieve in a manner consistent with our personality. Assessment of personality and its components is critical to evaluating complicated grief. There are many areas of assessment when considering a single grief reaction. Among those to consider are the nature of the loss, meaning of the loss, single or multiple losses, sudden or anticipated, grief history of the grieving person, support system, level of trauma around the loss, just to mention a few.

An area to consider, which is seldom discussed, is the area of our human personality. We have many different assessment devices to create a picture of our personality. This writing will consider and conceptualize our personality through an instrument called the Myers-Briggs Type Indicator (MBTI). The choice of using the MBTI allows a non-judgmental approach to personality and grief. There is no right or wrong way to grieve when seen through the lens of personality. Grieving is a way in which a personality expresses itself around the loss. Grief will tend to be consistent with the preferences of personality. Considering the variations in personality, it is safe to consider that there are an equal amount of variations in grieving. Using the type indicator, speculation about how a person in a grief reaction might respond can be drawn.

The importance of this exercise is two-fold. For the *caregivers*, a direction for care can be developed, along with appropriate suggestions

209

and interventions to help facilitate grieving for the bereaved person. For the *person grieving*, a baseline of what is "normal" can be developed.

THE EIGHT PREFERENCES

What Style of Rejuvenation is Preferred?

It is necessary for human beings to maintain energy. As time goes on our energy level will expand and contract. We have an energy bank account. As we live life, withdrawals and deposits for our account of energy are made. Unique to each of the first preferences we notice how the account flows. The MBTI looks at different ways in which deposits are made. Two broad categories are described. One area falls into what is called "extrovert" and the other category is called "introvert." There is no right or wrong way to manage the energy account. We only have to be sure that we know how it works and that we do keep a balance between withdrawals and deposits. It is the *how* of replenishing energy that is of importance to us. Contrary to popular belief there is a distinction between extrovert/introvert preference and sociability. Both the introvert and the extrovert can be gregarious and friendly. Gregarious and friendly, socialized appropriately to have social graces is not the point. The interest in this preference is how one becomes energized.

The extrovert preference (E) is one that will tend to move toward external interactions and experiences. The extrovert will revive by being with people. An extroverted person is more involved with people and things, the external world. Extroverted types may be more likely to see themselves primarily in relation to others and seek messages about their self-esteem from family and co-workers. The extroverted type may share more intimately with others without the benefit of being selective about the listener or material shared.

Consider the extrovert type grieving. This is a person most likely to show up at a support group, interested in sharing intimately with other members and upon leaving the group will state "I feel so much better now." There will be a lift in their step and a noticeable change in affect by sharing with others. The extroverted type will have difficulty keeping a journal, but will verbally share with another the details of their loss. This is also the person who is likely to be in numerous groups and other support systems after the loss of a loved one.

Pat came into therapy a few days after the death of her husband. She asked to be included in a group, if one was available. Finding an appropriate referral for her, she was asked if she preferred individual or group therapy. She said "Both." As Pat did her personal work in individual therapy she also went back to the monthly hospital support group where her husband died. This support group brought in speakers on various aspects of grieving and self-care. Pat stated this was the way she maintained her sense of balance after her husband's death. She wanted a place to talk, to learn, and to be with others. Pat also organized a weekly outing for breakfast for the support group at the hospital. This sharing, Pat stated, helped keep her going.

The introverted type (I) is more immersed in the inner world of ideas, concepts, and theories. In that world of the inner, an introverted person will begin to make energy deposits for their account by being alone with their experiences. The process of revitalization has begun when the introverted person takes time to be alone with ideas, concepts, and internal thoughts. An introverted type will seek out solitude as a place of refreshment. Thinking through thoughts and organizing their internal life is a prime concern for an introvert. The introvert type is less likely to rely on the positive reflection back from another to validate their value and worth. This valuing and affirming will come from within. Additionally, an introverted typed will selectively chose what to share, when to share it, and to whom the material will be shared.

In the grief process an introverted personality will journal without a problem once the technique of journaling is learned. This type will be less likely to be the first to speak, will leave a group as soon as the time is up, and share more intimately with one or two people rather than the group at large. Some introverted people will struggle to share much of their loss until it is organized in their mind and they have had time to sit with it alone first. Notice the introvert leaving a support group. Most often there is relief and an attempt to be one of the first at the door. After prolonged social contact, the introverted type has lost significant amounts of energy.

Jeri's family consisted of Jeri and her husband, two adult children, and her elderly father. At the time of the funeral of her mother she hung on tight to her husband and children. Several months later she came forward to be a part of a church sponsored bereavement outreach committee. Jeri noted that she was deeply moved by the outpouring of love and concern by her church. "Groups are not my thing" she stated, "but I want to help out other church members who loose a loved one." Jeri faithfully donates food and writes notes to families after they have experienced a loss. Jeri shared her grief with her family, tremendously benefited by the notes sent by people, and read everything she could about the loss of a mother. Maybe some day she will share her story with a group outside her family, but for now she prefers to stay right where she is.

What Type of Information is Gathered and Processed?

When entering a room, some people will notice the color, shape, and the condition of the room and furniture. Others will consider what possible uses the room could have, and whether it is metaphorically warm or cold (not measures of temperature). What information we take in, what information we consider first makes the distinction between the "sensing" and "intuitive" types.

The primary way to characterize this difference is to notice whether information taken in is relative to the five senses of touch, taste, smell, sight, hearing, or relative to the sixth sense of what is beyond. The sensing type (S) will notice details, live in a concrete world, and be highly aware of all that is present in a tangible way. The important moment is now. This is the scientist in the world. This is the type that notices and dares to see what is.

While grieving, an important part of the healing process is to hear the story about what happened. The sensing type will focus on the factual details and report the tangible pieces of the experience. Of significance are the concrete details, measurable by the five senses. The temperature of the room, the sights, sounds, and smells will be meaningful. This is the information that a sensing person will consider important to relate.

Paul came into the room filled with tears. "Her temperature has dropped and her blood pressure is low. The doctor said there is nothing more that can be done. She looks as white as a ghost and I don't know what to do." This is the sensing type.

The intuitive type (N) will live in the possibilities. Contingency, likelihood, probability, chances are all relevant patterns of information gathering. This is the visionary in the world. This is the type that dares to dream dreams and see what could be.

Grieving, the intuitive type will consider important the emotional dynamics present, the non-tangible material present in the experiences and the possibilities of how this might impact the other family members.

If Paul were an intuitive type his conversation might have included the following: "Her temperature has dropped and the blood pressure is low. We need to get the doctor to consider alternative methods of treating her. Perhaps we need to move her to another place. I do not know how I am going to share this with the kids. I cannot imagine what this will be like for them." Paul focuses on the world of possibilities, dreams, and non-tangible dynamics that are pending.

How are Decisions Made?

We are constantly faced with options and choices. From the moment we open our eyes in the morning to the time we close them at night, we are bombarded with choices and options. Picking out our clothing, choosing our breakfast, what do we begin first in our work, and whether to drive the speed limit or not. How we make decisions is the focus for this next discussion.

This preference of thinking or feeling is meant to examine how we come to conclusions and make decisions in our life. Our choices and decisions are weighted. Some choices are simple and less far-reaching, like the clothing we wear or the glass we choose to use at the breakfast table. Some are more complex like educational choices, places to live, and where we seek employment. Yet within that pattern of choosing and deciding we notice whether the final decisive move comes after our thoughts or our feelings have their say.

It is important to note another distinction in this preference. Both the feeling and thinking preference will experience emotion. Of concern is not the absence or presence of emotion but rather a preference between primarily considering the merits of consistency, logic, and rational decision making or considering the merits of qualifying factors, the context, anticipated outcome, and special circumstances.

A final vote for a feeling type (F) will come from values and context. A subjective view of the situation will be critical material to consider while deliberating a conclusion. The impact of a decision is an important component of the consideration process. Special circumstances and unique needs are of significance to the feeling type. As a result, the decision making process is colored by specific context and governing factors. The feeling type will tend to move from point to point in the process of decision making without the logical sequence that is noted with the thinking type.

The preference for decision making that we name the thinking type (T) will choose to have other factors come to the foreground. The thinking type will want consistency of outcome and logical, rational processing of impartial material. Congruence, integrity, and constancy are of great importance. A logical progression from the situation to the plan to the outcome is the protocol followed by the thinking type.

What Level of Closure is Needed?

The fourth and final question to consider is the level of closure needed for identification of personality preferences. This is also about level or definiteness, clarity, accurate portrayal, and definition coming from the individual.

The preference for judging (J) will prompt a person to seek order. Closure on things is settled upon sooner rather than later. Deadlines are favored and planning is important to a judging preference. Additionally, this type will use clearly defined language used in communication, seek to clarify any ambiguous information, and look for clear understanding.

The personality preference of perceiving (P) will include an affinity for the state of being open ended and take the opportunity to put off plans and decisions in order to gather more information. Trying to pin down a perceiving type to clarify, offer a commitment, or work to a deadline is to operate counter to the personality.

The person with a judging preference might say: "The air is cool, the leaves are getting their fall color, and this is my favorite time of the year."

A person with the perceiving preference, responding to the same picture would be more likely to comment: "It is a great day. Fall is wonderful."

Speculation about the judging/perceiving preference in the grief process brings us to consider several areas. The level of clarity around the message a perceiving preference will issue may be somewhat less defined than the judging. In working with a person with the perceiving preference, it may be noticed that there is some vagueness and ambiguity for the listener. The perceiving type is clear, but the listener may not be. This is the antithesis of the manner in which a judging preference will express.

Carl began to speak to his daughter about the loss of his own brother. When she asked Carl how he felt about this loss, Carl replied, "It's been many months and I hurt terribly. I am still not sure of how this is all going to be for me." This is coming from a person with a perceiving preference. The judging preference will be more likely to say, "I feel sadness and loneliness because I have lost my buddy." Notice the clearer definition with the J than with the P. Notice the openness around the kind of impact that the P states. The J is clearer and more wedded to a particular impact already experienced.

Another way in which the perceiving type will distinguish itself from judging type is in the comfort level of where they are. The perceiving will be in the moment with the journey and aware of the place they currently occupy. The judging will more likely have a checklist and agenda, ready to move on to the next piece of the grieving journey.

Table 1 illustrates the contrast among the eight preferences. It is meant to illustrate the way in which personality preferences will manifest themselves. The leap is the consideration of how personality preferences will play out in the grieving experience.

The Sixteen Types of Preferences for Personality

Consider your own preferences. Does the column under extrovert (E) or introvert (I) better describe you? This speaks to the question about your favored style of replenishment of energy or rejuvenation.

What type of information do you gather and process? Does the column under sensing (S) or intuitive (N) better describe you?

How do you make your decisions? Will the column under thinking (T) or feeling (F) better describe your patterns?

How much closure is needed? Listen to your language, consider your comfort level, and notice if the perceiving (P) or the judging (J) best describes you.

Each of the questions noted above can be answered with either of the two preferences. The preferences are on a continuum. A person may not neatly fall into one camp or the other. However, a person will most often have a preference. Doing the math on this process, we wind up with a total of sixteen ways to configure the eight different preferences (see Table 2).

Table 1. Key Words to Depict the Eight Preferences

EXTROVERT (E)	INTROVERT (I)	SENSING (S)	INTUITIVE (N)
External	Internal	Present	Potential
Interactive	Reflective	Scientific	Possibilities
Breadth	Depth	Actual	Visionary
Many Friends	Few Friends	Tangible	Abstract
Outgoing	Reserved	Concrete	Hypothetical
Talkative	Quiet	Practical	Creative
Thinks Out Loud	Ponders	Objective	Subjective
Life of the Party	Observant	Literal	Live from Guts

THINKING (T)	FEELING (F)	PERCEIVING (P)	JUDGING (J)
Objective	Subjective	Pending	Committed
Detached	Involved	Open	Concluded
Logical	Circumstances	Spontaneous	Established
Sequential	Random	Shapeless	Structure
Consistency	Relativity	Ambiguous	Defined
Law and Order	Values	Indeterminate	Clear
Processing	Responsive	Unsettled	Closure
Organized	Out of Order	Journey	Outcome Oriented
Regular Intervals	Haphazard	Inconsistent	Orderly

Table 2. What is Natural for Each Type

ESTP Conversation, Facts, Logic, Open-ended	**ESFP** Conversation, Facts, Impact, Open-ended	**ENFP** Conversation, Possibilities, Impact, Open-ended	**ENTP** Conversation, Possibilities, Logic, Open-ended
ESTJ Conversation, Facts, Logic, Orderly	**ESFJ** Conversation, Facts, Impact, Orderly	**ENFJ** Conversation, Possibilities, Impact, Orderly	**ENTJ** Conversation, Possibilities, Logic, Orderly
ISTF Reflective, Facts, Logic, Orderly	**ISFJ** Reflective, Facts, Impact, Orderly	**INFJ** Reflective, Possibilities, Impact Orderly	**INTJ** Reflective, Possibilities, Logic, Orderly
ISTP Reflective, Facts, Logic, Open-ended	**ISFP** Reflective, Facts, Impact, Open-ended	**INFP** Reflective, Possibilities, Impact, Open-ended	**INTP** Reflective, Possibilities, Logic, Open-ended

Extrovert, Sensing, Thinking, Perceiving is Noted ESTP

This open-ended realist notices the facts and logically follows the progression of the loss and grief reaction. This is the organizer and problem solver. Encourage this person to seek out and reflect on their feelings.

Extrovert, Sensing, Feeling, Perceiving is Noted ESFP

This open-ended information based sensitive person shares the facts and details with those around them. Encourage this person to think about, and reflect on, the long lasting impact of their experience.

Extrovert, Intuitive, Feeling, Perceiving is Noted as ENFP

Open discussions where possibilities are shared will characterize this personality. Details may be overlooked while the big picture is the focus of concentration. Encouragement to reflect on the important details of the loss will stretch this person into a fuller grief response.

Extrovert, Intuitive, Thinking, Perceiving is Noted as ENTP

Impact of the loss is not yet finalized but discussion of possibilities in a logical sequence is the preferred process in the grief reaction. Guidance to consider seeking and pondering the important details of the loss promotes healing for this grief-stricken person.

Extrovert, Sensing, Thinking, Judging is Noted as ESTJ

The reality of the loss described by its facts and events is the way in which this type will communicate. The subsequent grief reaction is discussed with clarity and sequence. This person benefits from reflection on the bigger impact of the loss, including the associated feelings about the loss.

Extrovert, Sensing, Feeling, Judging is Noted as ESFJ

An open discussion about the impact of a loss is a natural position for this preference. This type of person will tend to formulate an opinion as they speak. As a result, the grieving process will evolve in the conversations of this person. Ask this person to stretch in their typical way of doing things by thinking about and pondering their loss. Additionally, consider how to be personally expressive about the loss in a way that is creative and easy to understand.

Extrovert, Intuitive, Feeling, Judging is Noted as ENFJ

This personality sees the big picture through their feelings. Opinionated and persuasive, they will often promote open discussions about the loss. To promote personal growth, consider requesting the grieving person to engage viewing their loss through their thinking rather than their feelings. Encourage quiet internal reflection.

Extrovert, Intuitive, Thinking, Judging is Noted as ENTJ

The big picture will be shared with all the accompanying thoughts and opinions. Growth for this person will come by encouraging depth and range of feelings. Encourage deep internal reflection on the implications of the loss.

Introvert, Sensing, Thinking, Judging is Noted as ISTJ

This person will think about the details of a situation, before entering into conversation about the loss. An opinion will be formed and shared at a later time. Encourage this person to risk conversation and to consider the full depth and range of feelings and impact of the loss.

Introvert, Sensing, Feeling, Judging is Noted as ISFJ

The deeply sensitive, detail oriented person will focus on the facts of the loss. A leap toward growth would include conversation about the future impact of the loss.

Introvert, Intuitive, Feeling, Judging is Noted as INFJ

Sitting back, reflecting on feelings about the loss comes naturally for this personality. The big picture becomes apparent and opinions are formed. A deeper and fuller grief response would be experienced if this person would consider conversation about the specific details of the loss.

Introvert, Intuitive, Thinking, Judging is Noted as INTJ

This person will be in motion toward seeing the future possibilities due to this loss. Conversation about the current details around the loss will be a stretch for a person of this preference. Encourage exploration of feelings around the relevant information regarding the loss for a broader grief reaction.

Introvert, Sensing, Thinking, Perceiving is Noted as ISTP

This person favors the thinking part of their personality. As a result relevant information is readily available. What is missing is a conversation around feelings and the impact of this loss today and in the future. Encourage conversation, feelings, and impact for a full grief reaction.

Introvert, Sensing, Feeling, Perceiving is Noted as ISFP

High levels of feelings, experienced internally and related to the details of the situation, is a typical reaction for this preference. Feeling is the preferred part of the personality. As a result, a broader grief reaction includes thinking about the loss and drawing conclusions from that thinking, along with sharing this experience with others.

Introvert, Intuitive, Feeling, Perceiving is Noted as INFP

Deep reflection about the feelings and impact of the loss will be a natural state for this personality. Encourage conversation, details, and formulation of opinion for a wider spectrum of grief response.

Introvert, Intuitive, Thinking, Perceiving is Noted as INTP

A well thought out grasp on the full impact of the loss will be a natural spot for this preference. The missing pieces, that ensure a fuller grief reaction, include exploring feelings in conversation with another person and forming opinion about the loss.

SUGGESTIONS FOR INTERVENTION

It is considered appropriate for the grieving person to acknowledge and feel the full spectrum of the impact of a loss and also continue to *live* life in a new world without the presence of the person, place, or thing that was lost. It is also helpful to encourage what *does not* come naturally.

The extrovert is encouraged to reflect inwardly, the introvert is encouraged to speak the loss to another. The sensing is encouraged to notice the abstract along with current and future impact. The intuitive is encouraged to identify the factual aspects of this loss in the present moment. The feeling is motivated to engage the thought process and to consider the factual details of the loss. The thinking is encouraged to find the impact and meaning of this loss. The perceiving is guided to define their reaction to the loss and the judging is encouraged to just be with the loss without a checklist. Assistance for each of the preferences to move in this direction heightens the maximum possibility for full healing.

SUMMARY AND DISCUSSION

Personality and the preferences within personality are important considerations when working with a grieving person. Assessing the components of personality gives us the opportunity to consider the most effective ways to assist and support a grief stricken person. The optimal goal is to maximize the strengths of the personality while balancing support to stretch for what does not come with as much ease. This posturing by the helper supports the greatest level of recovery in the grief process for the grieving person. Knowing what tendencies come naturally for the individual, as well as areas to grow, will arm well-intentioned helpers to befriend, support, and guide the person grieving.

CHAPTER 15

Miscarriage in the Emergency Room: Meeting Parents' Needs

Diane L. Midland

When parents are confronted with the tragedy of their child's death, it is expected that they will grieve and mourn. Our society acknowledges the value of rituals as a means of saying "good-bye" and providing closure when a friend or family member dies. What happens when parents experience the death of their child by miscarriage? When the hopes and dreams of having a baby are shattered by the sudden realization that the pregnancy will not develop to term and eventual birth, what happens? Add to this the reality that early pregnancy loss is treated medically in an out-patient setting such as a physician's office, emergency room, or out-patient surgery area.

Oftentimes the personnel in these types of settings are not well trained or prepared to support the emotional needs of individuals who may be grieving. In fact, sometimes expectant parents encounter insensitive statements from staff who may view the "patient" as a "surgical candidate" and the "fetus" as a "pathology specimen." Well-meaning medical personnel may unintentionally minimize the pregnancy loss by making statements such as, "You can always have another baby." or "There must have been some type of deformity. This is nature's way of taking care of a mistake." These types of initial contacts with parents facing the loss of a pregnancy and, in many cases, a "wished-for child," can complicate the grief process for them throughout the months and years ahead. Davidson (1979) uses the phrase "death of a wished-for child" to describe the symbolic loss of hopes and dreams that parents experience with the death of a child through miscarriage, ectopic pregnancy, stillbirth, or newborn death.

For the purpose of this chapter the author will concentrate on early pregnancy loss in the emergency room (ER) setting. In many medical systems, women present to the ER when they experience symptoms such as cramping and/or bleeding during the first twenty weeks of gestation. Typically the ER is a fast-paced environment that lacks privacy. Medical personnel are accustomed to dealing with traumatic situations on a daily basis. They may not perceive a patient who is experiencing cramping and vaginal bleeding as a life-threatening case when in the next cubical there is a person in cardiac arrest.

How can personnel in an ER setting intervene and care for a woman (and her partner) who is experiencing an early pregnancy loss to assure that their emotional needs are met? Assessment is critical during this initial phase. Not only will the medical personnel want to determine the woman's physical condition, but it is vital that her level of attachment to the pregnancy be assessed as well. A common explanation for not acknowledging the grief of an early loss is that expectant parents have not attached or bonded to the child at this point. It's true that some individuals view pregnancy during the first trimester as merely a medical event, i.e., a union of cells. Others may have a strong attachment to the "baby" early in the pregnancy or, in some cases, even before the pregnancy is confirmed. Research done by Allen and Marks (1993) with one hundred women who had experienced a pregnancy loss between four and twenty weeks gestation, found that 71 percent of those interviewed felt that the miscarriage was the death of their child. A similar study conducted by Limbo and Wheeler (1986) concluded that of eighty-seven women they interviewed, 25 percent "felt their pregnancy loss was not significant: I view this as just another life experience"; 75 percent of the women perceived the loss of the pregnancy to be the loss of a baby. As a result, they grieved initially and over time for the lost child: "This is the worst possible thing that could happen to a family" (p. 5).

In assessing the patient's level of attachment, it is recommended that the term "pregnancy" (neutral) be used rather than "baby" (attachment) or "fetus" (cold, impersonal). This guards against implying that one should or should not feel a certain way about the potential miscarriage-loss or life experience.

The care provider can begin understanding the level of attachment to the pregnancy by asking for responses to the following questions and statements:

"When did you learn you were pregnant?"
"Tell me about what that was like for you."
"Whom have you told about your pregnancy?"
"What plans have you begun to make, if any?"
"How are you doing with all of this?"

As one listens to the responses, they will begin to obtain a sense of the level of attachment and bonding that may have started to develop. In situations where the miscarriage is viewed by the parent(s) as the loss (death) of their child, personnel in the ER setting are encouraged to adapt their approach accordingly. Some suggestions for appropriate intervention will follow.

Sometimes, however, women present to the ER with vaginal hemorrhaging and have their pregnancy and miscarriage confirmed at the same time. It cannot be assumed that just because the patient has not had time to tell people or make plans about the pregnancy that no attachment exists. Many females dream about having a baby from the time they are little girls and, as such, may experience loss of self image along with the hopes and dreams of being a mother to this child.

It is recognized that grief following a miscarriage can become complicated because of the following features:

- the suddenness and unexpected nature of the situation,
- there may be no visible "baby" to see and nothing tangible to grasp onto in an attempt to validate the pregnancy,
- there are few rituals for the death of a baby through early pregnancy loss,
- there may be little social support or acknowledgment that grief following perinatal loss is normal.

For parent(s) who have begun to define the pregnancy in terms of "having a baby" and the miscarriage as a loss of that dream, having guidelines in place can assure that the parent(s) are provided with options to meet their needs.

SENSITIVE CARE PROVIDERS

It goes without saying that care providers need to be sensitive and compassionate when encountering patients who are experiencing any type of loss. Additionally, they need to have knowledge of the grief that can accompany early fetal demise. If possible, pregnant care providers should not be assigned to patients who are miscarrying. When unavoidable, the care providers should to at least acknowledge that their pregnancy may be difficult for the patient but that they will provide the best care possible while assigned to them.

SUPPORT OF SIGNIFICANT OTHER

The patient needs to be given the choice of having a support person with them during their time in the emergency room. Although the father will usually be the person identified, it should not be assumed that this is always the situation. Rules should be flexible enough to allow for whomever the patient identifies as helpful to them. By involving support people early, personnel will begin to establish important links with resources for the individual that will provide ongoing assistance following discharge from the ER.

INTERDISCIPLINARY TEAM APPROACH TO CARE ·

In many settings an interdisciplinary team consists of physician, nurse, chaplain, and social worker. Facilities will differ in how they define the team for their unique setting. The team approach assures that the individual and their significant other(s) are treated in a holistic manner. It is unrealistic to think that one discipline is able to connect on all levels with a patient and her family. The interdisciplinary team approach provides a more thorough, complete service. Additionally, it protects from one discipline becoming overloaded or feeling isolated in their efforts to provide support. It is suggested that protocols direct that the interdisciplinary team be notified in all cases of perinatal loss so that each discipline has an opportunity to make contact with the patient and significant other(s). Generally, when a patient is asked if they would like the chaplain or social worker called, they decline. Not knowing how this type of contact might be of benefit to them, patients may state, "No. I don't want to bother them." Just as we do not ask a patient if they would like the physician or nurse called in to see them, it is felt that other members of the interdisciplinary team should be as standard in the care of the patient. A simple statement such as, "Many patients find it helpful to have some time with the chaplain and social worker who are also part of our team. I would like to contact them and let them know that you are here."

A key feature of interdisciplinary care is the collaboration that occurs between the disciplines. This assures that all those involved in providing services are informed of what is being offered and which discipline is addressing each identified need.

SEEING AND HOLDING THE TISSUE/BABY

Koziol-McLain, Whitehill, Stephens, O'Flaherty, Morrell, and Chapman (1992) found that a common theme reported by women was "What happened to me in the ER?" The underlying questions were "Was I really pregnant?" and "How far along was I?" The sudden nature of miscarriage, along with a lack of validation about normal responses following this type of experience, can make integration of the loss more difficult for the parent(s). As with other types of death, there is a need to see that which is lost, to have an opportunity to visually confirm that the loss has occurred. Parents are generally hesitant at first to view the "products of conception" since they feel as if this may be viewed by the medical personnel as odd or macabre. When staff are comfortable with and encourage the opportunity for viewing as an option available to everyone experiencing a pregnancy loss, parents tend to accept the practice as a normal part of their healing journey. With preparation of how the baby will appear and an explanation of how many parents find it beneficial to see and, when possible, hold their baby, this can be an extremely valuable opportunity for parents. Parents should be approached gently and on more than one occasion about seeing the tissue/baby. Parents risk the chance of saying "no" to something that they may later regret unless they are given adequate time and validation during their decision-making time. Whatever their final decision, parents need to be supported by those working with them.

OFFERING MEMENTOS

Memorialization of the deceased is quite common and needs to be considered when exploring avenues for assisting those experiencing the grief of miscarriage. Generally, parents value receiving anything that was in contact with their baby or reminds them of the child that they will only parent in their hearts. When an identifiable baby is delivered, pictures can be taken and offered to the parents. If the parent(s) declines the pictures initially, they should be informed of how the pictures can be obtained from the facility at a future date. Parents frequently change their mind after the initial shock of an early loss and regret not having pictures. It is very important to honor cultural variations in the area of picture-taking since some groups feel that this interferes with their spiritual tradition. Parents need to be encouraged to create mementos that will have personal significance to them. Some may have the ultrasound picture, others may find poetry, journaling, or writing a letter to the unborn child comforting.

When there is nothing tangible to see and/or hold, as with very early loss, it may be helpful for parents to receive assistance in finding symbolic mementos of their baby: a figurine, a charm engraved with the date of the birth/loss, a baby ring, jewelry, or a charitable donation in memory of the child are just a few suggestions.

NAMING THE BABY

Parents can be encouraged to name their baby as another means of making the existence of the child and their identity as a parent real. If the baby's gender is not known, parents may comment that they are unsure what name to give the child. Oftentimes parents will have an intuitive sense of whether the baby was a boy or a girl. It can be suggested that they name the baby based on their intuition, or select a name that is non-gender specific.

INVOLVEMENT IN TREATMENT DECISIONS

Usually patients entering the health care system feel as if they are entering a foreign land—procedures are unfamiliar, the language is difficult to understand, and the atmosphere is sterile and clinical. Add to this the emotional trauma of losing a pregnancy, and it is easy to see how parents might be intimidated. When possible, parents should be given clear explanations about what is happening and involved in deciding which treatment option is the best for them. One woman may prefer to proceed with a D&C when informed that she is beginning to miscarry; another may opt to return home and allow the miscarriage to occur naturally. Parents need to have information that is easily understood so that they can make the decision that is best suited to their needs and situation. They also need to be reassured that they will be supported in whatever decision they make and that they always have the option to reconsider their choices and select another form of treatment.

INVOLVEMENT IN DISPOSITION PLANNING

At the time of a miscarriage, parents seldom think of all the details that may surface once they leave the emergency room. Often it is days or weeks later that the parent begins to wonder, "What happened to my baby after I left the hospital? Where did he or she go?" Some parents call the facility to inquire about their tissue and/or baby and are shocked to learn that "it" was disposed of with the other surgical specimens. Needless to say, parents find this information quite distressing. Frequently hospital personnel are even unaware of what actually happens to the tissue following a miscarriage. All hospital personnel should be aware of the institution's procedures for disposal of the products of conception and miscarriage tissue. If the current practice does not assure respectful, compassionate disposition, a change may be required. Within recent years, some hospitals have begun the practice of having a periodic burial of all pregnancy loss tissue under twenty weeks gestation. Other facilities have developed memorial gardens where the ashes of cremated babies are strewn. Parents are given information about the ritual date and location and are invited to attend the brief ceremony that is held in conjunction with the disposition.

At the time of a miscarriage, parents should be informed of the hospital's manner of disposition. If tissue is incinerated, the term "cremation" offers a more sensitive description of the form of handling. Parents should be encouraged to consider whether they may want to arrange for the disposition of their baby themselves rather than rely on the hospital method. This need not be a costly venture. Parents may choose to bury their baby at the sight of a relative's grave, or may feel more comfortable with private cremation. Some parents may consider burying their baby on private property. They need to be reminded that this option runs the risk of some dilemma should they relocate or have renovation on the property. In any event, it is imperative that hospital personnel be knowledgeable about the statutes that govern burial within their area and are informed of the paperwork requirements for disposition.

FOLLOW-UP

Many emergency rooms call back patients within twenty-four hours of receiving treatment to assure that the discharge instructions are being followed and that the patient is progressing as expected. Follow-up with a patient experiencing a miscarriage is a key element of providing comprehensive care. Koziol-McLain et al. (1992) and Neugebauer et al. (1992) found that women who miscarried reported the follow-up phone calls to be very helpful. A therapeutic effect was experienced from having an opportunity to talk with someone who was either directly involved with caring for them or was able to answer questions regarding procedures and what had happened to them. The purpose of follow-up calls are these:

- convey concern
- answer questions
- provide resource and referral information (when necessary) (Heath & Gensch (Eds.), 1997, p. 189).

It is suggested that the patient be informed of the follow-up call protocol prior to discharge and asked if this would be convenient for them. Some women may not want calls from the ER made to their home. If unable to reach the parent by telephone after a couple of attempts, a note might be sent that explains that calls have been unsuccessful, but that they may call a contact person in the ER if questions arise. The importance of follow-up phone calls cannot be over-emphasized. When promising to call a patient, make follow-through the rule. It reflects poorly on the entire organization when this commitment is not met and adds to the parent's feeling of being isolated and unsupported. The ideal time frame for follow-up calls are these:

- within one week
- three weeks to four months
- due date/anniversary date (Heath & Gensch (Eds.), 1997, p. 182).

These dates coincide with the significant phases of grief as defined by Davidson (1984). Follow-up by a sensitive person who is knowledgeable about perinatal loss can help to normalize many of the responses that the parents may be experiencing. Additionally, parents who are struggling with complicated grief can be given information about resources or referred for further assistance (with their permission).

Often, with early loss, parents indicate that they do not require more than one call. Their request should be respected and information given about how they can reach a contact person at the hospital in the event that concerns arise in the future.

SUMMARY

This chapter has provided an overview of how grief can become complicated following the loss of a baby through miscarriage. Although some individuals do not view this medical condition as a loss, approximately 70 to 75 percent of the women studied felt that their miscarriage was the death of their baby. Since many miscarriages are treated within out-patient medical settings such as emergency rooms, it is helpful to look at interventions that are supportive and validate the loss. Some of these include the support of a significant other, being able to see and hold (when possible) the miscarried baby, offering mementos, involving parents in decision making, and providing follow-up. Obviously these types of options and interventions do not take away the grief a parent may experience with this type of loss. The hope, however, is that there will be less likelihood of one's grief becoming complicated when there are rituals for closure and opportunities for positive memories.

REFERENCES

Allen, M., & Marks, S. (1993). *Miscarriage: Women sharing from the heart*. New York: Wiley & Sons.

Davidson, G. W. (1979). *Understanding death of the wished-for child*. Springfield, IL: OGR Service Corporation.

Davidson, G. W. (1984). *Understanding mourning*. Minneapolis, MN: Augsbeurg Publishing House.

Heath, L. S., & Gensch, B. K. (Eds.) (1997). *RTS counselor manual*. La Crosse, WI: Bereavement Services, Gundersen Lutheran.

Koziol-McLain, J., Whitehill, C., Stephens, L., O'Flaherty, E., Morrell, M., & Chapman, M. (1992). An investigation of emergency patients' perceptions of their miscarriage experience. *Journal of Emergency Nursing, 18*(6), 501-504.

Limbo, R. K., & Wheeler, S. R. (1986, September). Women's responses to the loss of their pregnancy through miscarriage: A longitudinal study. *Forum Newsletter—Association for Death Education and Counseling, 10*(4), 4-6.

Neugebauer, R., Kline, J., O'Connor, P., Shrout, P., Johnson, J., Skodol, A., Wicks, J., & Susser, M. (1992). Depressive symptoms in women in the six months after miscarriage. *American Journal of Obstetrics and Gynecology, 166*, 104-109.

CHAPTER 16
Death at Birth: Inner Experiences and Personal Meanings

Janis L. Keyser

The death of a baby during pregnancy, at birth, or shortly after, is a deeply tragic loss affecting the well-being of the family. The far-reaching ramifications of the death are surprising even to the parents, who can be upset not only by the intensity of grief's confusing feelings and sensations, but also by the unexpected changes they find developing in their sense of self, the assault upon their beliefs and assumptions about life, and their struggle to identify who this person is whom they are grieving. In this chapter, the intricate movement through grief will be described using the powerful, moving, and passionate words of parents themselves from their private journals. The richness and intensity of the terrain of grieving a baby's death will be explored, conveying a sense of the internal experience unique to this type of loss.

As the experience of pregnancy and the birth of a baby is an inner journey for parents, as well as a rite of passage, so the tragedy of perinatal/neonatal death is an experience imbued with deeply profound, personal images of grief, as well as innumerable emotional, psychological, and social challenges. The intense feelings, thoughts, mental images, sensory experiences, and behaviors which follow the death can leave the parents traumatized, shaken to their inner core.

An enormous volume of research has suggested that the death of a child is one of the most difficult losses for an adult to sustain. The death of a child in the first year is particularly problematic in that the fusion of the experiences of birth and death complicates the already difficult process of grieving (Bourne & Lewis, 1984). Bonding can become strong during pregnancy, when anticipation of the baby's birth is high, with the formation of deep, powerful, and lasting attachments. In fact, bonding with one's child-to-be can begin, in an abstract sense, before a woman is even pregnant: it can begin when she is a little girl playing with her dolls, or upon anticipation of a pregnancy, or during frustrating fertility regimens. Once a pregnancy is achieved, hopes and dreams are further built and the child's identity is more intricately defined. Even early loss of the baby, through miscarriage or failure to achieve a pregnancy due to infertility, can be devastating in that it represents the loss of a potential child. Peppers and Knapp (1980) found many similarities in grief reactions in women who had experienced miscarriage, stillbirth, and infant death.

When the baby dies, so do the hopes, dreams, and all the plans that were never realized. Parents grieve for the baby who is missing from their lives, as well as a multitude of related losses. Lewis (1976) describes the bewildering nature of death at birth, an occurrence which places an enormous obstacle in the sense of a natural order of things. The mother and father have the difficult task of mourning someone whom they have not come to know through face-to-face interaction, who they cannot remember or for whom there are very few actually lived memories, and who they may, in turn, have difficulty "forgetting." They are grieving someone who is in many ways intangible. The wish to have and hold the child they lost and the opportunity to get to know *that* individual child, not just any child, is extremely strong (Kowalski & Bowes, 1976).

A special challenge for couples is what Peppers and Knapp (1980) have called incongruent bonding and grieving. Due to the physical realities of pregnancy, many times the mother finds her identity more strongly intertwined with that of the baby than does the father, resulting in differences in attachment. This, coupled with societal expectations of the father's role as protector and norms for men to refrain from the expression of feelings which may make them appear weak, sets the stage for strong differences in grief responses. The inability to share feelings with each other about a tragedy that so deeply affects them both, albeit in very different ways, can result in their grieving separately and alone. With virtually no one else in their circle of family and friends having gotten to know, or even see, the baby, the stress of this isolation can lead to complications in their grieving.

Leon (1987) summarized six factors that make the death of a baby particularly challenging to grieve. These include: "the narcissistic nature of the loss which is inherent in pregnancy-related death; the over-whelming self-blame and sense of failure experienced by the bereaved mother; the lack of concrete memories and objects which would make both the child and the loss real; the inability to anticipate the death; the prospective nature of the grief in which fantasies of future interactions must be mourned; and the stunning lack of social support and understanding."

It is the last factor in Leon's list, the lack of social support and understanding, that adds insult to injury for parents after a baby's death. Few people know how to listen to the griever's experience because it is, in fact, so intense, so deeply personal and painful, and so imbued with confusing images for which parents struggle to find expression. It is difficult for others to imagine this baby whom the parents are grieving—to even catch the essence of who that child is to its parents—let alone validate the many layers of their grief, each with its own set of intricately woven feelings, thoughts, and images.

In order to develop a deeper understanding of the profundity of this very internal experience, it is necessary to consider the words and contemplate the images shared by bereaved parents themselves. Some of our most meaningful learning can occur by our empathic listening, taking their stories in, and allowing their meanings to resonate within us. It is through this process that we can gain a sense of the remarkably rugged terrain of parental grief after a baby's death. And as we learn to vicariously walk the territory with them, letting them be our teachers, we build the capacity to more fully understand and support them through this most difficult of times. We then become witness to the resiliency of the human spirit which can accommodate to and even grow through deep psychic pain to emotional renewal.

In the pages that follow I will share the inner experiences and personal meanings of several mothers who kept journals through the period of their most intense grief. The women are: Sarah, whose first child Ricky was stillborn; Emma, whose first child Zachary was stillborn and whose second child was lost through miscarriage; Mary whose second child Helen was stillborn; Maureen whose first and second babies were lost through miscarriage and ectopic pregnancy and who also experienced infertility; Elisa whose first child Emmy lived seven weeks; Eleanor whose first child Jonathan lived thirty hours; and Cyndi whose third child Christopher lived seventeen hours. In addition to their journals, the women and their partners further described their journeys through grief during in-depth interviews. They shared from their hearts, conveying the texture and fabric of their grief with the hope that they might make it easier for family members, friends, hospital care givers, and others to support grieving parents who are similarly suffering.

Through content analysis of the journals and interviews, a number of themes emerged as characteristic of the journey through grief when a baby dies (see Keyser, 1993, for detailed description). The themes are: 1) grief reactions, including emotional aspects, physical sensations, and behavioral expressions; 2) changes in the self-image of the griever; 3) challenges to belief systems; 4) the personhood of the baby and their place in the family; 5) desire for a subsequent pregnancy; 6) reaching a degree of "recovery"; and 7) the personal meaning of the loss experience.

As some of the journals from which this material has been drawn were over 300 pages long, what will be described here is not the actual journey, not even the travel diary, but short selections from the travel diary through grief. I have chosen passages which poignantly illustrate the emotions, thoughts, sensations, images, and experiences which are an integral part of grieving a baby's death.

GRIEF REACTIONS

After a baby's death, grief reactions are innumerable and intensely felt by the parents, permeating the entire life of the griever. Eleanor said that after her son Jonathan died, "I couldn't understand why this little baby would have so much of an impact on me, why this little baby's death would make me feel so sad. I never knew what sadness was until Jonathan died. I almost felt like someone was ripping my heart out. I hated to wake up in the morning because the pain would smack me in the face. I hated to see the night time come because it felt so lonely." This deep pain was described by Emma as "wordless pain" and by Elisa as being "lost in misery." Maureen said that after her miscarriage, she felt emotional pain like she had never known. "We were so happy those weeks I was pregnant. It just brought a whole new dimension into our lives. Then it all came crashing down. Nothing is important after that." She wrote of feeling pitiful, just wanting to crawl into a cocoon and not come out. "Everything is changed. Nothing is important. I just want our baby back, our happiness back, our plans back, our family back. We were so happy then and so awfully empty now. Everything we had invested is lost."

In a poem, Mary described the images that carried great pain for her—the memories of Helen's silent birth. "Still. Looking back, I know why they call it stillbirth. After the commotion of pushing, she came. 'It's a girl.' The doctor quietly checked his routine joy. Then it was so still. As if in a silent movie, he gave her to us. Silently they worked around us, and we gazed at her perfect body, fingers, toes. Her dad choked back quiet tears into frightened eyes. We beheld her. The quiet passed too quickly. He never held her, he would later sob. They took her away. I looked back. She lay on the ohio, disheveled, alone. Was this our only good-bye? Only a few silent moments? Are life and death so far removed? The horror of that silent quickness plays back like an uncomprehended dream from which we were forced to awaken. Still, no one heard the screaming inside me."

Emptiness and aloneness is so much a part of grieving a baby's death. Filled with hopes and dreams, Sarah used to sit in the rocking chair in the baby's room while she was pregnant. After her son died, she sat and rocked as she grieved the few memories there were. "There is a rocking chair where I would sit on hot spring days and hum to him, and dream of rocking him here in my arms. But now my rocking chair is not for my baby, but for me to cry and mourn and long for him, rocking his teddy instead of my baby. The rocking chair that we shared is now to remember when he and I were one, for rocking my lonely heart with emptiness in my arms."

As well as the emotional emptiness of birthing a baby who dies, there is an immense sense of physical emptiness. Mary, whose daughter Helen was stillborn, expressed her pain in both literal and symbolic terms, a few weeks after Helen's death. "My belly is empty and it aches. I still caress it wishing you were still there and half waiting for you to kick in response. My womb aches to feel you move inside it again. My heart aches for you. My flesh aches for you."

Cyndi wrote, "The day Christopher died was the first time in my life I wanted to be anyone but me. The pain was unbearable. Sleep was fitful and unsatisfactory; after all my pain was still there when I awoke. Joe was numb and struggled through the day just as I was. We had nothing to say. There were no words that I could give him or he could give me." She said that every morning she woke up and thought she was still pregnant and was shocked to find out she wasn't. She had a lot of phantom movement. She just couldn't shake the anticipation of the new baby, couldn't accept the fact that her baby had died. She felt like she was losing her mind. Another mother said that for six to eight weeks she didn't really understand what happened and mulled around in a fog. Nobody talked about her baby's death, which made the unreality even more intense.

Adjusting to the emotional and physical sensations, the loss of prospective memories and confronting the reality of the loss takes an incredible amount of effort. Four months after her son's death, Sarah used her journal to recount the many physical aspects of her grief and her adjustment to the reality of her baby's death. The fact that she had to adjust to the hormonal changes after giving birth added to the already difficult task of grieving. "I remember when I first came home from the hospital. My head was empty. I slept about fifteen hours a day. I had to hold a pillow close to my body because I had a big empty ache in the middle of my body where my baby used to be. That ache used to keep me up at night. After two or three weeks it gradually went away. I would go into the nursery in the mornings after Rick left for work and just sit and look at the crib filled with presents. Sometimes I cried, sometimes I didn't. I thought maybe he just had jaundice and they'll send him home soon. Or maybe he's downstairs in the bassinet and he's sleeping. Or maybe I'm in the wrong house. I must be in the wrong house because there is no baby here. Or maybe I woke up as the wrong person, because there is no baby here. This can't be me, because I was just pregnant a few days ago. I was just pregnant, and I just gave birth, and my milk just came in, so there must be a baby nearby. I must be the wrong person if I don't have a baby. I dreamed once that my little boy was crying, and I picked him up to put him to my breast because they hurt from being full, so I knew it was time to feed him. But then I didn't feel any relief and I looked down, and I was holding a doll with no face. And it was the cat next door that was crying."

The struggle to adjust to the reality of the death is a daunting task. Eight months after her son's death, Sarah wrote, "I am tired of fighting the tide, but if I don't I'll drown. I just want to stop all this torment and turmoil so I can act and feel as if none of this ever happened. But it did. My whole life is shadowed by my baby's death, my joy of living is eclipsed by my grief, and people wonder what I'm making such a big deal over." Maureen, who had experienced both a miscarriage and an ectopic pregnancy worried that people might not even believe she was pregnant. Both worrying about others' perceptions and dealing with the invalidation of the loss, i.e., "What's the big deal?," complicated the already difficult process of grieving.

Self-blame, guilt, and shame can be a most difficult aspect of a mother's experience when a baby dies because the death, whether through miscarriage, ectopic pregnancy, stillbirth, premature birth, genetic anomalies, or other causes, is so intimately connected to the mother's body, so physically a part of her. There is frequently the irrational, but heart-felt belief, that there must have been some measure of control over the baby's fate which was not properly exercised. "If I had been a good enough mother, this wouldn't have happened." Sarah wrote, "I am so sorry for my baby. I am so sorry that I couldn't help him, I'm so sorry that my body killed him. I remember laying on the delivery room table after they put my baby boy up on my chest, screaming that I was sorry. Sorry is too late. Everything was too late. He was dead. My body killed him. God, what did I do wrong? I thought I was taking such good care of him."

A month after her son Zachary's death, Emma wrote of the sadness and loneliness for what her life was supposed to be, but wasn't. "I start to feel myself swirl down into panic and dark, and I just have to get a hold on myself." Sometimes the feelings are turned outward with the anger so great that in some cases parents fantasize massive acts of destruction, like blowing up a subway, or dream of revenge on a doctor whom they felt had been grossly negligent. Sarah wrote in big letters across her journal pages: "I HATE THIS."

Anniversaries are predictably difficult times. Sometimes there are anniversaries of significant, but initially unrecognizable, events—the date the pregnancy was discovered, the first ultrasound, first kicks, due date, date of death. Images of these occasions can return with striking, startling vividness. Sarah experienced deep pain on the days leading up to the first anniversary of her baby's death. "Has it really been a year? If it has then why does the loneliness in my heart feel so big? Why does the ache in my arms feel so heavy? Why can I see my little boy's face so clearly? Remember Rick's crying, the sound of the tear of the episiotomy, the print of the wallpaper on the delivery room ceiling, the silence of my hospital room, the weight of my son in my arms, the silkiness of his skin to my touch, like it was yesterday? Has it not been forever that my longing heart has wept over that brief moment when our lives touched? How do I extinguish the burning anger, the hot tears, the flames of longing for my child?"

The strength of the images that are recorded deep in the parents' hearts, and their duration in time, is incredible. Eleanor's husband Dave said, "Almost six years later those images are so powerful still. I can remember what he looked like, the hospital room, those thirty hours. I can get back there like that."

Differences in partners' responses to the loss frequently become obvious. Cyndi wrote in her journal, "The world came crashing in around us when Christopher died, trapping us together yet apart." Cyndi said, "The difference between Joe and me was that he was out there everyday. Sometimes you have to 'turn off' to function in your role at work. I never left it. I could talk about it everyday constantly. He had to leave it. His grief seemed more painful because he had to do it all in a short time period. So during the whole first year, it outwardly looked like I was coping so much better. His grieving looked much sadder than mine, even though he didn't cry a lot." Joe described his way of coping: "I would think in the shower—that's where I tended to process the loss—and have private conversations. I would compose poems for the newsletter, but was not much of a talker." They had differences in their need to visit the cemetery. Joe would have "agitated weekends," as Cyndi called them, and they'd find themselves driving around and ending up at the cemetery to visit Christopher. Cyndi viewed the cemetery as a brutal place, while Joe found comfort there. Other couples noted the stress of grieving together, yet alone. Sarah wrote about the strain on their marriage and "the hole in our hearts that lets the passion drain." Mary's husband John said he felt jealous when he saw his wife get support from her friends, but got little concern from his.

When siblings were involved, another dimension was added to the equation of grieving. In her journal, Cyndi noted a conversation she had with her young son. "Joey asked about Christopher today. It hurts when a child of five must learn so young about death. He asked if I prayed. I said yes, I do. Then he asked me if I prayed for our baby, and if I did, why didn't God let him live? He had been angry at me for not fixing things with God. He said he felt so bad he never got to see him. But he did say that he liked to talk about him, that it felt good. Oh, I ached for him. How cruel life can be. I'm sorry, Joey, that mommy couldn't make it go away." Cyndi regretted that her preoccupation with her grief kept her from being as good a mother as she wanted to be for her boys. She said that for a time, the effort it took to make a peanut butter and jelly sandwich for them seemed too much to ask.

So many emotions make up the kaleidoscope of grief. Sarah summarized some of them in a poem. "I am frustrated that there is no way to change the fact that my little boy is dead. I am angry that there is no one to blame for the fact that my little boy is dead. I am sad that there is a loss of a little person I love because my little boy is dead. I am lonely for my baby who was with me, reminding me of himself and now he's not with me because he's dead. I am hurt that my own flesh was taken away so abruptly because my little boy is dead. I am tortured by the fact that I wanted him so much but I can't have my little boy because he is dead." She wrote, "Our lives are so permeated by our son's death that there is virtually nothing we do or think about that is not affected by our grief."

IMPACT UPON SELF-IMAGE

Who am I as a mother, if my baby is dead? This is an especially challenging question when a first child dies. Maureen worried that others would not only doubt she lost a baby, but even feared they would doubt the legitimacy of her once pregnant status. She wrote, "Now I feel like a fool, like I was playing a black charade, as if people will point to me a say, 'I knew you were never pregnant.'" Her worries about others' judgment was more a doubting of herself. She equated the loss of her babies as very much a failure as a mother, and she was angry at her body and herself. Emma wrote about crying over her loss of what motherhood would have brought her and her lack of identity in the world of parents. Even Cyndi, who had two other boys at the time of Christopher's death, said that her initial reaction when he died was that she wasn't a mother, as though she wasn't deserving of that special status.

The grievers found that their images of themselves as women had changed, also. After Helen died, Mary felt ugly. She felt that she and her body had failed, and that she had done something bad and dirty, not measuring up to femininity. She felt like a freak of nature because babies just don't die inside of women. Two months after Helen's stillbirth she wrote, "Once in a while I get that horrible awful feeling that I am not a woman—that people look at me and see a man. I look in the mirror and see something freakish—a unisex person, someone without any sex, and that frightens me more than anything. It's worse than depression. When I'm depressed I just feel lazy but when I get this feeling, I feel self-destructive—like I can't hide from myself anywhere."

A month after Zachary's death, Emma expressed her self-doubts in her journal. "I had thoughts of being a horrible monster that gives birth to dead children, due to some deep terrible flaw at the center of self, a flaw translated into physical failure." But she noted that with time her perspective had shifted, remembering that, "Zachary was of a time when I stopped believing bad things about myself. I realize that interpretation is just not true."

The struggle of fathers was often a lonely one, infrequently articulated, but deeply felt. Joe, whose son Christopher died after seventeen hours, captured his feelings of helplessness in a poem he wrote three years after Christopher's death. "It's hard to believe that almost three years have passed since the day you were born. The time sure went fast. It's hard to imagine you running around, playing with your brothers, tumbling to the ground. It's hard to accept that if you hadn't died, your sister wouldn't be here. And we wouldn't have cried. It's hard to get across that this deep dark hurt is still only tolerated by the will I exert. It's hard to swallow that one of my children is dead. I think that rather than you it had been me instead. It's hard to go on. No, that's not quite true. It's just hard to live, living without you."

ASSAULT ON BELIEF SYSTEMS

Beliefs are turned upside down after a baby's death. Sometimes the tragedy leads to a reversion to childhood thinking. Maureen said, "I used to try to bargain with God, 'If I get pregnant, I promise I'll go to church.' You laugh at yourself because you're like a ten year old. I'm jealous of the people who can pray, go to church a lot, read the Bible, or things like that. They believe that there will be good to come out of it, that there is hope, that there is a plan. I still believe in God, and I still believe that He's basically good and kind. But I have no idea what God has in mind, and I guess I'm afraid to think what He has in mind if it's that we're not meant to have children. I don't really want to accept that because that's not what we want. So I kind of leave Him out of the picture."

Sarah wrote to her baby, "Your death has rocked everything we ever believed to its foundation. That you aren't here anymore proves our reasons to doubt." Emma wrote that she didn't believe in "sweet wonderful things anymore. Good things don't last. You only get a minute between hard things." She found she had "lost belief in the fairy tale that life is good."

Mary had relied on her faith for everything. She became angry at church members for their failure to be there for her, leaving her very alone in her grief. She and her husband were also disillusioned and angry with their pastor, feeling abandoned by him when Helen died, as if they were an embarrassment to the church. Mary feared she had at some point in her life done something wrong in the eyes of God to deserve her daughter's death and the subsequent pain. She struggled to find meaning, writing to her Helen, "Even as I begin to accept God's plan, there are tears in my eyes. I still have a very human heart and right now that human heart needs to mother you."

Sarah wrote of her anger at having the rug of her comfortable beliefs pulled out from under her. "I'm angry at myself because I didn't know anything was wrong. I'm angry with myself that I am a wretched person who probably deserved this. I'm angry at myself that I keep depending on others for their support, and when I don't get it, I'm afraid that I won't be able to stand this by myself. I'm angry at my weakness, my dependency, and my inability to give life to my son. I've depended on people and God when they've let me down and I was left floundering. I had so much faith in them, I gave my own power away. No more will I give that power to anyone not even God. I cannot pray for a healthy baby next time. I just have to hope I beat the odds that were dealt me this time. God isn't a magician. This is a natural world where things go wrong, not always, but on a regular basis." Emma expressed that it was her belief in randomness that helped her put perspective on things—that God, or whoever/whatever, was *not* doing things to *her*.

PERSONHOOD OF THE BABY

Who is this baby, this little person, who has died? That is a huge question confronting parents. Though physically present for only a short time, the hopes and dreams for this child run deep. Sarah was grieving the loss of future interactions and who her baby would've been, noting in her journal, "It's a gray dreary day. On a day like this, I would want to have my little Ricky dressed up warm, and rock him, and maybe play with a rattle, and I would love to hear him laugh. Ricky would be five months old. He would roll over. I think he would sit up. He would be a happy baby, because he would be with me all the time. I believe that gives babies confidence and security, and when he gets a little older then he wouldn't be upset if I had to be away from him. Maybe he's upset that he's away from me now. I'm certainly upset that he is away from me. Before I had a baby, I never really understood why parents made such a fuss about leaving their kids at a babysitter. But this is the ultimate separation anxiety."

On the struggle to maintain closeness, Sarah wrote: "He's so far away. I feel such a huge chasm between us." It was a couple of days later that Sarah wrote about her feeling of closeness to her son. "I was hanging laundry yesterday, and happened to look across to the other hill. To the north I saw the cemetery, the white marble gleaming in the sun. My heart jumped to think my little Ricky is just across the valley. I thought, I wish I could shout, 'Ricky come home! Ricky, we're waiting for you. It's time to come home now!' I wanted to call him, to think he might come running at the sound of my voice. I stood on tiptoes, to see around the trees better, to catch a glimpse of my son but the hill is too far away, and my son is very tiny yet. For the first time, my baby doesn't seem light years away. For the first time, I felt happy to think he might be nearer than I thought. For the millionth time, I miss him."

Mary expressed that there was a "Helen-shaped" vacuum in her heart, that no one else or nothing else could fill. All of the mothers and fathers cherished the uniqueness of their child who died, even when others' comments and reactions tended to invalidate this specialness. Dave wrote a poem to his wife Eleanor about the personal meaning of Jonathan's life. "We lost something grand, you and I. Something that cannot be measured—a lifetime. Jonathan's memories are in hours and not in years as we had hoped. Just an instant, an eternity of emotions grasped in a handful of time. Our lives are not the same now. We have lost a part of ourselves, a gift to each other, to mankind, to time. For children are a gift, a promise, a sign of man's longing to continue. The reminders will always be with us, but not in the things we remember; his life was too short. But in the things that will never be—no first steps, no words, no baseball gloves or scraped knees, no

Christmases or Halloweens. Just a marker and the memories of a handful of time the three of us shared. Thank you, Jonathan, for giving us the time you had. We will always love you for it. Rest easy, Jon. You will *not* be forgotten, just missed." Over time, after incredibly hard work, the special and unique personhood that parents find in their babies' lives becomes a link to making meaning out of their suffering.

SUBSEQUENT PREGNANCY

Hopes for a subsequent pregnancy are accompanied by strong fears of another loss. Emma wrote about "aching to get pregnant again to fill the scathing emptiness." She also acknowledged, "Trying to get pregnant again will mean moving into a fresh layer of mourning—afraid of having to relive the horror of Zachary's death as I grow this new baby." Some of the mothers expressed that on an unconscious level they hoped that getting pregnant again meant bringing back their child who died. Sarah wrote, "If we had a choice between Ricky and a new baby, we'd want him. We only want a new baby because we can't have him." Parents struggled with loyalty issues as they realized that it wasn't possible to get their baby back. Getting pregnant again felt like leaving their baby behind. Mary wrote to Helen, "When I try to think of the new baby, my thoughts always end up with you." But the drive to bring forth new life is strong. Maureen wrote, "I've come to the realization that I would get pregnant ten times to have a baby in our arms."

The sense of vulnerability during subsequent pregnancy is immense. When Cyndi was twenty weeks pregnant with her subsequent child she wrote, "My heart sings! I rejoice this baby." Then she added, "I have been missing Christopher a lot lately. I tear up at the slightest. God, why did he have to die? I always feel his absence. I am so scared this baby will not live. Sometimes my intense desire for this baby scares me. How will I survive the loss of another child? I feel I barely survived Christopher's death. How could our marriage make it? I'd like to think that we could make it, but I also know how deep the cut goes."

During her subsequent pregnancy Mary wrote, "The closer I get to this baby, the more I fear. It's as if some dark shadow were saying, 'Be careful—don't get too close—you'll get hurt again.'" She added, "Many times I just lie back and savor the baby's movement as though these will be the only memories I ever have. I wish I had done that with Helen."

The parents were very clear about their dead child's place in the family. Eleanor wrote, "Jonathan, you will always be a special part of our lives. You will always be our first child. We hope to have other children; they will never take your place. Your brothers and sisters will know they had an older brother who their mommy and daddy love so much. We will share with them your footprints, your bracelet, your pictures, and our memory of you." The term "forever baby" was used by many of the parents to describe their child's permanent place in their lives, even when others seemed to forget about their child or invalidate their grief.

RECOVERY

At various points throughout the grieving process, the spiral of grief allows glimpses of the elusive goal of recovery. Emma knew that her grief work was going somewhere when she wrote, "I am moving out of the shadows. Other senses are returning. I'm moving into the world of the living. I had forgotten that roses have fragrance and some babies live." Mary wrote, "With this new year I feel like a new person. I like me. Somewhere deep inside, God is working out a gift in me."

Sarah described her sense of recovery using rich imagery, "I am very excited! I've felt truly expectant, like when you know something good is going to happen. From somewhere, it's coming to me here. Like a warm soft rain on a wilted garden, I can feel it gently, slowly reviving me. My life is coming back now. I feel it, like morning sunshine on a frost encrusted landscape, like summer rain after a drought. I feel my life creeping back in. I know I'm not who I was. But I am who I am. And that's okay." Nearing the first anniversary of Ricky's stillbirth, she wrote, "I told mom that my grief work feels fairly complete, because I allowed myself to feel the sadness, to be immersed in the grief at the time it was most powerful, and I didn't try to push it away or pretend it wasn't there. Finally, I feel my life again."

It might not be long after such a "break-through" that a parent is once again plunged to deeper levels of their grief. Elisa wrote, "I know I've done a great amount of resolution, but that's not where I'm always at. Even by my calling it 'My Emmy Experience' as I do, tries to separate it, objectify it. But it isn't separated from my life. It's incorporated. There are times I still find myself torn apart emotionally and it's powerful learning for me." Emma wrote about the uneven process of recovery. "At moments when I feel okay, I look back on Zachary's death and my miscarriage as a tunnel of time that is covered over for me but which remains intact to be re-experienced and redigested. Much like the ice on the river in the winter, the absolute horror of that period is crusted over. But I will always go back and fall through." Despite the setbacks, it was undeniable that progress toward reclaiming their lives was being made.

Mary said, "Resolution is incorporating it into your life, realizing how it's changed you, and then going on from there. There is a hole, a loss, and nothing will make it as before. Everything is different, the whole landscape is different. But you can't not go through life because it is different." She wrote in a poem, "Time passes; It does not heal all wounds but binds them in the bandages of the past. Time eases the pain; But it does not erase the memories, only frames the special ones out of the attic clutter. Time's forced march orders us to follow, and we limp beneath the baggage of grief. Time changes, and times change, forcing us to emerge only ourselves."

UNCOVERING MEANING

Movement to a new normal is accompanied by a search for meaning in their child's brief life. Meaning emerges, painstakingly, bit by bit, as feelings are uncovered, explored, and expressed. Elisa described Emmy as "a giver of gifts," someone who had enriched her life beyond compare. She said, "Emmy was the first hint of what love—unconditional love—was like." Sarah said that even in death, Ricky was the light of her life. In a poem called "Imperfect Grief," she wrote of finding life in the midst of grief. "Pain of my heart: the imperfect grief of crying out to be heard, but finding there are no words to say it like I can feel it, like my tears can pour it out. So hush, my heart. Don't try to tell what can only be felt. Through your tears, look. See the beautiful here now. Look through your imperfect grief to life, like through a crystal to the sun. From your imperfect lens shines this moment's gift. Take it."

Emma captured her feelings about the meaning Zachary had for her life. "You have redrawn my internal country, uprooted trees and changed the course of lanes, here with a soft curve, there with a sharp angle. You moved mountains, sowed orchards in my hair and made me beautiful. You laid new boundaries, tumbled down walls, and taught this land to be still and fertile. You quieted the harsher winds and steadied me with the warm sun and the moon's wakeful presence. And in the heart of this new country, you carved out a deep lake, unplumbable, dark and safe. A place of abundance and unfailing life."

Using the metaphor of a tree, Emma described her new sense of self. "All through my life as a tree, I have lived at the tips of my branches, reaching and reaching for others, toward them, trying to bring them to me. Zachary was the beginning of my me-ness. I lived in myself for the first time during my pregnancy. Now I'm down in my roots learning about who I am."

Sarah's poem, "The Phoenix," described the transformation that was the result of her grief work which moved her from looking for reasons for her son's death to searching for meaning in her son's life. "For the love of him she rent her heart, her life and her spirit lay wasting in sackcloth and ashes. For the love of him from the ashes of death with no reason she now rises as me because his life holds true meaning."

Asserting the uniqueness of their child and having others understand the specialness of their baby's brief life is an important part of the process of making meaning. Eleanor's husband Dave captured the feelings of many other bereaved mothers and fathers in his writing, which he entitled "Private Lessons." "Don't think my loss was greater than my gain, because it will take a lifetime to gauge. Grief is a teacher, an emotional lesson. Grief is a journey. Duration—undetermined. Destination—understanding. Don't say it's good you didn't get a chance to get attached, because my heart knows that's not true. Love doesn't understand time. Don't say you're young, you can have more children, because we don't take things for granted anymore. Besides babies cannot be replaced. So if you don't know what to say, I understand. But please don't deny my son's existence."

Sarah said, "I still need to talk about him and probably always will for ever and ever. I'll always need to validate his existence by acknowledging that he happened. The kindest thing that anyone can do for me is to allow me to show them this part of my life."

CONCLUSION

The death of a baby is a deeply personal and painful experience. Moving through grief is a process of becoming aware of and giving expression to the many layers of conflicting feelings, confusing thoughts, and intense images which compose the internal landscape of the bereaved parent's reality. This winding path includes the work of figuring out who this little person was and would have been, redefining their own identity as a parent and as a person, discerning what to trust when everything they believed in has been turned upside down, and through it all to discover the lasting meaning of their child's life and the special place in their hearts which their baby will forever hold. This difficult journey is necessary in order to reach some degree of accommodation to the whole experience. But one other component must be in place in order for a sense of recovery to be felt. To have the meaning of their baby's life validated and their grief empathically understood by others is at the heart of healing for parents.

When we walk with parents through their grief, listening with our hearts to the stories they tell us, taking their words and images into our own beings, and allowing their meanings to resonate within us, we help bereaved parents heal. This is not easy to do—it is extremely difficult and painful to "sit in the mud" with another who is hurting so deeply. But in doing so, we not only help them heal, we become witness to the resiliency of the human spirit. In the process we are changed, ourselves. We are healed also.

REFERENCES

Bourne, S., & Lewis, E. (1984, July). Pregnancy after stillbirth or neonatal death: Psychological risks and management. *The Lancet*, 31-33.

Keyser (Heil), J. (1993). *The grief recovery process after the death of a baby: Inner experiences and personal meanings.* Unpublished doctoral dissertation. Temple University.

Kowalski, K., & Bowes, W. (1976, October). Parents' response to a stillborn baby. *Contemporary OB/Gyn, 8,* 53-57.

Leon, I. (1987). Short-term psychotherapy for perinatal loss. *Psychotherapy, 24*(2), 186-195.

Lewis, E. (1976, September). The management of stillbirth: Coping with an unreality. *The Lancet,* 619-620.

Peppers, L., & Knapp, R. (1980). Maternal reactions to involuntary fetal/infant death. *Psychiatry, 43,* 155-159.

CHAPTER 17
Partners in Complicated Grief: National Grief Reactions to Disasters and Grassroots Memorialization

Hannah Sherebrin

In recent years we have seen a rise in spontaneous outpouring of community grief in the form of letters, flowers, crying, and candlelight vigils as a reaction to violent deaths of public figures or innocent bystanders. Community grief reactions in cases of unpredictable terrorist attacks or large scale disasters are examined through events of the last ten years in Israel. The phenomenon of mass public outpouring of grief is examined by employing the stage model of personal grief, as well as through a cathartic event, leading to reliving and revisiting of personal traumas. The structural approach to trauma is discussed in order to understand the dynamic relationship between external and internal pressures acting on an individual. It is postulated that the grass roots creation of a new visual language of commemoration is a viable alternative to official government commemorative rituals. The personal nature of this commemoration vastly enhances the process of healing.

When a community is faced with terrorist attacks which are unpredictable in time, place, and scope, or when faced with disasters of large scale, what are the expectations of the immediate families of the victims, the bereaved, from the society they live in, in terms of support, compensation, and being partners in their grief? Is there a universal pattern as a society reacts to terrorist attacks, or is the Israeli society different in the way it reacts from other societies that experience frequent terrorist attacks?

I have moved back to Israel after thirty years of living in Canada, and the first thing that struck me was the intensity of feeling everyone has as soon as there is a disaster. People get involved in every incident, and immediately try to find out the names of those killed or injured. Invariably they will find a personal connection since the country is relatively small, and even the newcomers of recent years have served in the army together with those born in the country. There is virtually no extended family that does not know grief. One or more members in most families have been killed or disabled in the wars, terrorist attacks, or mass accidents. There is a feeling of a shared destiny when you have to stand in line for a Gas Mask like we had to do in the fall of 1997, and the people remembered the sealed rooms and Scuds of the Gulf War. Anxieties have been revisited, and not only those of recent events. Within the adult segment of the population most have experienced up to five wars in the last fifty years.

In Israel, where the army is highly valued as a necessary means for survival, male identity is strongly linked to military functioning. Most men over the ages of eighteen have seen combat, and many have experienced more than one combat situation. Much has been written about war veterans, and the general consensus is that there is an association between catastrophic trauma, less adaptive personality structure, and greater difficulties in coping (Sutker et al., 1989). Moreover, a significant association has been found between duration of combat exposure and the prevalence and persistence of Post Traumatic Stress Disorder (PTSD), (Buydens-Branchey, Noumair, & Branchey, 1990). Solomon (1987) cited extensive reviews which contend that traumatic experiences often render the afflicted individual vulnerable in the face of future adversity. Israeli men are regularly exposed to military stimuli which serve as continuous reminders of their combat, since, after their three years of mandatory active service, they continue to serve in the reserves for about thirty days per year until they reach the age of fifty-five. Follow-up of combat veterans who had suffered from PTSD and successfully negotiated subsequent combat, showed that they had a higher overall level of psychiatric distress and more intrusive war related thoughts and imagery. They also had a greater tendency to avoid war-related stimuli. Solomon et al. (1990) have remarked that these results indicate that "men who sustained CSR (Combat Stress Reaction) are unlikely ever to completely regain their former equilibrium."

The same theory may be postulated in regard to the survivors of concentration camps. The older population in Israel consists of many Holocaust survivors who live with the memory of those horrors. Many women have also served in the army, are survivors, and live with veterans. Thus we have a situation in which the majority of adults carry with them memories of traumatic events. As in other parts of the world, so here in Israel one can observe an increase in seemingly spontaneous outpouring of grief in the form of flowers, candles, songs, and just gathering together whenever disaster strikes. Princess Diana's death, bombings in Ireland, the events of Jamestown in the United States, as so many other events of violent death seem to trigger a pattern of reaction which seems to be universal. The media, especially television, is responsible for showing in real time how people react in different countries, thus encouraging "copying" behaviors. Yet we do see some unique cultural differences in the way the Israeli public reacts.

TRAUMA AND COPING

Witztum and Malkinson (1998) contend that the term trauma always alludes to changes of internal construction following an external, sudden, unexpected, and unwanted event. In order to understand the dynamic relationships between external and internal pressures, I would like to propose the structural approach to trauma advocated by Benyakar, Kutz, Dasberg, and Stern (1989). They state that the maintenance of wholeness in human systems is reflected in the capacity to retain a sense of identity, continuity, and internal consistency in the face of relentless external and internal pressures. This is an operational definition of autonomy in humans and it implies that the self, like all other structures, must be adaptable.

In evaluating stressful situations, any violent and sudden attack on life, such as war, terrorist actions, or a mass accident, is generally considered to be an environmental event. That type of environmental event is defined as a catastrophe, which causes an overwhelming external assault on the individual (Saigh, 1984; Steele & Cox, 1986). Figley and McCubbin (1983, p. 6) define catastrophes as sudden life-threatening events, to be looked at in terms of their impact on individuals and families. They state that the a catastrophic event "due to the circumstances renders the survivors feeling an extreme sense of helplessness." Our attention is drawn to similarities in the emotional experiences of survivors of war combat, prisoners of war, hostages of terrorism, rape, or natural disasters. However, we must be cautious not to define traumatic stress exclusively from the perspective of an environmental event. Most recent literature acknowledges that the evaluation of a potential stressor should also take into consideration the person/environment interaction model, which takes into account individual coping mechanisms (Heimberg, 1985; Solomon et al., 1987, 1989; Chimienti et al., 1989; Sutker et al., 1989).

In an extensive review of studies of stress and coping styles, Roth and Cohen (1986) point to two concepts—approach and avoidance— which are central to the understanding of the response to trauma. These concepts are considered to be metaphors for cognitive and emotional activity, oriented either toward or away from the threat. Two core areas of stress studies exist. One concerned with anticipating events which create stress, the other with recovery from trauma. It is not always easy to differentiate clearly between the two conditions, but Roth and Cohen established that the same approach/avoidance processes were central to coping with both anticipation and recovery from trauma. Thus, while each individual may have a particular style, both approach and avoidance strategies can be successfully employed in trauma resolution. In any given situation the key to coping lies in evaluating the potential costs and benefits of approach and avoidance. The authors conclude: "It seems clear that a lack of flexibility in regard to the use of both approach and avoidance strategies is not adaptive."

Flexibility seems to be the key. Benyakar, Kutz, Dasberg, and Stern (1989) define psychic trauma as: "the collapse of the structure of self along all four (of its) referential planes resulting from an encounter of a catastrophic threat and a chaotic response." They describe the four planes of reference which form the base for the system, and propose a continuous exchange of action between the structure and its environment to create a state of equilibrium. Thus the structure must be adaptable. This concept is based on Piaget's notion of structure, which consists of three key ideas: wholeness, transformation, and self-regulation. Within the structure, the planes of reference are utilized as descriptive analytical tools in order to study processes and events.

Using the structural approach, we may view any event in any given time as occurring simultaneously along all four referential planes. The two structural planes define relationships between elements in the psychological structure. The psychostructural plane is devoted to the relationship of elements within the psychic structure (defence mechanisms, ego, superego), which may be conscious or unconscious. The sociostructure defines the relationships between the self and members of a given social unit, such as a couple, family members. The psychofunctional plane defines activities within the psychic structure such as anxiety, anger, or apathy, while the sociofunctional plane is devoted to activity between the representations of the self and of its social environment.

Any threat which overwhelms all four structure planes and endangers the integrity of the relations and functions which maintain the functional whole is a catastrophic threat. As a result of a threat, adaptative activities have to take place within the system. If the system can reorganize its internal order by accommodating and assimilating the threat, then the threat is transformed into an integral part of the human meaning-system, allowing growth and development to occur.

An unsuccessful attempt at reorganization, or a total inability to reorganize the inter-relationships into a meaningful whole, is a chaotic response which characterizes a traumatic experience. When we picture the structural collapse, we can see the initial stage of the traumatic experience as a forced-open state in the structure. The inability to terminate this unstable state by closing the boundaries is accompanied by intense emotions such as fear of death and horror that the world will never be the same again. "What causes the traumatic experience is not merely the presence of mounting unacceptable emotions, but the perception of the diminishing ability, or even loss of ability, to perform the essential autonomous functions that define the human system" (Benyakar, Kutz, Dasberg, & Stern, 1989, p. 442). In an examination of the nature of threats which could lead to a structural collapse, Benyakar, Kutz, Dasberg, and Stern (1989) stated that four factors stand out as essential in specifying the traumatogenicity of an event. Loss, Unpredictability, Proximity (to the self- structure), and Suddenness, in various combinations of intensity, endow the threat with the potential for becoming a traumatic experience. Other researchers, such as Figley and McCubbin (1983), Rosenthal, Sadler, and Edwards (1987), and others, who see war events as uncontrollable and to some degree unexpected, life threatening, and likely to continue over long periods of time, have put forward the same idea. Shaw (1987) goes even further, stating that "war is a vast laboratory that provides opportunity to observe how individuals adapt to an actual psychic trauma inflicted from without in the form of continuous threats of injury and death."

RELIVING, REVISITING, RE-CREATING

The phenomenon of reliving and revisiting personal and communal traumas of the past, triggered by the current traumatic event, whether a personal one or as a result of a public disaster, is a crucial element in understanding the outpouring of public grief. Commemoration, whether public or private, is both a cognitive act and an act of seeking to learn and preserve memories of the deceased. These acts are a part of our natural defense and survival mechanism. Creating memorials and myths, collecting and preserving pictures, writing, preserving, and creating articles of importance to the deceased help us re-live and rearrange within ourselves the events of our losses while enabling us to continue in our daily life tasks, and even in fulfilling our life's mission, each according to his/her beliefs.

In his film "Out of Love, Be Back Soon," Dan Katzir (1997), a student studying film production at Tel Aviv University, accidentally stumbled onto an example of a current traumatic event reactivating the process of reliving the trauma of a past event. He was filming his grandmother, the wife of the late scientist Aaron Katzir who was massacred at Ben Gurion airport in 1972 by Kozo Acomoto, a Japanese Red Brigade terrorist. During the filming, she received a phone call telling her about the terrorist attack on a bus in Tel Aviv. Watching the film one can see her grief surging. She then invited her grandson to see the scrapbook she created, and until then never shared with a soul. In it was his blood soaked passport, newspaper articles, the doll he brought back for a granddaughter, photos, and other memorabilia. With the showing came the sharing of memories, stories, and sharing the grief. Witztum and Malkinson (1998) claim that rumination is an identified act known to assist the person in grasping the new reality. In fact, it is the very beginning of a cognitive understanding of this new reality. Rumination has also a cathartic effect emerging from the repetitious pattern of going through the details of the death event. Thus Dan, by including this segment in the film and by later showing it on national television, helped people to understand the need for personal journeys of commemoration.

In order to remember and commemorate, we employ different commemorative devices—headstones, monuments, houses, statues, commemorative books, albums, poetry, gardens, trees, videos, music, naming streets, organizing memorial lectures, sports events, and many more creative commemoration rituals. These symbolic acts and creations help change the reality of the events they commemorate. Ochana (1998), in his article "Myths, Memory, History," writes that we understand a phenomenon by giving it a symbolic shape. The different manifestations which we employ help us shape the event. Language gives it a name, science provides laws with which to examine it, religion provides meaning, and art gives it form and shape. History arranges the "facts" in time and myths give it a particular angle from which to view it. Therefore, collective symbols show a particular world view of a group, creating a collective mythology. We, as humans, need to create our private and collective myths, since we tend to understand the language of myth. We can then take both, the act of creation and the myth, and use them in order to integrate the traumatic events and heal. Sometimes we even re-write a person's biography and regenerate him to suit our needs. Examples of this can be seen in the reactions to the recent assassination of the late Prime Minister Yitschak Rabin. The historic Rabin is assassinated, the mythical Rabin lives. Witztum and Malkinson (1998) discuss how television reinforced the image of Rabin as a leader and a strategist through interviews with family members, friends, and colleagues. Comrades and opponents alike helped reinforce the image of the leader who fought and fell in the battle for peace. The myth is created of one who's life is synonymous with that of the nation. This is not unlike what happened in the United States after President John F. Kennedy was assassinated. The most telling comparison according to Witztum and Malkinson (1998) is that of the massive television coverage after the assassination that was watched by almost all the nation. This massive media coverage marked the beginning of the media as a tool which not only delivers information in real time, but also shapes the "here and now" and has an impact on its viewers and readers. However, they also draw our attention to a symbolic analogy that can be drawn between the individual process of bereavement and the chain of reactions that took place socially. Using the "stage model" of grief, analogous reactions to an individual's grieving process could be observed in the behaviors displayed by the Israeli society at the time. Shock, disbelief, idealization, and devaluation, accusations and counter accusations, and the controversy over memorialization procedures were coupled with efforts to return to a routine at the public level. The stage model of grief alerts us to observe similar reactions in an individual who is grieving.

A NEW VISUAL LANGUAGE

Hundreds of "memorial candles" were lit spontaneously even by adolescents at the assassination site of the late Prime Minister Rabin, leading to the coining of a new idiom in the Hebrew Language "Candle Children." From the television coverage of the Rabin Square, it appears as if this phenomenon of spontaneous outpouring of grief was inaugurated only after the Rabin assassination. However, the spontaneous unofficial public outpouring of grief used folk-art codes which were created and perfected in previous traumatic events. The first creation of instant folk-art started in March of 1993 at the Aliya St. in Tel Aviv where two men were knifed to death by a Palestinian. The same occurred at the Dizengoff bus explosion of 1994 which was shown in the Katzir (1997) film. Perhaps the occasion afforded an opportunity to individuals to transform their individual grief to public rage. Memorial candles arranged in the shape of a Star of David after the explosion at Beit Lid, January 22, 1995, were followed by candles arranged in the shape of the number 18 after the explosion on the number 18 bus in Jerusalem shortly thereafter.

Besides candles, which are a temporary, self consuming memorial, people started to erect more permanent, not officially sanctioned, memorials. One of the first was after the disaster in Beit Lid. David Shabat, a blacksmith from a small town, and Yehuda Blazer, an electrician from another town, have created a monument which was erected by them with volunteer help of friends without official sanction. Their motive was, in their words, "to make a frame for what people brought to the place." Indeed, the monument (Figure 1), which features a combination of a cut down tree and leaves on which the names of the victims appear, became a focal point for people who brought to it plants, pictures, even poetry. The meaning which Blazer wanted to convey is that "we will not be cut out of here, and the trunk will remain." The need to create order in the chaos of the universe, order in time and in the world, is one of the first impulses in any creative art form. The need of bringing order into a chaotic, traumatic event is served well by using an artistic symbolic language.

As the fear of becoming the next victims to an unpredictable attack grows, and as the trust in the protective power of the establishment lessens, official commemorative sites are no longer fulfilling the needs of the public. They were never conducive to private empathic outpouring of grief by people who are not directly connected to the bereaved families. I remember as a child, being always the wreath carrier to the official monument commemorating my brother and his company on the anniversary of their death every year (Figure 2). The bereaved families and some officials were the only ones present, and there were never any signs of others using those sights as places of commemoration (Figure 3).

The winter of 1996 brought with it a wave of terrorist attacks which increased the number of families who were personally involved. This struck a deep fear in the population, and was expressed by solidarity commemorations in the affected communities. A variety of cultural and local symbols were employed in the commemorative gatherings. A forgotten stone pile in a neighborhood in Jerusalem became an instant memorial. The stones were painted in every color but black by a group calling themselves "the neighbourhood kids." The stone pile was made to resemble the colorful Mimuna table, a Sefardic tradition of celebrating the end of Passover with a table of colorful foods signifying renewal and fertility. However, after the second explosion of bus number 18, the same neighborhood lit torches decorated by black ribbons.: black ribbons, which are made of impermanent material, but not black stones which are enduring. What we see here is an act of spontaneous grief and commemoration, employing a language which receives approval by society as legitimate and normative.

Private commemorations, while creating a link to the loss and becoming a personal journey, are nevertheless culturally dependent. A Druz (a religious sect living in Israel and Syria) woman's

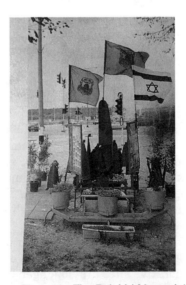

Figure 1. The Beit Lid Memorial.

commemoration of her husband who was killed in action in 1996 fighting a terrorist attack, consists of having his picture placed on his favorite chair, airing his clothes weekly, and waiting. A Druz legend says that the soul of the deceased will migrate into a child, who will come to announce to the family that he is the reincarnation of the deceased one. That is what she is waiting for.

The need to share the pain of loss leads people to create a variety of objects. A recent exhibition (March 1998), "Memory Design" at Ascola Gallery in Tel Aviv, had ample examples of people's use of objects large

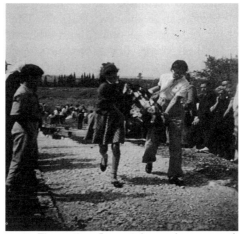

Figure 2. The author (in pants) carrying a wreath.

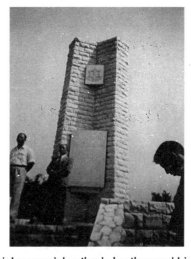

Figure 3. Official memorial author's brother and his company.

and small to express and share their grief. What struck me particularly, as an art therapist, was the natural way in which people turned to creative means in order to relieve their pain and grow and integrate their experiences. There was the Torah Scroll, written painstakingly so that the Torah will live on after the victim dies. The ceremony of bringing it into the Synagogue is likened to the wedding ceremony. The symbolic link is not hard to understand. In my work with bereaved individuals I often observe symbolic transferences in the use of common materials, and use them to enhance the healing process. I encourage people to create boxes, or even use envelopes in order to have internal spaces within which to store important objects of memory. On the outside I encourage them to display items that they wish to share with others. The activity of creating the spaces, choosing what to keep inside and what to display, reaffirms the need of the individual for privacy as well as sharing. The therapist is seen as respecting the pace with which the individual is able to take items from inside the box or envelope and display them on the outside, thus legitimizing the internal reorganization process. The flexibility mastered by the process and the ability to create new "realities" may aid in the process of becoming more flexible and in the reorganization of the self.

At the exhibition, I was impressed with a special pendant fashioned exquisitely. It was designed to be worn by a mother and two sisters as their way of being able to talk about their loss every time someone remarks about it. This answered a deep emotional need to talk and share the pain. Myrim Berman memorializes his son, Gabriel, who was born and died during Hanukkah, with a collection of Hanukkah menorahs he has been creating for twenty-five years. One was given to President Clinton, who used it to light the first Hanukkah candle in the traditional White House Ceremony (Haaretz Newspaper, December 30, 1997). A strong, emotional direct symbolic link exists between death, earth, and nature. The planting of trees as a living and growing memorial has been encouraged by Jewish tradition, and has been accepted into other cultures as well. Arela Tal chose to commemorate her brother by building a special space of wood, gravel, and concrete steps in a forest near her community. The place serves as a permanent site for people to come and communicate with nature. Friends who came to help in the building of the site commented that the act of creation helped relieve the pain of the loss.

One of the newer forms of private-public sharing are the privately produced music CDs and videotapes. They combine a celebration of the life, which has ended, and the special talents of the person commemorated thus. People use their talents, to express and to share their grief, via various art forms, as well as to link it to a collective grief. "Akedat Aran" (Aran's Sacrifice) is a poem written by Eitan Peretz (Peretz, E., 1997), Aran's father, during the time of the Shiva (the 7 days of mourning after burial). It was put to music and sang on the Shloshim—the commemoration service occurring on the thirtieth day after burial. It talks about a private sacrifice, but links it symbolically to the biblical sacrifice and to a national sacrifice.

Akedat Aran—Aran's Sacrifice

My father built an Altar
And to me he said:
"Go chop some wood
the sacrificial lamb
will appear in the bushes"
And I said "I am here, take me . . ."

My son Aran
lies bound,
his eyes gazing at the heavens
too simple to ask and understand.

My father hands the blade to me
And to me he said:
"God will provide us with solace
May his Name be Hallowed"
And I said "I am here, take me . . ."

My father built an Altar
And I mended its cracks,
Fixed its stairs
and my son, Aran, on top
lies wallowing in his blood
not knowing whether tears or earth his fists contain.

And I cry out: "My son! My son!
would only I died in your stead"

Aran, one of seventy-three young men killed in a helicopter accident (February 4, 1997) over Shear Yishuv, a village in Northern Israel, became a symbol for the tragedy. The whole country was in shock, and the grief code of candles, flowers, poems, etc. became almost institutionalized—even commercialized. "Hamashbir Latzarchan," a chain of twenty-two department stores, has instructed all its branches to create a memorial window display. The code was known by now. Candles, strewn flowers, and hand written signs in black ink. The motivation was undoubtedly the same strong feelings which drove many private citizens without direct connection to the disaster to express their grief. However, the connection between commercial interests and the need to identify with the national feelings of grief seems more than tenuous. Shefi (1998) discusses the bi-lateral direction of the new visual language of grief which people created. The symbols were created by ordinary people in the community. Therefore she contends that the influences came first from the grass roots "below," then the symbols were integrated and used by the establishment "above." In time they became entrenched as a new accepted language, which people embellish and build upon.

It was inevitable that political and national interests will also add their interpretation to the developing visual language of commemoration. The long held traditions of commemorating fallen soldiers by means of monuments, street names, songs, and commemorative books, according to Feiige (1998), facilitate the connection between the individual sacrifice and the national interest and give another meaning, a more noble dimension, to death. Victims of terror, on the other hand, become often "martyred" by nationalistic political movements. Here too we can see a different visual commemorative language evolving, incorporating the road side monument with the building of a new community. The Rechelim settlement was established in the place where Rachel Druk, a passenger and mother of seven, and Yitzchak Rofe, the bus driver, were killed in an ambush. Women have taken up a vigil, and finally were successful in establishing in the national consciousness a connection between the biblical Rachel who died in childbirth "on the road," and the contemporary Rachel Weis, who was burnt to death with her three children when a Molotov Cocktail was thrown into her car near the same place where now Rachel Druk was killed. A yearly pilgrimage to Rechelim, the new community, has become a metaphor for the road which the entire nation is undertaking—a process of constant ascent toward a place which has a rich meaningful past. Thus we create a familiar image out of an unknown stranger, and conceive an icon. Rachel Druk has become a conduit into a collective Jewish memory of other "Rachels," and re-connects that memory to the present and the future.

CONCLUSION

The ultimate grief, however, is still the one the immediate family endures. After the public has expressed its solidarity and has used the occasion to further its own private grief work, the family is left alone again to continue with life. They are left with the memories, the pictures, sometimes writings, film, video, and any other tangible creations and objects belonging to the deceased loved one. They are left with the need to remember, not forget. In the silence of the passing time we sometimes find new courage to grow in spite of, or dare I say because of, the loss.

I conclude with a poem by Aran Peretz, the boy who was killed in the helicopter disaster. He says it better then I ever could. His mother sent me a booklet she published (Peretz, S., 1997) to mark the occasion of a year passing since his death and in celebration of his life. In it are precious photographs taken of him and by him, portions from a personal diary, and poetry no one knew he wrote. The poem I chose is titled ironically, "Akeda?"—"Sacrifice" which he wrote without any knowledge of his father's poem by the same name. It was written February 9, 1994, before joining the army. It was triggered by the incident in Lebanon in which Tal Cohen, a friend, was killed.

Akeda?!—Sacrifice?!

Marching, marching, wet boots
young children, dressed in green.
Fierce rain is pouring, all is water logged
and the road twists, the end is still far.
A silent march, long hours
There, in the gates, an enemy waits . . .

Mother—
Till when will you send me, while he holds the knife?
You know—they will not always find a ram to sacrifice!

Marching, marching, red boots
Young children, clad in white.
Fierce rain is pouring, all is full of tears
Weeping cries are rising—the world darkens.
A silent march, yes—their road is done
And the mother stands mourning her son . . .

Oh, my dear sons—
I guard you even while sending you to face the knife
Only thus will you protect me, the homeland,
Only through weapons—blood and tears.
If only you were the last sacrifice
that we give to pay for peace!

The translations are mine, but I am not a poet. I am merely a catalyst, trying to bring together elements which might work to create a chemistry of healing. By observing and adapting the processes which people naturally create in order to become whole again, we may learn how to help those who's capacity to function, heal, and reorganize their inner self has been impaired by trauma and grief. Unfortunately, as I am concluding the writing of this chapter, the situation in the Middle East is unstable again. The American Embassy has ordered their nationals out of Israel, and Gas Mask distribution centers are open again around the clock. What we have learned may need to be implemented too soon. Today, the clouds have dispersed, and a beautiful sun has been shining. Let us hope the war clouds will similarly disperse.

REFERENCES

Benyakar, M., Kutz, I., Dasberg, H., & Stern, M. J. (1989). The collapse of a structure: A structural approach to trauma. *Journal of Traumatic Stress, 2*(4), 431-449.

Buydens-Branchey, L., Noumair, D., & Branchey, M. (1990). Duration and intensity of combat exposure and posttraumatic stress disorder in Vietnam veterans. *The Journal of Nervous and Mental Disease, 178*(9), 582-587.

Chimienty, G., Nasr, J. A., & Kahlifeh, I. (1989). Children's reactions to war-related stress. Affective symptoms and behaviour problems. *Social Psychiatry and Psychiatric Epidemiology, 24*(6), 282-287.

Feiige, M. (1998). Myths, memory, history. In *Memorialization Design,* Part 2, Askola Gallery of Design Ltd., Cat. #21/98, Achad Haam 84, Tel Aviv, Israel, 652006 (in Hebrew).

Figley, C. R., & McCubbin, H. I. (Eds.) (1983). *Stress and the family, Vol. II: Coping with catastrophe. Catastrophes an overview of family reactions* (pp. 3-20). New York: Brunner/Mazel.

Heimberg, R. G. (1985). Defining traumatic stress: Some comments on the current terminological confusion. *Behaviour Therapy, 16,* 419-423.

Katzir, D. (1997). *Out of Love, Be Back Soon.* Film and Video, Israel Television, Channel 1.

Ochana, D. (1998). Myths, memory, history. In *Memorialization Design,* Part 2, Askola Gallery of Design Ltd., Cat. #2 1/98, Achad Haam 84, Tel Aviv, Israel, 652006 (in Hebrew).

Peretz, E. (1997). Akedat Aran. *Akedat Aran,* Music CD, self-produced, Degania A, Israel.

Peretz, S. (Ed.) (1997). *Aran,* Peretz family and Degania family production, Degania A, Israel.

Rosenthal, D., Sadler, A., & Edwards, W. (1987). Families and post-traumatic stress disorder. *Family Therapy Collection, 22,* 81-95.

Roth, S., & Cohen, L. J. (1986). Approach, avoidance, and coping with stress. *American Psychologist, 41*(7), 813-819.

Saigh, P. (1984). Pre- and Post-invasion anxiety in Lebanon. *Behaviour Therapy, 15,* 185-190.

Shaw, J. A. (1987). Unmasking the illusion of safety. *Bulletin of the Menninger Clinic, 51*(1), 49-63.

Shefi, S. (1998). Myths, memory, history. In *Memorializing Design,* Part 2, Askola Gallery of Design Ltd., Cat. #21/98, Achad Haam 84, Tel Aviv, Israel, 652006 (in Hebrew).

Solomon, Z., Garb, R., Bleich, A., & Grupper, D. (1987). Reactivation of combat-related posttraumatic stress disorder. *Journal of Psychiatry, 144*(1), 51-55.

Solomon, Z., Avitzur, E., & Mikulincer, M. (1989). Coping resources and social functioning following combat stress reaction: A longitudinal study. *Journal of Social and Clinical Psychology, 8*(1), 87-96.

Solomon, Z., Oppenheimer, B., Elizur, Y., & Waysman, M. (1990). Exposure to recurrent combat stress: Can successful coping in a second war heal combat-related PTSD from the past? *Journal of Anxiety Disorders, 4,* 141-145.

Steele, K., & Cox, T. (1986). Psychological and physiological reactions to visual representations of war. *International Journal of Psychophysiology, 3,* 237-252.

Sutker, P. B., Thomason, B. T., & Allain, A. B., Jr. (1989). Adjective self-description of World War II and Korean prisoner of war and combat veterans. *Journal of Psychopathology and Behavioural Assessment, 11*(2), 185-192.

Witztum, E., & Malkinson, R. (1998). Death of a leader: The social construction of bereavement. In E. S. Zinner & M. B. Williams (Eds.), *When a community weeps: Case studies in group survivorship.* Philadelphia: Brunner/Mazel.

CHAPTER 18

Viewing the Body and Grief Complications: The Role of Visual Confirmation in Grief Reconciliation

Richard J. Paul

From the perspective that grief is a natural human reaction to any loss, it is the circumstances of the loss and/or the world view of the bereaved that causes complicated grief. Loss by death of a traumatic or tragic nature can facilitate complicated grief. The perspective and the choices of the griever at the time of death can cause later complications in grief reconciliation.

"I want to remember him alive," "Viewing the body is barbaric." Statements such as these are growing more common in response to viewing a dead person's body as part of the funeral rituals. Resistance to viewing the dead body as part of the funeral process has gradually increased over the last fifty years to the point where a closed casket, or no casket, is becoming more and more a part of a standard funeral practice.

Perhaps it is not a coincidence that during the same period of time, death and dying have become more institutionalized, less visible, and isolated from the day-to-day experience of the general public. Lack of experience with the realities of aging, dying, and death have caused these subjects to become unfamiliar, engendering a fear of the unknown. Naturally, the body is the most powerful symbol of death and, therefore, the object of the "fear of death."

The procedure of viewing the dead body of a significant person is a ritual that predates human history. Although viewing the body has been an integral part of the survivor's adaptation to the death of another human being, across cultures and throughout time, during the last half of the twentieth century North American Funeral Directors have seen the practice rejected by a small but steadily expanding number of the bereaved.

The funeral service in North America has evolved to specialize in serving the practical, social, emotional, and spiritual needs of those affected by a death. This vocation arose from the simple root of an individual in the community, often a cabinet maker (who made caskets) or livery owner (who provided a horse-drawn hearse). This person, through repetitive exposure, came to know the local customs, procedures, and legalities related to funerals and would be consulted by the recently bereaved for assistance. As our society has become increasingly industrialized, nuclear, faster-paced, and specialized, the funeral director continues to provide many services based on this original, simple concept of acting as a resource to be consulted.

Funeral Directors offer both information and facilitation around the subject of viewing the body. To continue as a resource for the grieving client, modern Funeral Directors and other counselors are challenged: to understand the objections of those who resist viewing; to identify the purposes and benefits of viewing the body; to communicate these purposes and benefits effectively, without pressure.

The questions, rationalizations against, and objections to viewing that are most frequently heard are these:

1. What's the point of viewing?
2. It was his/her wish.
3. Promoting "Viewing the Body" is self-serving for the funeral director.
4. Viewing the body is primitive and barbaric.
5. I want to remember him or her as healthy/alive/as he or she was.
6. But he or she has failed/was injured so badly.
7. With the long illness we have suffered enough.
8. We just want private viewing.
9. The emphasis should be on God/the spirit, not the dead body.
10. Viewing the body is unnecessary or irrelevant.

These ten positions, whether self-created or instilled by socialization, do introduce obstacles to viewing during the funeral process. In my frustration with being unable to consistently convey the value of viewing the body to every client, I reached out to my fellow funeral directors as well as to clergy and others. I wanted to establish a consensus as to whether or not viewing had value. I also wanted to learn from funeral directors: what they thought those values were; some of their examples that demonstrate these values; how they had successfully conveyed this information to their clients. As seen in the responses to this survey, many funeral directors have first-hand experience with how not viewing the body has perhaps unnecessarily complicated the grieving process for the bereaved.

Surveys were sent out in Ontario to 200 funeral homes and twenty local clergy. There were fifty-eight Funeral Directors, twenty-three Student Funeral Directors, ten Clergy, four Secretary/Receptionist/

Assistants, and two Bereavement Counselors for a total of ninety-seven respondents. Many respondents shared examples of clients, or of a very personal nature, that were both moving and compelling.

The survey was composed of three open-ended questions which made it necessary to identify common themes in the answers in order to quantify the responses. Within each individual survey, where a specific point or answer was given in response to one question and then repeated in another answer, that point was only recorded once. Following the separate tally of responses by each segment of the respondents, the responses of each were blended into a total for each point. The resulting lists of responses to each question are ordered by the frequency of their appearance. For the purpose of this chapter only the first five responses to each question are included.

1. In your opinion, in general, is viewing the dead body of a loved one helpful, unhelpful, or irrelevant to the grief recovery process. (96 of 97 respondents specifically said it was helpful). Explain your answer.

71 Promotes accepting the reality/seeing is believing/helps cut through shock and denial

33 Helps to begin the grief recovery process

32 Facilitates saying good-bye/helps with closure

27 Helps to see the deceased at peace

13 Those who don't view have most difficulty during funeral and later

2. From your experience would you please briefly share one, or more, examples of funerals which you recall that clearly demonstrates your answer above.

26 Families thanked funeral director for chance to view/giving them back their loved one

15 Sudden and/or traumatic deaths, i.e., car accident, suicide, when grievers indicated viewing helped

14 Related professional or personal experiences where viewing was helpful or missed and regretted

14 Had examples of families who didn't view and are still waiting for deceased to come home

11 Reported families wanting closed casket, changing their minds and glad they left it open

3. If you were called upon by a family to counsel them about viewing or not viewing, what reason(s) or point(s) would you offer for their consideration?

34 Viewing facilitates seeing, touching, sharing, crying, laughing, resolving unfinished business, and good-bye/closure

26   Seeing is believing/moves family past disbelief and denial/starts the grieving process

16   Informed consent is the goal

16   It is reassuring to see deceased at peace, dressed and prepared in a dignified manner

15   Said they use previous true examples relevant to the situation at hand

Throughout the responses there is a near absolute certainty that if the family chooses viewing, they find it helpful. And on the other side of the equation where either viewing is not possible, or not chosen, the respondents indicated from their experience that these survivors had a higher frequency of complication in their grieving. Every response helped shape and build my conviction that viewing should be considered by the bereaved, and encouraged by the professionals, in almost every situation. In those circumstances where resistance or objections are expressed, the client should never be pressured but the specific objections should be explored as thoroughly and diplomatically as possible, so that additional information and alternate perspectives may be offered in the client's best interest.

Funeral directors may have the initial exposure to the complications associated with not viewing the body, but the real work of dealing with complicated grief often begins long after the funeral and often involves the professional assistance of grief counselors. In her article, *The Value of Viewing in GriefWork Reconciliation: A Psychotherapists Perspective,* Kelly Osmont (1993) describes some of her experiences which have led her to believe in the value of viewing the body. She also relates a rather unique method of supporting those experiencing complicated grief where the body has not been seen.

In one support group where every member had not seen the dead body of their loved one, Ms. Osmont obtained their permission to gather any photos taken by the various authorities and agencies attending the death scene. In careful detail Kelly Osmont relates the procedure by which she introduced these photos to her clients and in each case when they saw the photos, "It was as if they were being told for the first time about the death, and we were viewing their intense grief reactions encapsulated in a 20 to 30 minute time-span."

Dr. Earl Grollman and Todd Van Beck are both authors and educators in the areas of death, grief, and funerals. Immediately following the bombing at Oklahoma's Federal Building, both rushed to the city to offer whatever support they could. Both men have since reported their individual experiences with the bereaved who wanted, needed, and were grateful for the opportunity to see any part of the body of their loved one. This same experience was reported by several funeral directors in the survey confirming the maxim, "Beauty is in the eye of the beholder."

Therese Rando (1993), in her book *Complicated Grief,* described her model of grief recovery called "The Six "R" Processes of Mourning in Relation to the Three Phases of Grief and Mourning." In the Avoidance Phase, the first process, Recognize the Loss, involves two sections, Acknowledge the Death and Understand the Death. Dr. Rando says that the initial acceptance of a death is on an intellectual level. "It will take much longer to internalize this fact and accept it emotionally" (p. 44). According to Rando, when people have either been unable or have chosen not to view the body, problems may occur. "A high percentage of mourners who experience complications either have not viewed the body or have failed to participate in funeral rituals" (p. 46).

However, it was in her *Grief, Dying and Death, Clinical Interventions for Caregivers* (1984) that Rando most clearly and succinctly validated the practice of viewing the body.

> Viewing the body is often quite helpful as it challenges the normal desire to deny the loss while promoting acceptance of the death. Participating in the funeral ritual—standing at a wake and repeatedly looking at the deceased in the casket, attending a funeral service, accepting the condolences of others, witnessing the casket at the grave—graphically illustrates to the bereaved that the death has indeed occurred. Even if it cannot be emotionally accepted at that time, the memories of the experiences will later help to confirm to the bereaved the reality of the loss of the loved one. Viewing the body has been criticized in recent years, as some mourners have wished to avoid the painful reactions that seeing the body can engender. However, it is precisely the impact of the finality of the loss that viewing seeks to promote. Clearly the body of the deceased is the best symbol of the individual and therefore the most effective one to focus upon in attempting to perceive the deceased in a new relationship, as someone who is no longer alive and will only exist in memory. The custom of viewing the body not only promotes realization of the loss, especially after sudden or accidental death, but also, through proper preparation and restoration of the body, assists in recall of the individual prior to any disfigurement from pain, accident or violence. This preparation is not designed to make the deceased look alive, but to provide an acceptable image for recollection of the deceased. The presence of the body provides an immediate and proper climate for mourning and is a natural symbol to stimulate discussion and expression of emotion about the deceased. (pp. 180-181)

The "real experts," as Dr. Earl Grollman describes everyday people dealing with their grief, validate what the clinicians and the educators have found to be true. In a *Woman's Day* magazine article, Lois Duncan described how in her family children were always spared the rituals of grief and, "The first funeral I ever attended was my mother's. I was an adult and the mother of three at the time." Having no previous experience with funerals she insisted the casket remain closed and her children were not involved. She found that for her children, "Their grandmother's death is not a reality for them." After attending her mother-in-law's funeral, which included an open casket, she concluded, "I now believe that I did our children an injustice by not giving them the opportunity to come to grips with the death of their grandmother at her funeral. In my effort to shield them from pain, I may have left open an emotional door that they'll have to struggle for years to close."

During the introduction period of a workshop I presented on this subject at the 1998 King's College conference on Complicated Grief, a participant related the experiences she had had following her first and second husbands' deaths. At the time of her first husband's death, the family arranged for an immediate cremation of his body without a funeral. During the ensuing years they discovered that the choices they had made had not been helpful. The woman began to do research into grief and had viewing and a funeral following her second husband's death. Her question to me was, "Why didn't anyone at the hospital or the funeral home talk to us about the decision we were making when my first husband died?" Her question reiterates the point that a Funeral Director is a consultant, an expert in the area of funerals, and has a professional obligation to offer alternatives and discuss the pros and cons of each.

Drawing from the examples and comments shared by the respondents to the survey conducted for this chapter, the next portion of this chapter includes verbatim responses which help to demonstrate various points being made. For me the following anecdote was the most moving and demonstrative illustration of the need for visual confirmation of the death, and the funeral director's role as an advocate and facilitator of this process.

[A] young woman killed under an industrial type lawnmower. (Worst condition I've seen in 15 years!) Body was unviewable, due to pieces only we had. Mom/Dad and husband were adamant about their denial and it escalated until funeral day. They would not allow the funeral to happen 'till they saw her. All fellow funeral directors said "No way!" From grief standpoint, I knew they had to! Convinced my boss: brought clergy and investigating detectives in and the coroner to sit with all of them. I had the father stand next to me—knowing that in grief our mind plays crueller tricks than what reality is. I touched him on his head, arms, legs and body to show what parts we had of her. The mom and husband backed off in insisting to see her—Dad's anger and disbelief were as strong as ever. So into the visitation room to open the casket we went—with cops, clergy and doctor. When he saw her hand and some of her hair—immediately his disposition changed and the reality helped him to relax—he hugged everyone of us and his wife and son-in-law cried in trust of him. The funeral home received a *great* thank you note about *me* and how I was the only one who would listen to them and they brought me flowers afterwards. I follow-up with them extensively, too.

With all the insight provided by the survey, related readings and my personal experience, it becomes much easier to respond to the resistance and objections to viewing the body.

1. What's the point of viewing?

The primary reasons for viewing are these:
Seeing is believing, the more senses involved in assimilating the reality the better. It cuts through the shock, the disbelief, the denial, and sets a foundation upon which to do grief work.
Viewing helps to bring closure to the physical relationship, allows saying good-bye.
Viewing initiates the grief process for most people.
Viewing offers the opportunity to see the deceased at peace, not suffering.
Viewing avoids the possibility of later regret about not seeing the deceased.
Viewing after professional preparation of the body is never associated with complicated grief, but the experts (clinical therapists) say that many complicated grieving patterns involve not having seen the body.
Viewing provides the simple reality of death for children; otherwise death is an abstract subject that children have trouble dealing with.
"Clearly the body of the deceased is the best symbol of the individual and therefore the most effective one to focus upon, attempting to perceive the deceased in a new relationship, as someone who is no longer alive and will only exist in memory."

Imagination will work to fill the gap of sensory information, often thwarting the progress of grieving. A funeral director related,

[My] most vivid recollection is of a service where a young husband was a professional truck driver killed in vehicle mishap and consequent fire in his truck cab in a S.W., U.S. state. His remains were not recognizable. Parents accepted requirement for casket to be closed. Young widow of deceased went into "full" denial. Parents suggested that the casket be nailed shut because widow said she was going to open—"no matter what!" We turned casket backwards. At conclusion of each visitation we would have to clean smeared fingerprints from wife trying to open, and others having need to "see" the body. Widow figured dead husband was trying to defraud insurance company and was in hiding only to call her when it was "safe" to come out.

A bereavement counselor observed, "Although viewing the body may be an emotionally painful event, grief is a painful event. Unfortunately, avoiding the pain is not usually an effective way through grief." And a funeral director, who is also a certified grief educator, observed, "I have also noticed the emotional chemistry in the visitation room following the first viewing is much less charged and anxious as opposed to the closed casket visitation. Once the family has viewed their loved one, they seem to settle down."

2. *It was his / her wish*

This is perhaps the most frequent and challenging issue the funeral director must respond to regarding the open casket and viewing. The challenge is to help the client sort out what they want in the face of the deceased's request for a closed casket, and then to validate their decision.

My primary method of responding to this statement is as follows:

1. Ask, "Do you know why he/she said that?"
2. Ask, "How do you feel about that?"
3. If there is no uncertainty by those in attendance, I ask if there is any family member not present or at a distance who has expressed a desire, or may wish, to see the deceased. If there is none, then the issue, and the casket, is closed.
4. If the client indicates any regret or hesitation about not having viewing, I ask, "If the deceased hadn't made the statement about a closed casket, would you wish to see him/her?"
5. If the answer is affirmative, I then ask, "Was the person deliberately cruel or hurtful?"
6. The answer is always, "No!"
7. Then I say, "Perhaps the deceased made the statement not knowing two things:
   (i) That you would want and need to see him/her once more and it would hurt you if you couldn't.
   (ii) That viewing the body is very important to the grieving process for the survivors."
8. I then make the statement that, "The funeral is for the living, not the dead, and the survivors are responsible for taking care of themselves so that both today and years from now there will be no regrets." If the deceased did love them, and was not being intentionally cruel, then the survivors must make the decision to view or not to view based on their needs.
9. I then offer them the suggestion that they view privately prior to the public visitation but I remind them that there may be others either in the family or friends who may also need this opportunity for their grief journey.
10. Often after the private viewing, the casket is left open for everyone else.

One Funeral Director shared this story,

A man wanted to be cremated immediately following death. His wife came in to prearrange [the funeral] about two weeks before he died and explained this to me. I asked if all the family were satisfied with this (11 children). She said most were, but [all] wanted to follow their father's wishes. She then told me about a granddaughter who went into the hospital room, saw her grandfather hooked to tubes, and went into hysterics. She would not go back in the room. I suggested that they consider having a short visitation after death, if not for [the] public, at least for family. After discussing this, she left, discussed options with [the] family. When the granddaughter in question came to the funeral home, they practically dragged her into the room. When she left, she came up to me, hugged me and thanked me for giving her back her grandfather. He now looked like himself and wasn't hooked up to all the machines. It was truly a satisfying experience.

The uninformed desires about no viewing expressed while alive can be an altogether unnecessary additional burden for the bereaved to shoulder during grief. A funeral home receptionist recalled, "One young lady held the rail of her mother's closed casket for two days visiting. It was just heartbreaking to see her sitting there hour after hour, holding onto a piece of wood. How much better it would have been for her to touch the face or hand of the mother she loved and mourned."

3. *Promoting "Viewing the Body" is self-serving for the funeral director*

Funeral directors did not invent the practice of viewing. All that funeral directors have done regarding the practice of viewing the body is facilitate the experience. They do recognize the enduring value of viewing the body as part of the grieving process. And one of the key services provided by North American funeral homes is the option of sanitation, preservation, and restoration of embalming the body for viewing.

The embalming process preserves the body for the period of the funeral proceedings. Embalming renders the body safe and inoffensive to be near. By this method the body is restored to a familiar, composed, dignified, "at peace" appearance. All of this only helps the planning of the funeral, the travel of distant friends and relatives, the social support for, validation of, and the reality of the loss, and the celebration of the life of the one who died. As viewing the body was practiced before there was an occupation known as funeral director, it is no more pertinent to say that funeral directors facilitate viewing the body for their own gain than it is appropriate to say that surgeons perform surgery expressly for the profits.

When I am asked if I like embalming, my response is, "It's not that I like embalming but I like doing it well." In the short period of time that a funeral director has with a bereaved family, a strong bond and desire to help in any way possible very often develops. A funeral director shared these two examples. "We had one case where we were told by the family that they absolutely expected to see their son who was literally severed in half by a portable saw mill. It took a lot of time and effort but this young man was showable and you could just tell that this family needed that in order to go on." "Another case was a husband and wife who both passed away following a motor vehicle accident. Their three children were also in the vehicle, but they all survived but watched their parents die. It was crucial for the eldest child to see his parents. I remember doing hours of wax work and reconstruction, but in the end it was all worth it. The children were able to see and say good-bye to their parents which I felt couldn't have been more necessary."

4. *Viewing the body is primitive and barbaric*

Certainly the custom of viewing the body predates recorded history, and could therefore be called "primitive." It is precisely because viewing serves our most basic needs and methods of understanding and adapting to the reality of a death that this practice has survived.

The charge of barbarism is simply misplaced. The barbarians roamed through the countryside raping, pillaging, and murdering, leaving not only their victims, but also their fallen comrades, where they dropped. In contrast, the practice of treating "the last earthly remains" of our fellow human beings with a degree of dignity and reverence would seem far more civilized than barbaric.

During the reign of Queen Victoria, British Prime Minister Gladstone responded to a cartoon criticism of funeral directors which ran in the January 1885 issue of London's *PUNCH* with the statement, "Show me the manner in which a nation or community cares for its dead and I will measure with mathematical exactness the tender sympathies of its people, their respect of the laws of the land and their loyalty to high ideals" (Van Beck, 1993, p. 35).

The receptionist of a funeral home responded to the survey with several stories including this one.

> My sister's family considered viewing "barbaric," and at her husband's sudden death only agreed to viewing to conform to custom. After two days of viewing and visitation they were constantly commenting on the helpfulness of visitors' comments as they viewed. Because of the suddenness of death no one had been given a chance to say good-bye. The several trips to the casket, the good-byes after each successive viewing helped them so much to realize their loss and say their good-byes in their own ways and times. They were glad that they had chosen viewing.

Sometimes, the discomfort or lack of understanding about viewing by some family members or friends can make them quite self-righteous and cause them to interfere with the rights of the bereaved. A case in point was shared by this Funeral Director, "I can think of one mother who had a stillborn child. All of her family and friends had discouraged her from seeing the baby. Throughout the funeral the mother was very distraught. After the service while everyone was gathered at a reception the mother returned here [to the funeral home] alone and saw her child. Finally, she had some peace of mind and left feeling much calmer than she was earlier."

The efforts to prevent viewing are usually well-intentioned, if misguided. However, the goal of preventing pain from bereavement is doomed to failure because grief will find expression. Grief is only frustrated, and complicated, when viewing is thwarted. Another Funeral Director shared,

A young family lost their son of only 10 days, he had never made it out of the hospital. The mother really wanted to see her son. The father did not. Both the father and his side of the family felt the mother was very weak, overly emotional and not excepting their child's death. The mother also wanted to dress her son, because she never had the chance to do that while her son was alive. The father's side of the family did not think anyone should see the child let alone help dress him. The mother's side of the family did want to see the child. The mother did come in to help dress her son. Her husband waited outside the building. The mother did very well helping to dress her son (doing most of it herself) and seemed somewhat calmer afterwards.

The next day the family was to come in to the funeral home for private visiting before going to the church for the funeral The casket was only to be open for the parents and the mother's parents. None of the father's family wanted to the see the open casket. The father was only going into the room to give support to his wife. Once the father saw his son and spent some time with him, he went to his parents and suggested they may want to see him as well. End result was the casket remained open till it was time to leave for the church. All members of the family did see the baby.

A week or so after the funeral I received a phone call. The father's brother, who at the time of the funeral told me in no uncertain terms that it was very wrong for me to have allowed the mother to help dress her son and that I should have told the family that for an infant the casket should have been closed for everyone. This same man was calling me to thank me. He could not believe how much it meant to the mother to have been given the chance to dress her son and be a mother to him. He told me that even for himself it helped to see the baby looking like a baby rather than being in the hospital hooked up to all those machines. He apologized for saying that I was not doing my job and realized that by allowing the family choices and making them aware of their options I was doing what was in the best interest of the family.

5. *I want to remember him or her healthy / alive / as he or she was*

Of course, it is the goal and hope of everyone who has experienced the death of a loved one, that we will be able to hold onto the best memories of that person. The premise of this argument seems to be, "If I see him/her dead it will wipe out any memory of him/her alive." The contrary is more likely.

The challenge is to move from a relationship based on the physical presence to a new relationship based on the spirit, or memory, or love of the person who died. It would seem most efficacious, therefore, to acknowledge at all levels (sensory, emotional, intellectual, social, spiritual) the end of the physical in order to mark the beginning of the memory relationship.

One story from my own experience demonstrated for me not only the real need to see the body, but also to remember that indeed, "Beauty is in the eye of holder." Following the suicide of a young man in his late thirties by gun shot to the head, I spent six straight hours just trying to put the pieces back together because the family wanted to see him. Finally, I was finished but unsatisfied with the results so I called one of the deceased's siblings and asked him to just come and identify his brother before I placed his body in the casket and closed it.

The brother came into the embalming room alone and saw his brother dressed and prepared to be seen the best I was able, and after a few moments asked if it was all right if he went home to bring his mother into the funeral home. To make a long story short, within a short while there were sixteen people in the embalming room. After about forty-five minutes, I told them that I now needed to place his body in the casket and indicated they were welcome to either leave, stay or assist me with this procedure. Thirty-two hands lifted his body from the dressing table and gently placed him in the casket. The last remark I heard from a brother before I closed the casket was, "Doesn't he look beautiful."

6. *But he or she has failed / was injured so badly*

With the intervention of modern medicine, the last days of an individual's life can be drawn out for a long period of time, often involving intravenous tubes, breathing apparatus, medication, monitors, and other undignified and intrusive paraphernalia. The individual's body often ends up gaunt, dehydrated, in a coma with mouth agape and eyes staring blankly. The last view of the person alive can be quite disturbing and hardly how we would like to remember them. Thus the phrase, "Doesn't he/she look good!" arises from the peaceful appearance of the loved one's body after the funeral director has removed the unnecessary and restored the familiar in repose.

In the accidental or traumatic death, although the Funeral Director cannot make something from nothing, through the embalming and restorative process part or all of the deceased's body can usually be seen by the survivors in a familiar and inoffensive appearance.

As one Funeral Director related,

I had a wife whose husband died tragically and reconstruction was not an option. Disfigurement to his face was too extensive. The wife said to me that she had to see him, any part of him so she could come to terms with him dying We were able to show his hands with his wedding band on. I was not sure of her reaction to this, but after viewing just his hand, she told me she was now at peace with herself and could let herself mourn.

7. With the long illness we have suffered enough

With medical intervention, death can often be delayed long past what we once might have expected. Psychologists comment that this delay can afford the opportunity to begin some preparatory or anticipatory grieving. However, there is an optimum length of time for doing grief work determined by the relationships, the dynamics, and the situation beyond which the anticipated loss becomes like a Chinese torture. Work in anticipatory grief shows that the stress following a protracted period of dying can complicate the grieving process. Grievers can be emotionally and physically fatigued and have been shown to possess symptoms similar to those suffering from post-traumatic stress disorder. Research in this area reveals that the bereaved in this type of circumstance cannot begin their grieving until they have unwound from the stressful ordeal of the extended dying period.

The logical timing of the funeral following a death presents itself when the primary need of the survivors may be to debrief from their ordeal. However, the bereaved will benefit down the road from having gone through the rituals of viewing and a funeral ceremony following a death. In the months that follow, as the shell-shock of helplessly watching the long illness begins to wear off, those most affected by the death will have the advantage of remembering the funeral to help them finally begin the grieving process.

From my own experience I share a technique for doing grief work which, when used, often helps cut through the numbness and shock. We knew for almost five months that my father was going to die from his cancer. However, growing up in a second generation funeral home did nothing to prepare any of us for dealing with his impending death. When my father died I was unaware that I was left with lingering and, for me, important issues of unfinished business. Attending a course for Funeral Directors five years later, the instructor suggested that perhaps I did indeed have unfinished business with my father and gave me an assignment which I have developed into the following formula and share with every family I serve.

Amendments (then write below it)
"I'm sorry for . . . (and fill in whatever comes to mind and repeat it) . . . and I forgive myself."

"I'm sorry for . . . (do it again and again until nothing comes out) . . . and I forgive myself."

Forgivenesses (then write below it)
"I'm angry about . . . (fill it in, but add at the end) . . . and I forgive you."
"I was hurt when . . . and I forgive you." (repeat it until nothing comes to mind)

Other Significant Statements (then write whatever else is important to say)
"I love you" or "Thanks for . . ." are frequently sentiments that are left unexpressed.

When you have completed the list above, try saying out loud, "Good-bye."

Using this formula during the visitation period helps the bereaved to cut through their fatigue and focus on the matter at hand, saying good-bye to the physical relationship which has finally ended. People have stood by the open casket during private times and talked out loud to their loved one, and many letters have been placed in the casket following my suggestion of the formula above.

As one Funeral Director responded in the survey, "Because death interrupts relationships, people need to be able to say "good-bye." They want to see the physical person, not just look at a casket, a piece of furniture."

8. *We just want private viewing*

It may be a function of the myth of independence that says one should bear all one's own pain in private. It may arise from the very personal nature of grief which may cause all one's focus to turn inwards and disregard the pain of others. Whatever the cause there is an increasing sub-group of those opposed to viewing who will opt for allowing only the immediate family to see the body.

This decision should take into consideration the following points:

(i) Oftentimes the bond between people is stronger among friends, co-workers, than some family members. For these people their grief may well be frustrated by the lack of opportunity to visually confirm the death.

(ii) The poet John Donne (1986) wrote,

No man is an island entire of itself every man is a piece of the continent, a part of the main. If a clod is washed away by the sea, Europe is the less, as well as if a promontory were, as well as if a manor of thy friend's or of thine own were. Any man's death diminished me, because I am involved in mankind. (p. 1107)

To a greater or lesser degree everyone's death affects the community where that person lived.

(iii) The phrase, "A burden shared is a burden lessened" describes the very real process which occurs during viewing the body. Funerals, or memorial services, which seek only to "celebrate" the life without also acknowledging the loss do not provide a balanced perspective of the situation. Primary grievers do gain real support from the contact, the hugs, the handshakes, the smiles and tears that arise from sharing the reality of the loss with others during the viewing.

One Funeral Director responded to the survey in this manner,

> I will draw on my most recent personal experience. When my son-in-law died very suddenly at age thirty-three, it was devastating to our daughter (married 3 years) and of course to the rest of our family and his family. We were relieved when the decision was made to have the casket open and to have ample time for visitation. The benefit to the immediate family is often more obvious; but I will not forget so many of his colleagues standing for so long by the casket. They obviously needed this time to come to terms with this death of someone they had been working with just a few days prior. They lingered in the visitation room for long periods of time, chatting and sometimes laughing over some of the pictures which we had displayed. Because he was still visibly with us, it seemed like he was a very real part of what was taking place that day. I cannot imagine not having had the opportunity to share this with his friends.

9. The emphasis should be on God / the spirit, not the dead body

Cultural, religious, or family perspectives that hold no value or even discourage viewing can override any inclination to see a loved one's body. Rabbi Earl Grollman, in his response to this survey on viewing the body, stated that Judaism discourages viewing the body and this is generally accepted, but that, "Those who opted for viewing were grateful for (the) opportunity to say 'Shalom.' "

There are those who argue that as soon as a death has occurred the focus should immediately shift from the physical aspect of the deceased person to their spirit and to the comfort that comes from faith in God. However, this position equates the transition required after the death of a loved one to a simple, intellectual adjustment. In a way this position actually supports viewing because only the dead body confirms on all levels that the transition from physical to spirit has indeed occurred.

> It is important for us to realize that the rites and rituals that we use to mark the end of life are our efforts to say a significant and appropriate "Good-bye." We don't just dispose quickly of the bodies of those we love as if they were worthless. Some remnants of our love are still attached to them, whether we want to admit it or not. We cannot treat what we have loved without loving care without doing damage to all of the other loving relationships in life. (Jackson, 1966, p. 32)

In John (20:19), the disciple Thomas demonstrates the human need for empirical evidence when he demands to see the nail holes in the hands of the risen Christ, giving rise to the phrase, "doubting Thomas." The honest doubting of Thomas only led to his certainty about Jesus as his Lord and Savior when he could see with his own eyes. In the same way, the opportunity to use our senses of sight, touch, and hearing during the viewing of a dead body logically assists in accepting, and adapting to, the new reality created by the death of a loved one.

Author Doug Manning relates his experience on a religious talk show where the host repeatedly came around to the same issue of faith in the face of grief. Finally, Doug Manning realized the intent was to demonstrate by his testimony that those of faith do not need to grieve. His response was to say that God has built into each of us a method of dealing with loss and that is our ability to grieve.

A clergy person responding to the survey wrote,

> One's senses (touch, sight) should be given opportunity to agree and support what you know—that your loved one is dead. If your senses are denied this stimuli, an important source of information is lost (which is unfortunate as many people's greatest method of learning is through visual information) and a tension and conflict develops—your lack of sensory information contradicts the information your brain knows to be true. The result is your feelings are drawing from two contradictory sources. I am confident that this conflict can only result in a less gentle road for the "griever" to travel.

Following a death, the funeral activities that ensue serve a number of purposes on the physical, cognitive, affective, and spiritual levels. Among the most obvious are the celebration of life, and this includes not just the individual who has died but God, as understood by the survivors, as the source of all life, comfort, and consolation. However, just as we are in the world but not of the world, our humanity that experiences loss and suffers also provides us with the means of assimilating and adjusting to the death. With a deeper understanding and appreciation of life that can only come from a full-frontal confrontation with how fleeting and precious human life is, we also have the opportunity to glimpse the unseen, the energy that binds us, the undying nature of love.

In the face of contrary cultural, religious, or family perspectives, the practice of viewing can only be offered as being considered a benefit by many, experts and grievers alike. The funeral director, or other counselor, can only present information and choices as is deemed appropriate without any investment in the outcome. The old adage; "You may lead a horse to water, but you can't make it drink" is especially applicable here.

10. *Viewing the body is unnecessary or irrelevant*

This argument can originate from at least two sources:

(i) In situations where the survivor had no cathexis, or no love invested in the one who died, it may very simply be true that seeing the dead body is irrelevant because there was no relationship which needs decathexis, or to be formally ended, in order for a memory relationship to begin.

(ii) The rational perspective maintains that following a death the adjustment is simply a logical one and viewing is irrelevant to this process. In our society, the dominant view of reality is that the rational mind is superior to the physical, emotional, and spiritual aspects of our humanity. For individuals who maintain that the mind should rule the heart, it would appear on the surface that there is no point in pursuing the subject, and occasionally that may be the case.

However, it may appeal to the logical mind to reflect upon the observation of Italian physician and educator Maria Montessori (1870-1952), who said that our best learning experiences are ones that connect our senses with the learning process. The role of the senses in learning was further validated by Columbia University research (1982) which determined that we remember 10 percent of what we hear, 25 percent of what we see, and 90 percent of what we do. An enduring piece of wisdom is the 2000 year old Chinese proverb, "I hear and I forget, I see and I remember, I do and I understand" which reminds us that seeing and being involved in the changes of our lives helps us to internalize them.

The reality that a loved one has died is one of the most significant facts we have to learn in our lives. To enhance our acknowledgment and understanding of the reality of the death, it only makes sense to involve our senses.

Dr. Thomas Frantz, in his 1988 King's College lecture, made the statement that he had a theory which he could not prove, but which he believed to be true just the same. He suggested that as humans we are all very simple emotionally. He described his theory by saying that it is like we all have one conduit through which we express and perceive emotional experience, when we try to block one emotional event, to a greater or lesser degree we partially block up our ability to feel or express any other emotions. I believe Dr. Frantz's hypothesis applies directly to this discussion about viewing the body. Viewing the body is perhaps the most effective way to unblock the resistance and the emotions arising from a death.

I also have a theory that I cannot prove, but which I believe to be true just the same. It is my belief that behind whatever objection is stated for not viewing the body, fear may be the real cause of rejecting this confrontation with reality. It may be fear of the unknown, i.e., How bad will he/she look? How will I, and others, react? It may be the fear of the anticipated suffering which may attend, and follow, viewing of the body.

In our world suffering and death are both abhorrent subjects. Dame Cecily Saunders, the founder of the modern hospice movement, observed that in our society, "Death is an outrage." The suffering which could well follow confronting death by viewing the body, is too often mistakenly considered just as outrageous, and perhaps infinitely more avoidable.

One response to suffering is to close the heart and shut out the cause. Thus, by not viewing the body we might expect to avoid suffering. However, when we push something away out of fear, we entrench and validate the fear. At the same time when we close our heart to pain, we are making an enemy of the heart and imprisoning it. The Russian philosopher, Gurgeef, said, "In order to escape from prison, the first thing you have to do is realize you are in prison." Confronting death by viewing the body is one sure way of pushing past the fear of suffering which can confine and constrict our hearts.

Avoiding viewing the body is a manner of pushing away the reality of death. When we push anything away it throws us off balance and we are not content. The only way to be in balance and content is by being with what is, which means in this case, being with death.

When the tendency is to pull away and shut down from death, the best method for dealing with the suffering is, ironically, to move toward it, to "lean into grief" as recommended by Dr. Alan Wolfelt. At the 1996 Kings College conference, Dr. Terry Tafoya related the Pacific-Northwest native legend of Dashuaya, who had gathered children, bound and blinded by sap over their eyes, around an open fire where they were to be cooked. It was by leaning in toward the very fire that was there to kill him, that one boy melted the sap from his eyes so he could see to free himself and the other children from their tormentor. Dr. Tafoya asked the question, "But you wouldn't lean towards the very thing that could kill you, or would you?"

Lawrence LeShan said, "Two of the best kept secrets of the twentieth century are that everyone suffers, and suffering can be used for growth." In a culture that is dedicated to developing medications and diversions to avoid suffering, it is indeed a challenge to re-educate people that the suffering which may arise from confronting death provides part of the balance and the growth of our human experience. In order to be fully human we have to embrace suffering, as well as joy, when it appears. Our joy cannot be rooted in the denial of suffering. Our joy has to be rooted in being fully with what is in the present moment.

In his book *The Prophet,* Kahlil Gibran (1983) comments on people who "would seek only love's peace and love's pleasure" (p. 12) out of fear and would try and avoid experiencing the pain and grief from love lost. He suggests that these people end up in a "seasonless world where you shall laugh, but not all of your laughter, and weep, but not all of your tears" (p. 12). In my ignorance about the power and influence of grief, and how to work with it, I shut down emotionally for five years after my father's death and I would describe my emotional life as a "seasonless world." I would not wish this existence on anyone. It is truly not living in the full sense of the word.

My apprehension is that without the healthy balance of joy and suffering in our lives, we not only reduce the valleys and sorrows, but also the peaks and joys, in our lives. I believe that the inability to tolerate suffering creates a very shallow existence which might be described as "low-grade, chronic depression." This state of mind robs us both of the fullest experience of life and of our humanity.

Avoidance of viewing the body is not the cause of this increasingly pervasive fear of suffering. However, the inclination to avoid viewing the body may be a symptom of this fear. Not viewing the body may actually promote this unbalanced approach to living of demanding the positive and denying the negative. It is only with the ground of pain that we can clearly see and appreciate the figure of joy; we need the contrast.

Viewing the body can be considered a critical event, a "moment of truth," which facilitates not only the expression of the acute grief but also allows vent of our lifelong accumulated pool of grief. On the other side of suffering is joy and, from this perspective, viewing the body can be considered an essential method of moving through grief toward the relief and appreciation of life that makes living worthwhile.

Everyone who deals with grieving people is in effect "in counsel" with them and is, therefore, a grief counselor. Funeral directors, doctors, nurses, social workers, palliative care volunteers, clergy, pastoral care workers, teachers, police officers, and all others who find themselves in this pivotal situation with grieving people have an obligation to be informed, and to inform the bereaved, about the subject of viewing the body.

My current personal mission statement is: "To grow in my wisdom, and in my ability to love, through service to grieving people." I can think of no greater opportunity to fulfill this mandate than in the profession of funeral service, and especially in the area of educating, serving, and supporting people to confront their suffering by viewing the dead body of their loved one.

From my own experience, the experience of others, and the writings of experts on the subject (Gibran, 1983), I now feel certain that viewing the body is helpful, not unhelpful or irrelevant, to the grief process. The memory picture of a loved one dead helps the transition from a physical relationship to a memory or spirit relationship. Of course, a pre-judgment that viewing is unhelpful or irrelevant will color the choices people will make. As professionals, the obligation remains to offer insights that will assist the bereaved in making an informed decision. If the path is chosen of confronting the reality that has befallen them, the bereaved will have a solid foundation upon which to base their mourning and eventual reconciliation of their loss.

REFERENCES

Donne, J. (1986). Devotions upon emergent occasions, Meditation 17. In M. H. Abrams (Ed.), *The Norton anthology of English literature* (5th ed., Vol. 1). New York: W. W. Norton & Company.

Jackson, E. N. (1965). When to talk about death. In *Telling a child about death* (p. 32). New York: Channel Press.

Gibran, K. (1983, October). *The Prophet.* New York: Alfred A. Knopf (originally published September 1923).

Osmont, K. (1993, November). The value of viewing in griefwork reconciliation: A psychotherapists perspective. *The Forum Newsletter, Association for Death Education and Counselling, IXX*(5).

Rando, T. A. (1984). Funerals and funerary rituals. In *Grief, dying and death: Clinical interventions for caregivers* (pp. 180-181). Champaign, IL: Research Press Company.

Rando, T. (1993). *Treatment of complicated mourning.* Champaign, IL: Research Press.

Van Beck, T. W. (1993). *Ethics handbook for funeral service practitioners.* Covington, KY: The Loewen Group.

CHAPTER 19

It's Never Easy! Children, Adolescents and Complicated Grief

Robert G. Stevenson

Childhood is a time filled with potential, a time that looks to the future. It is, as Robert Kastenbaum has said, the "Kingdom where nobody dies" (1972). As a death educator for over twenty-five years and a parent for almost thirty, I have read countless articles which began with those or similar words. Childhood was a time of only good thoughts and events. Why spoil it with unnecessary worry or fears related to death and grief? After all, wasn't there plenty of time in a child's life to learn of such things? They could be dealt with tomorrow. Here we see one of the chief "complications" in the grief experienced by children. There are some who must first be convinced that these young people are even capable of grief. As recently as the early 1980s, while presenting a research proposal on sibling grief to hospital administration, the head of the psychiatric service of that major New York medical center actually stated in the meeting that he believed children and adolescents were "incapable" of grief since the superego was not sufficiently developed in young people. He was stating that grief did not occur in young people at the same time that researchers were studying grief reactions in animals and finding responses which they identified as grief in species as diverse as gorillas and dolphins. Since key hospital personnel did not believe there was grief in childhood, there was nothing to study and the project was abandoned. Here is the first complication for young people in grief. Unlike most bereaved adults, their first task is to convince others that they are actually grieving after a death.

In the time since that unfortunate experience, research on childhood grief has progressed quickly. It is fueled by a need to find appropriate responses and interventions to assist grieving children and adolescents. Some interventions only seem to make things worse. How many children have tried "play therapy" as a way to deal with their grief only to be told, "Stop that! How can you play when your grandmother just died?" Unless someone answers that question, the need of children to use play as one means of externalizing their inner pain may never be met. Since, in many cultures today, grief is never to touch the life of a child, every death they encounter can be seen as traumatic and the resulting grief, often with lack of needed support, complicated. Grieving children face fears of their own dreams and even conscious thoughts related to the death, apathy and diminished interest in life, changes in or detachment from existing relationships, fear, anger, acting out or punishment seeking behavior, somatic complaints and sleep disturbances (Nader, 1997; Stevenson, 1995). They do not have the access to treatment that most adults have and may even "bury" their grief so as not to hurt surviving adult relatives. They are told to "be strong" for mommy or daddy.

Children may also take on responsibility for a death. The blurting out of an angry, "I wish you were dead," or the silent thought of those same words, has caused some children to believe they actually were an active cause of the death they now are grieving. In a high school death education course in 1988, a seventeen year old stood to tell the class of an experience in his own life. He had been getting ready for school and thought he heard someone call his name. He finished dressing and went downstairs to find his father dead of a major coronary. Doctors had told him that death was almost instantaneous and that there was nothing he could have done. As tears ran down his cheeks, he told his classmates that, since he had not responded immediately to his name, for eight years he had believed that he had killed his father. The death education class became a safe place where he was finally able to externalize thoughts and fears that he had kept hidden inside for years. Increasingly it is the school that children, and their parents or other family caregivers, turn to for assistance with their grief.

THE ROLE OF THE SCHOOL

In classrooms throughout the United States in the 1950s and '60s, there were mandatory lessons that showed ways to "cope" with disaster. The case in point was how to survive a nuclear attack. Students learned warning signals that ranged from an intermittent blast on a siren to a sudden flash of light. Response varied from moving to a prepared fallout shelter to simply crawling under desks and covering one's head. Recovery was discussed only briefly. It described where radiation might be less intense, the need to wash off any possible contamination, and what food and water might be less contaminated. I still remember that beer in brown glass bottles could become a beverage of choice. In 1967 when I began teaching, these lessons were still a part of public school curricula. However, times had changed and so had technology and the amount of available information.

We learned that the plans which we had taught so diligently to students were now, and perhaps had always been, of no real value. The detonation of a twenty kiloton bomb over some nearby metropolitan area might have been "survivable" in the 1940s. However, the Soviet Union now had bombs that exceeded one hundred megatons in size. To equal that force, a bomb like the one dropped on Hiroshima would have to be dropped every day of the year for thirteen years. I was teaching New Jersey students how to survive fallout when, after such a blast, they themselves would have been fallout. In addition, we now know the Soviets had over a dozen of these warheads targeted for aerial detonation over the New York metropolitan area. The schools where I taught would have been part of ground zero. After looking at these facts, our social studies curriculum shifted its emphasis from fallout survival to "war prevention" and included ways of coping with more readily "survivable" crises.

This example is a useful one when we examine the plans which educators have developed for dealing with grief in schools. A number of educators have developed protocols for helping grieving students. These include suggestions of how to inform students of a loss (Stevenson & Powers, 1987), of responses to "community grief" (Grollman, 1995; Stevenson, 1994), and of ways to support students as they grieve (Grollman, 1995; Stevenson, 1996; Worden, 1996). Teachers now receive in-service programs on how to help a student who is grieving a loss. The information provided is good as far as it goes. Typically, it provides a model to represent the typical grief process that follows a loss. That, however, is also its shortcoming. Students may not be experiencing the grief of one loss, but from multiple losses that may extend back over a period of months or even years. Then there are those individuals who experience special difficulties with the grief process. They pose a special challenge to teachers, counselors, and school nurses when the grief they experience is complicated by factors that they and the teachers who seek to help them do not understand. There is little or no support for teachers and counselors who must work with students experiencing complicated grief. Thus, when we say that a school has prepared to help each of its students to cope with a loss, this may not be a useful model. What can educators do when losses are multiple or when one or more students is coping with complicated grief? Are we repeating the mistakes made in the example of crisis response to nuclear attack presented above? Are we preparing for a "theoretical" loss that bears little resemblance to what will actually occur in the lives of many of our students? Are the models and procedures we present already inadequate when confronted with the real needs of our students?

It is said that "No decision can be better than the information on which it is based." If we have provided students and educators with incomplete information or incorrect generalizations about the grief process, we should not be surprised if the decisions they make or the plans they develop are also inaccurate or incomplete.

EXISTING PROTOCOLS

Most schools have had to deal with the impact of the death of a member of the school community (student, educator, parent, or support staff member). Educators are less likely to view such an event as isolated and unique . . . a one-time occurrence that will not repeat and, therefore, does not necessitate any change in school procedure. Existing school protocols have several features in common:

- They describe procedures for notifying a student, class, or entire school community of a death.
- They provide educators (and sometimes parent groups) with a basic understanding of the grief process.
- They allow for the development of rituals related to a death to help validate the change experienced by the school community.
- They identify one or more "safe places" where students can go if they need to grieve (or to be apart for a time from other students), typically a counselor's or administrator's office or the school nurse's office. The faculty room has also been used for this purpose in some smaller schools where space is limited.
- They typically identify key personnel (administrator, counselors, school nurse, and one or more teachers).

Most such plans call for a period of special attention to the needs of students for a period of one to two weeks after the loss. However, such plans may also make some key mistakes. These "problem" measures include:

- Depending on one individual to coordinate all response plans. This can lead to overload for even the most competent professionals, and what if the death in question is that one individual?
- Assigning the school nurse one or more tasks (such as visiting classes to tell of a death) which prevent her from being available to carry out her primary responsibility—caring for the health-related needs of the students.
- Attempting to "minimize" the impact of the loss by identifying groups to whom it applies to receive special support, while at the same time identifying others who should not need such support. This approach, although often well intentioned, ignores the needs of individual students and can trample on their feelings. An example would be the principal who brought all students to a school assembly in the gym to announce the death of a student (the 3rd junior to die in that private high school in 1 year). He then told all juniors to remain in the gym for a bereavement support program, with no chance for any student to absent himself should he wish not to participate. The students in the remaining three years were sent back to class including all those students who had known the young man and might have wished to stay.
- Referring "problem" students to members of intervention teams from outside of the school. This may provide the student with emotional

help, but may not be effective in assisting the student (or the staff) with ongoing issues in the classroom.

- Assuming, in true—if unconscious—paternalistic fashion, that what is planned is the best thing for each student. Some students may want to see changes take place in a classroom when someone they love has died; however, other students may want to go through a school day with few or no changes to reassure themselves that some things are still stable in this time of change.
- Addressing each bereaved student according to a model based on "simple" or uncomplicated bereavement. A student may actually be attempting to cope with a series of losses or with a number of losses that occurred simultaneously. Losses seem to "travel in groups."

Although the need was identified for educators several years ago (Doka, 1996), educators still seem unable to identify the signs associated with grief that is extreme in behavior or emotional distress. The protocols that do exist are good as far as they go, but the time has come for educators and schools to move beyond that first step in responding to student bereavement.

BETTER DECISIONS

To develop improved responses to student needs there are several points that must be considered. Although there are similarities in all grief, the grief process can be different after different losses. For example, divorce and death can both represent the forcible loss of something precious. They each are a type of bereavement. However, it can be more difficult for students to obtain closure following a divorce; self-blame is higher and learning difficulties are higher for children in a family going through a divorce (Worden, 1996). These problems seem to affect boys more than girls when the bereavement comes from divorce. However, when a death occurs, it is girls who suffer more disruption related to learning and school.

The cause of death can present special problems. An AIDS-related death complicates the grief process for all grieving loved ones, and students are no exception (Stevenson, 1991). Suicide also causes special problems that are not effectively addressed in school procedures. One New Jersey administrator travels throughout the country telling schools that they should never memorialize a deceased student or teacher, because they might then have to do so following a suicide and that could cause other deaths. This simplistic answer plays on educators' and parents' fears, but it is based on misinformation about the effect of recognizing the change that a death causes in a school community. To do nothing can actually be more harmful to many students. School routine goes on, not acknowledging any change caused by the death of a member of the school community. That is to say to many students—the deceased did not matter and neither do you! For still other students, the grief process can be especially painful and drawn out. This is the type of reaction referred to as "complicated grief."

COMPLICATED GRIEF

The description of complicated grief is not new. It was outlined by Eric Lindemann in 1944 (cited in Sanders, 1989). Those coping with complicated grief showed over-activity with no apparent sense of loss; physical symptoms related to deceased's last illness; medical problems that were psychosomatic in origin; changes in relationships with friends and family; angry outbursts against specific people; changes in patterns of social interaction; at times, a stoic appearance seemingly devoid of emotion; harmful or punishment-seeking behavior; and agitated depression with feelings of guilt and regret. Most teachers can remember one or more students who could have been described by many of these points after the death of someone they knew or cared for.

A visiting teacher who was presenting a death education class to middle school youngsters reported in an article about her experience that three of the boys in one class appeared apathetic, uncooperative, spoke rudely to her, and engaged in repeated punishment-seeking behaviors. They disrupted a story-telling session dealing with grief and sadness despite repeated warnings. The teacher had the three removed from the room and summed it up by saying, "boys will be boys." But was that really the explanation of their behavior? Has there been a history of loss? Was there something going on in each of their lives that raised feelings which these lessons aggravated? Were they simply misbehaving or was there an element of complicated grief present? The teacher never tried to find out and no follow-up, other than detention, was offered. There are certainly times when the misbehavior of students is simply that, testing boundaries or "letting off steam." However, if problem behavior is due to complicated grief, or if it requires referral to a school counselor or psychologist, how is an educator to know?

CLUES TO COMPLICATED GRIEF

There are signs which educators can look for when one of their students is grieving a loss. A number of writers have commented on changes that educators may witness.

Classroom Teachers may observe the following:

- expressions of guilt feelings.—students may say that they do not deserve to be happy or to be successful,
- panic attacks or episodes of school phobia that have not appeared before,

- themes of loss expressed in student writing or art,
- changes in relationships with classmates or teachers,
- withdrawal from clubs, teams, or other extra-curricular activities or when the students still attends, a lack of enjoyment of activities which previously gave the student pleasure,
- appearing tired, or sleeping in school, alternating with periods of apparent high energy,
- signs of alcohol or substance abuse—this may be an attempt at self-medication to deal with grief.

School Nurses may observe the following:

- physical complaints that relate to the deceased,
- physical distress in the upper half of the sternum—feeling as if something is "stuck" there,
- repeated visits to the nurse without a specific reason,
- reporting "choking" with no apparent physical cause,
- an inability to speak about their loss—this is especially noteworthy if over a year has passed since the death.

School Counselors may observe or have knowledge of the following:

- symptoms of depression after the death of a friend or loved one,
- a student's history of delayed or prolonged grief,
- recurrence of problem behaviors on anniversaries of loss, or on special holidays,
- feeling like the death JUST took place, even after some time has passed,
- unwilling to move material possessions of the deceased or to allow any physical changes in surroundings connected to the deceased— such as the classroom or other school facilities (Lazare, 1989 quoted in Sanders, 1989; Stevenson, 1998; Wordern, 1996).

A student, or students, undergoing such a difficult grief reaction may have little ability to focus on school work or to "learn" anything meaningful from a typical day's lessons. As time passes, if this situation is not addressed, it becomes increasingly difficult for students and teachers to make up for lost ground. What then can educators do for students who are experiencing complicated grief?

Positive Interventions

Many of the interventions which are beneficial to students coping with complicated grief can be beneficial to all students. These can be included within six main principles.

1. Communicate to all students what has happened.

Use clear, accurate language and avoid "platitudes." Tell the students what has happened in an age-appropriate way. Provide enough information to allow them to have answers for their questions and information to calm their fear of the unknown. Be careful not to over-whelm them with more information than they want or need.

2. *Create or implement rituals to acknowledge the reality of this "change."*

To see external changes can assist students in dealing with their internal issues—a flag at half mast, a change in the school schedule, a moment of silence. Be sure to include students in decision making related to these rituals whenever possible. Do not close the schools following a death. For some students this is their only support network during the day. For a few it may provide their only positive support at any time. When a popular school principal died on a Saturday evening, the students of his high school gathered on the school steps and sat there all day Sunday. They felt they had nowhere else to go with their grief. School counselors arrived and opened the school for them. If students are sent home, it may only be to an empty house to be alone in their pain. In school they can be with their friends and with caring adults in a familiar, supervised atmosphere.

Procedures for deciding on a ritual and how to include all interested parties can be standardized; however, the ritual itself should be specific to this loss. An elementary school principal in Canada was faced with the task of telling very young students about the death of a classmate. He had the students sit in a circle on the floor, and he lit a number of candles in the center of the circle. The candles were of all shapes and sizes and gave off a beautiful glow. Soon some of the smaller ones, birthday size, began to go out. He explained to the students that each of us is like a candle bringing light to the world. Some candles do not burn for a long time, but we can remember how beautiful their light was when they did shine for us. He then told the students that their friend had died and answered questions they posed about what happened. After a few minutes, he asked the students to tell what they saw as their friend's "light." This simple ritual helped make a very difficult task easier for all those who participated in it . . . even the principal.

3. *Acknowledge and validate the feelings of students. Explain that what the students feel, or don't yet feel, is a part of the grief process.*

Everyone experiences grief in a personal manner. Some students, even older students, sometimes feel that they are the only one who ever felt exactly this way. Others may worry that they do not seem to feel the same emotions as others around them. They wonder "What's wrong with me?" Encourage them to speak about their fears and explain where some of these fears come from. If we help grieving students to "understand" their feelings, it can help to make those feelings less frightening or strange. Provide reassurance that they are not to blame for the loss. There is an episode of Sesame Street which helped to tell the children of America about the death of the show's character Mr. Hooper. One of the segments of that hour long show dealt with the fact that, even when we plan and do everything to avoid them, sometimes bad things still happen It does not have to be someone's "fault."

It is important to listen to the students. They know that something is not right, and they can provide the best clues to help identify just what they see as the problem. By speaking about feelings, students can be helped to feel less overwhelmed by them. An excellent resource in this regard is the book by Jack Kent (1975), *There's No Such Thing As A Dragon*. Its lesson is that speaking about problems can make them smaller, even if they never go away entirely.

4. Help students to externalize thoughts and feelings about their situation.

Reading, drawing, writing are all ways of externalizing things that students may be holding inside. Have students tell a story. Simply start, "Once upon a time . . ." and see where it leads. Another exercise is the Burning of Secrets. This was originally based on work done with college students who were asked to write down and then to burn something which they were holding in and did not believe they could share with anyone. I explained the task to my students and had each one write something on a piece of paper. It might have been a secret, a source of shame, or simply the words "This is a silly assignment." That way, no one was singled out. The students then crumpled the paper and placed it into a ventilated coffee can. They accompanied me out of the school building, and we burned the papers. Students were told they might want to share what they had written with someone, but they did not have to. It was their choice. Starting with the next semester, new students began asking when we could "burn the secrets." It has continued to be an important part of every class since then. It has also worked with grieving students in counseling. Whether we use books as bibliotherapy, writing, art or the power of a flame, each of these techniques allows things that are building up inside to be externalized and privacy to still be maintained by those students who need it.

5. Help to give abstract concepts some "concrete" form.

Students respond well when presented with an amulet or talisman to help them cope with their loss. An amulet is intended to ward off evil. A talisman helps the bearer to accomplish great deeds. One object can be both. These symbols of loss and caring can be almost anything to which someone connects a special meaning and the feeling of caring they wish to convey. In my work with grieving students I have used religious symbols, lenses, stuffed animals, dragons, stones, and even broken sea shells. It is not the object that has power in itself. It serves to remind grieving students of their own abilities to handle difficulty and reminds them that someone thought enough of them to give this to them.

I first used broken sea shells with two young children whose parents were going through a very difficult divorce that was painful for the children to see. We walked along a beach, and I said that some of these bits of shell had special power. They had come through the turmoil and trials of the surf and now rested here. I told them they would know "their" shells when they saw them. As they ran up with different colored shells, I used Jungian color symbolism to describe the "power" of each shell. From that day on, the children kept their special shells with them. They would take out a shell and use it to speak about being in a difficult situation (orange), feeling that things were out of control or that they wished they could have more control over their lives (purple), feelings of anger (red), or feeling sad (light blue). The shells acted as an amulet by helping them to feel "protected" against perceived threats and against their fears. They were talismen because they helped them to speak to others—teachers, counselors, and their parents—about their feelings. It is the process that is important, not the object chosen.

6. *Help students to overcome feelings of helpless or worthlessness by encouraging them to find things that they can do for others.*

Students have volunteered to help grieving families—cleaning, preparing food, even "house-sitting" to answer the phone while the family was at the wake or funeral. They have raised money for charity (chosen by the students) and given the money in the name of a deceased loved one. They have written articles as a "legacy" for future classes on topics from stress and grief to suicide prevention. They provided a nearby faculty with a list of things that they would want from teachers if they had been the grieving students. Finally, they wrote a discussion of the pros and cons of young children attending a wake, shiva, or funeral. A number of these articles were published in the journal, *Illness, Crisis and Loss.*

After an initial mourning period, continue daily routine when possible, and when the students desire it. Once the changes occasioned by the loss/death have been acknowledged, things can start back to a regular routine. However, it is important to remember that individuals do not grieve at the same rate and this creates a need for flexibility as some students resume their routine while others are not yet ready or able to do so. It is valuable to have a "safe" place (in the nurse's office, library, or some other spot in the school) where students can go for a "time out" if they need to. They should have adults present in that place at all times for observation and, more importantly, for support if needed.

There should be opportunities for students to remember the deceased, even when school observances have ceased. Students sometimes place a memorial in their yearbook when the class moves on to another school, typically at the end of eighth or twelfth grade. Here it is best to keep things simple. Acknowledge but try not to overly romanticize the loss. It can be even harder to grieve the loss of someone we now come to visualize as "perfect." It can make it harder to say good-bye to the "real" person who is gone.

Students facing multiple losses can be helped, but the classroom may not be the best place. A school counselor, school nurse, or school psychologist can ask the student to list the losses he/she believes he/she has suffered. These can then be placed by the student in order of severity and the student picks which one he/she will work on first. The issues can then be dealt with one at a time in a less overwhelming fashion.

NO PROBLEMS

Special note must be taken of students who show no apparent sense of loss. This form of coping can become a heavy burden for a student to carry, especially as time goes on. Educators should speak with the family to see if the student is acknowledging the loss in other areas of his/her life. We must be careful not to praise the "courage" of a student who is in denial. This can make later grieving seem to be a loss of courage. Again, it is not the brave front that is the problem, but what it may be concealing inside. Our society praises those who hide their feelings and "get on with it." We must be careful to allow students to grieve, if that is what they need to do. The single most popular elective in one high school for twenty-five years has been a course on grief and loss. Literally hundreds of students have said that they shared the notes from that course with family members as a way to open up a topic that no one had wanted to discuss previously. Sometimes all that a caring adult need do is listen and let the young person say what they need to. A curriculum is a statement of priorities. If that is true, there should certainly be a place there for the things that students see as most important in their lives.

BEEN THERE, DONE THAT

Death education and bereavement support have existed in school for well over two decades. However, this brings us back to our initial example. Curricula that have been working successfully in a school for a quarter century have, in many cases, never been updated or reevaluated. The teacher/teachers who created the course have moved on to other schools or retired. New teachers may know only the basic course outline, but lack the broad knowledge or experience of the instructors who made the original course so effective. A "complication" that now exists for students is twofold: a stagnating curriculum and a new faculty that does not yet have the expertise to strengthen and update it. Courses about death and loss are not requirements. There is a real danger that worthwhile courses with proven value may start to disappear because no one is quite sure what to do with them..That would be a real loss for students, educators, parents, and the entire community.

COMMUNITY RESPONSE

It is important to remember that educators and schools cannot take on this task alone. The student should be encouraged to draw on family, religious, and community support. Students do not exist in a vacuum and neither must schools. All of the caring adults in a student's life should communicate with each other and work in a way that is in the best interests of that young person. This may take time, since the grief process is neither on a time table, nor is it automatic. Lines of communication among educators (teachers, counselors, school nurses, social workers, and psychologists), parents, and community mental health centers should exist NOW. Then, if grief becomes complicated, destructive, or simply too much for one person or group to deal with, referrals can bring many helpers together to deal with this important task. These would be people familiar with the school and, ideally, already known to the students.

When a student faces complicated grief, the greatest benefit will be to have a school that is seen as a caring place rather than an additional burden. If this is to happen, there is much to be done and the time to start is now. Helping prepare students to cope effectively with the losses they encounter, or to learn to live with those already in their lives is a difficult task for any caring adult, whether parent or educator. It seems to be yet another job, although certainly an important one, added to the load already placed on teachers. For most educators, teaching is a challenging, rewarding, fulfilling profession. For those teachers who truly care about their young charges, it is never easy.

REFERENCES

Doka, K. (Ed.) (1996). *Living with grief after sudden loss*. Washington, DC: Hospice Foundation of America.

Grollman, E. A. (1995). *Bereaved children and teens: A support guide for parents and professionals*. Boston: Beacon Press.

Kastenbaum, R. (1972, November 23). The kingdom where nobody dies (pp. 33-38). *Saturday Review*.

Kent, J. (1975). *There's no such thing as a dragon*. Racine, WI: Western Publishing Co.

Lazare, A. (1979). Unresolved grief. In *Outpatient psychiatry: Diagnosis and treatment*. Baltimore: Williams and Wilkins.

Nader, K. O. (1997). Childhood traumatic loss: The interaction of trauma and grief. In *Death and trauma: The traumatology of grieving*. Washington, DC: Taylor and Francis.

Sanders, C. M. (1989). *Grief the mourning after.* New York: John Wiley & Sons.

Stevenson, R. G. (Ed.) (1994). *What will we do? Preparing the school community to cope with crises.* Amityville, NY: Baywood.

Stevenson, R. G. (1995). "I thought about death all the time . . ." Students, teachers and the understanding of death. In E. A. Grollman (Ed.), *Bereaved children and teens: A support guide for parents and professionals.* Boston: Beacon Press.

Stevenson, R. G. (1998). ΘΑΝΑΤΟΣ ΚΑΙ ΣΧΟΛΙΚΟ ΠΕΡΙΒΑΛΛΟΝ. IN ΤΟ ΠΕΝΘΟΣ ΣΤΗ ΖΩΗ ΜΑΣ (ππ. 97–106). Athens, Greece: Merimna (Not available in English).

Stevenson, R. G., & Powers, H. (1987, May). How to handle death in the school: Ways to help grieving students. *Education Digest, LII*(9).

Stevenson, R. G., & Stevenson, E. P. (Eds.) (1996). *Teaching students about death: A comprehensive resource for educators and parents.* Philadelphia: Charles Press.

Worden, J. W. (1996). *Children and grief when a parent dies.* New York: Guilford Press.

CHAPTER 20

Complicated Grief: Family Systems As a Model for Healing

Stephen J. Hoogerbrugge

The primary purpose of this chapter is to discuss how family dynamics can hinder adequate grieving, often resulting in complicated mourning. It is intended to relate basic concepts of family systems theory to the treatment of complicated grief and to assist practitioners from different disciplines to support grieving families effectively.

The term "complicated grief" suggests reactions to loss that become inhibited in their expression, denied, exaggerated and chronic, unresolved, even pathological. All grief is difficult and complex to a degree. As one person put it recently, "All grief is complicated" (Silverman, 1998). Without turning grief reactions into pathology and recognizing that all grief should be taken seriously, some characteristics of grief reactions deserve thorough evaluation.

There are four general categories of complicated grief. Prolonged or chronic grief persists over a long period of time (more than a year), and the grieving person is aware of the problem. Delayed, inhibited, suppressed, or postponed grief suggests itself when a person becomes aware that a current, moderate loss has created an overly intense reaction. The intensity points to an earlier, more serious loss. Grief masked as somatic or behavioral symptoms suggests that the person is unaware of the impact of the loss and its importance and meaning. Exaggerated grief response ("I deserve to die, too!") is characterized by deep depression, anxiety, or other symptoms that make the person dysfunctional, suggesting a psychiatric diagnosis (Worden, 1991).

In each case, one or more of the four tasks of mourning have not been completed. Worden (1991) explains these four tasks as follows: 1) accepting the reality of the loss (instead of denying it); 2) working through the pain of grief (instead of not feeling); 3) adjusting to an environment in which the deceased is missing (rather than failing to adapt); 4) emotionally relocating the deceased in one's personal view of the universe and moving on with life (instead of refusing to love others).

The history of family therapy demonstrates a neglect of family bereavement and its influences on the grief process. In the past, family systems theorists often regarded grief and loss issues as merely the content of intrapersonal feelings. Walsh and McGoldrick (1991) describe this historical split between systemic thinking and individual psychology, resulting in a dearth of systemic analysis of family bereavement. J. William Worden (1991), noting this distinction, says, ". . . most significant losses occur within the context of a family unit, and it is important to consider the impact of a death in the entire family system."

The concept of family systems rests on the belief that people are shaped and influenced by families. Families are characterized by multiple dynamics and interactions that are understandable when viewed from a systemic point of view. Nobody lives in a total vacuum. All members of a family influence all the others. Family members affect one another's emotional and mental health for good or ill. A family's reactions to loss needs assessment just as much as an individual's (Davies et al., 1986; Worden, 1991). When a family member complains, "I've heard all the crying I can stand out of you," the other family member may decide never to cry again.

Unresolved grief may be a key factor in family pathology. Treatment professionals benefit themselves and the families they serve by recognizing the forces affecting complicated grief. Spark and Browdy (1972) point out that unresolved grief in a family of origin may impede experiencing emotional loss within a current family. Family grief reactions affect everyone in the family and unresolved grief reactions may be passed from one generation to the next. Therese Rando (1998) says, "Grief is to mourning what infancy is to childhood." If unresolved grief turns into a longer unresolved mourning process, it is likely to be passed to several succeeding generations. Grief is both an individual and a family process that may affect an individual over many years and a family over many generations.

FAMILY SYSTEMS CONCEPTS

Writers in the field of family therapy show an increased interest in the individual and the system, the processes of independence, and the dynamics of mutuality or interdependence (Friedman, 1985; Olson, 1988; Sugarman, 1986; Wachtel & Wachtel, 1985). Family therapy considers the family the unit of treatment. Just as a physician would regard the color of the skin as likely related to the functioning of the liver, a family therapist would regard a troubled adolescent as a family problem. The human family is an organism like the human body. If only the symptom receives treatment, the underlying problem returns to cause pain. As Friedman (1985) affirms, "Trying to *cure* a person in isolation from his or her family . . . is as misdirected and ultimately ineffective, as transplanting a healthy organ into a body whose imbalanced chemistry will destroy the new organ as it did the old." Family therapy aims to treat the whole organism, as well as its parts.

Homeostasis

When someone dies, a family's balance is disrupted. A family's unique balance is the way the family functions and how it handles its anxiety. Homeostasis is the term used to identify how a family operates from day to day and generation to generation. Like any system, a family has a structure and functions for its various parts. Families have leaders and followers, gender and psychological rules for functioning. If the family patriarch dies, homeostasis is disturbed and a new person must fill the role of leader, or a new way of operating must be adapted. This process is normally unconscious. Any death of a family member creates a structural void or a systemic imbalance that requires homeostatic adjustment (Bowlby-West, 1983; Crosby & Jose, 1983).

Homeostatic adjustment includes displacement of feelings through scape-goating. It is a form of blaming someone in the family for all the pain and problems of the family (this person is called the "identified patient" in systems theory). Displacement of feelings may result in increased enmeshment or over-involvement in each other's lives, idealization of the deceased, infantilization, parentification, role reversals, and creating family secrets. If family homeostasis includes a tradition of denial of feelings and the expression of feelings, these adjustments are used in greater proportion (Bowlby-West, 1983). The bereavement counselor or family therapist can facilitate more open communication and encourage the family to make use of social resources, such as the churches or synagogues, bereavement programs at hospitals, and support groups.

Homeostasis functions to keep a family's operational balance. The influences of homeostasis can produce a new, healthier way of functioning, or push the family to revert to old habits (e.g., not talking about negative feelings, or blaming a family member for the death). Every grief counselor, therapist, clergy member, chaplain, or social worker can assess the homeostasis of a family. The forces of change (i.e., the death) and the forces of maintaining a familiar homeostasis create an opportunity for significant and positive change. Conversely, homeostasis creates the likelihood of returning the family to a familiar but less healthy way of functioning. The bereavement counselor can intervene by normalizing intense feelings of grief and assisting in redirecting any blaming or scape-goating.

If a family tradition (homeostasis) includes alcoholism and the alcoholic dies, a new person may be influenced, no matter how indirectly, into that role. Edwin Friedman (1985) tells the story of Karen. She was the youngest of five children from a poor family. The father, an alcoholic, was alienated from the family and considered a drunk and a bum. When he died the family refused to have a funeral or to acknowledge the man in any way, not even with a marker for his grave. Karen called it "a lousy way to die." She became increasingly obsessed with thoughts of her father and could not let go of her grief. As she entered adolescence, she acted out, got in trouble in school, and was often told by family members, "You're just like your father." In her later adolescence and into her twenties, Karen increasingly abused alcohol. Fortunately, she entered treatment for alcoholism and discovered the connection between her complicated grief reactions and her drinking. She also began to learn about family homeostasis.

MULTIGENERATIONAL TRANSMISSION PROCESS AND THE IDENTIFIED PATIENT

Families transmit to each new generation their particular ethos, values, benefits, traditions, problems, and pathologies. Each new generation lives out these family characteristics often without awareness or choice. Included in this process is a sense of family loyalty, which may come into conflict with the values and traditions of other families merging into the first one by marriage. Sometimes ignoring grief, or shaming mourners for openly expressing sadness, emerge as factors in complicated grief. Other clashing family values can create high anxiety, distrust, conflict, and divorce, especially at a time of transition and stress when a family member becomes ill and/or dies.

Karen, the young woman who became an alcoholic following her father's death, demonstrates the process of multigenerational transmission and the identified patient. Like child abuse, family dynamics, traditions, and pathologies are passed from one generation to the next. Child abusers received abuse as children. It is eerily accurate how family strengths and family weaknesses and problems are passed effectively to succeeding generations. In the case of Karen, a counselor trained to think in systems concepts could assess the family, not just Karen. The counselor could see the whole, not just the part. This wholistic approach becomes a powerful tool for assessing and then intervening in the grief process, even when it is complicated grief.

The systemic approach avoids pathologizing the patient. The identified patient (IP) is a systems concept. In a family with high anxiety, one person is often identified as "the sick one," the one really troubled person in the family. If only that person would get cured, then everything would be okay. In systems thinking the identified patient is the person ". . . in whom the family's stress or pathology has surfaced" (Friedman, 1985). We are each part of a bigger whole, a living system that influences and shapes us. Becoming more aware means increasing the possibility of exercising more choice. While assisting the patient to take responsibility for his or her own identity, it is also helpful to identify the powerful influences affecting our development as persons. The family genogram (Friedman, 1985; McGoldrick & Gerson, 1985), which symbolically illustrates a family's history of births, deaths, marriages, and divorces, can assist counselors and clients in gaining an intergenerational perspective on the identified patient and the multigenerational transmission process.

The genogram is a formalized way of taking a family history which elucidates family realities without judgment or labeling family members or experiences as "sick." The family of origin passes health and illness, weakness and strength to each new generation. A strictly individual model of helping people tends to focus on what is sick or weak in a family, i.e., the identified patient. The systems model enables people to see their family of origin as a source of strength, as well as weakness. It enables people to seek relationships in their family of origin, perhaps helping to create a healthier, stronger family, without having to identify the "sick" person. Sometimes the old, negative problem behaviors, habits, and traditions are replaced with positive and healthy ones. The chain of problems passed down to the next generation can be broken.

Emotional Triangles

The main concepts of systems or family therapy represent dynamic processes that intermingle and overlap. When self-differentiation is low and anxiety is high in a family, emotional triangles form to cope with the anxiety (Bowen, 1976; Friedman, 1985; Olson, 1988; Shapiro, 1994). When two people (a "dyad") become unstable in their relationship, a third party is brought in to help stabilize the relationship. The third party can be a person or a problem.

Father becomes gravely ill, but a son, who is alienated from and fears the father, pushes mother to speak on the son's behalf. Mother attempts to help father and son reconcile, especially at this moment of transition in the face of the father's impending death. Mother and son fight over what to say to father and how and when to say it. Mother becomes severely distressed and hopelessly locked in a fruitless effort to "make peace" between the two. Father dies before mother can make her own peace with him. Triangles can be therapeutic, but often they function to create new problems and tensions. Such conflicts and anxieties develop situations ripe for complicated grief.

Triangles can exist when a problem (instead of a person) is the second part of a dyad. An alcoholic cannot face the truth, i.e., denies his or her problem. An "enabler" is the third point of the triangle, attempting to stabilize the other two, i.e., help solve the alcoholic's anxiety and drinking problems. The enabler's efforts are inevitably doomed. Triangles grow out of anxiety and result in the third person failing repeatedly. Triangles usually create new problems and defeat the third person. Similarly, when a marital dyad is stressed, one or the other of the partners may seek an "amateur therapist," i.e., an affair. The third party of the triangle unwittingly gets used in the process of stabilizing the stressed relationship.

Triangles are evident in grieving families. "Don't say anything to grandma about how Dad really died. She couldn't take it. It will just upset her." Now the grandson fears talking to grandmother about his own father's death. The grandson/grandmother dyad faces the stress of grieving. A third party imposes herself in an attempt to keep grandma from the truth and any resulting anxiety. The grandson is pressured to keep secrets from his grandmother. Whether or not the grandmother could handle the facts about her son's death, the grandson cannot experience a genuine relationship with his grandmother. They lose each other as resources for dealing with the grief they share.

An emotional triangle can occur as the result of a death. Robert was a patient in an alcohol rehabilitation program. Deeply depressed and uncommunicative, Robert had a five-year history of prescription drug dependence, depression, and alcohol abuse. He could not work. Attempts at direct drug and alcohol rehabilitation had failed repeatedly. He felt hopeless and helpless. In a group therapy session focused on grief and loss, Robert finally disclosed the death of his daughter in a tragic accident to which he had been a witness five years previously. His daughter was eight years old at the time of her death.

Robert was haunted by mental images of his daughter's death scene. He took prescription drugs and drank alcohol to relieve his pain in a vain attempt to forget the memories. He suffered guilt that he was somehow responsible for the accident, an irrational perspective when evaluated in the light of the facts. As part of his therapy, Robert was asked to write a letter to his daughter. In it he was to tell her all of his feelings, worries, guilt, and struggles since she had died. A triangle had been created: Robert, his daughter and alcohol/depression. The dyad of father and daughter was highly stressed by the daughter's tragic death. Robert was still in the shock of grief and trauma, even though it was five years later. He abused alcohol to stabilize his guilt- and anxiety-ridden relationship with his dead daughter. What Robert needed was to address his grief directly with his daughter. He had to let go of the third party in the triangle, his drinking problem, and deal directly with the source of his pain.

In a powerful group therapy process, Robert read his letter to his dead daughter, an excruciatingly painful exercise. He was also asked to imagine what his daughter might say to him in a letter. Robert prepared such a letter and read it to the group: "Dear Daddy, I know how sad you have been, but I am okay. I am here in heaven. I miss you. Please get better and I will always be here for you. I love you. Chrissy." The emotional catharsis that resulted from this part of his grief therapy stabilized Robert's relationship with his deceased daughter. Robert was able for the first time to let go of alcohol and drugs, instead of trying to "let go" of his daughter and her death.

The process of moving from traumatic grief to the tasks of mourning had begun. Robert's healing began as a direct result of a counselor's use of emotional triangles. Robert's symptoms (depression, alcohol abuse) needed to be assessed in the light of the whole family system in which he lived. Direct treatment of depression and alcohol dependence had failed repeatedly. Esther Shapiro (1994) sharply notes this process when she says, "As with most symptoms, a family's triangulation of the dead represents a family's best solution to a psychological dilemma." Creating and using a triangle was Robert's best solution to his psychological dilemma, but it created more problems than it solved.

Triangles result as an attempt to control anxiety (Bowen, 1978; Friedman, 1985). To the extent that one person feels responsible for protecting another person from his or her pain, to that same extent a triangle is likely to be created. In grief work a counselor or therapist can get "triangled" if he or she attempts to get between a grieving family and their pain. All the comforting in the world cannot substitute for the work of mourning a loss. Indeed, in a vain attempt to help others "let go" of the dead, any grief counselor or therapist may actually help stabilize a family in its complicated grief reactions of denial, depression, or other serious symptoms.

When the therapist's own anxiety about a person or family's loss increases markedly, it is a sign of potential triangle trouble. Every person who works with grieving families should explore his or her own history of losses. It is important to identify any unresolved grief issues that may be present from prior losses. If similar losses exist that are not adequately resolved, a helper may create more confusion. Sometimes feared losses can place us in a triangle, e.g., a counselor/therapist who is an over-anxious or overprotective parent counseling someone whose child has died (Worden, 1991). Any bereavement counselor can easily lose his or her way without clear understandings of emotional triangles.

Self-Differentiation

About forty years ago, Murray Bowen (1978) of Georgetown Medical School and one of the fathers of family therapy suggested a key concept for understanding how change occurs in families. He hypothesized a scale of self-differentiation which describes the capacity of a family member to establish and maintain an individual identity, while maintaining an emotional connection to the family.

Families attempt to clone themselves and survive over generations, extending their influence, values, and identity into the future (multi-generational transmission process). Self-differentiation is the process of becoming a whole person, an adult who can live in a family as an individual without being a mere family "clone." It is the capacity to listen to a family's advice and still make decisions independently. As Edwin Friedman puts it, "Differentiation means the capacity of a family member to define his or her own life's goals and values apart from surrounding togetherness pressures, to say 'I' when others are demanding 'you' and 'we'" (Friedman, 1985).

Some families support this process, while other families resist it mightily. One could call it a process of maturation. Self-differentiation includes the ability to maintain a relatively non-anxious presence in the midst of anxious systems. A more self-differentiated person can take more responsibility for his or her own direction in life and for his or her emotional well-being, without blaming or whining about family influence.

This maturity is partially measured by the repertoire of emotional responses a person exhibits when confronted by a crisis, such as the death of a family member. It is the capacity to keep one's wits when everyone else is losing theirs. It is the capacity to settle down, stay grounded and focused, to be an "I" while maintaining emotional contact with one's family. Self-differentiation means making choices about values and one's destiny that may be different from one's family of origin, but does not require abandoning the family in the process.

Members of a particular extended family, like the whole human family, can be placed on a continuum of more or less maturity or self-differentiation. Conflicts and anxiety are intensified during periods of family stress over grief and loss. This key concept of family systems helps to assess both individual and family behavior when in crisis and how to use family maturity level to intervene in problems of complicated grief.

The case of Mary, an adolescent hospitalized for a suicide attempt, illustrates the use of family systems concepts to assess and intervene in complicated grief. Mary had been seen by a social worker for three years. The enmeshed family had sought counseling for their daughter because she was acting out with screaming and some violence at home and school. During therapy Mary's social worker was triangled in between Mary and her family. The therapist allied with her against the family and became her "friend." The family was rarely allowed into the counseling sessions. Losing most of her objectivity, the social worker unwittingly maintained Mary's "stuck" position in the family system. Mary's condition slowly but steadily worsened.

Following the suicide attempt, Mary's family sought out a different therapist. This therapist approached counseling from a systems point of view. Mary was depressed, on home schooling because of debilitating migraine headaches, and subject to angry outbursts. Her parents feared she would fail her senior year at high school and lose a scholarship to college. Mary was falling further and further behind in school and had become increasingly isolated.

During the intake the counselor assessed the entire family system, looking for triangles, attempts at family "cloning," any significant disturbances to family homeostasis, i.e., any major losses or problems in the family history. It became clear that a major loss had created deep-seated and unresolved grief reactions in this family. About eight years previously, the father had been in a serious car accident and sustained some brain damage. He nearly died and was faced with critical losses of speech and brain processing functions.

The impact on the family was severe. The father lost his career. He faced years of agonizing physical rehabilitation. The wife was forced by circumstances to become the primary caretaker and breadwinner. The children lost the father they had known and depended upon. They lost the warm, articulate, and confident father, who was replaced by a needy, insecure, depressed, and inarticulate, home-bound patient named "Dad." In the family's attempt to pull together, they did not grieve this tragedy and its consequences. In a loving but vain attempt to get between her husband and his emotional pain, his wife told the children not to talk about his accident or his current condition. No one in the family wanted to upset Dad. He had enough emotional and physical pain. The truth was sacrificed for an attempt to protect another from pain.

The family anxiety was high and self-differentiation was very low. Unresolved grief and loss issues overwhelmed the family members, but no one had the support or the courage to speak up. Then Mary started acting out the family anxiety with temper tantrums, failure at school, migraine headaches, failure in therapy, angry outbursts, and then a suicide attempt.

The traumatic grief experienced by this family after the father's accident was similar to that of a family member's death. Mary had become the "symptom bearer" for the family anxiety and its unresolved, complicated grief. She became the "identified patient," the person who is triangled in between the family and its unresolved grief. As long as Mary needed all their attention, no one in the family had to deal with the agonizing loss and pain of the father's brain injury.

It is often the case that the identified patient in a family is attempting to be more self-differentiated. Mary was somehow refusing to go along with the family value of silence in the face of loss. She raged unconsciously against the family pain that was unacknowledged and festering in every heart. In a sense, she was willing to sacrifice herself to get the family to face the truth and deal better with their pain.

Using the premise that the identified patient is more self-differentiated than other family members (Friedman, 1985), the therapist began to work with her, but only in family therapy with her parents and two siblings present. She would be most likely to respond to support for her journey toward self-differentiation. She identified the real issues surrounding the father's injury and led the family in facing their pain. She courageously shared her own hurts of losing a close and warm relationship with her father after the accident, her frustrations with his inability to communicate well, and her resentment about never talking about these realities. She led her family in acknowledging and grieving their losses in some heart-wrenching and brutally honest sessions. Then healing began.

Finally, the family looked at itself. Triangles were identified and truth was honored. The family began a journey of healing itself rather than trying to fix either the father or the adolescent daughter. In their wholeness as a family, they learned to accept more self-differentiation in each family member. Mary was challenged by the therapist to claim openly her newly identified (through the diagnostic prism of systems thinking) maturity and courage to move her family toward the truth and self-differentiation. Before long her migraines disappeared, she went back to school, finished her semester and was able to enroll in college.

Family Secrets

Many families are riddled with family secrets, i.e., information that might cause pain or anxiety in the family. Sometimes we call them "family skeletons." Most children know the fear and confusion of someone saying, "Oh, you were adopted. You're not really your parents' kid!" Adoptions, abortions, incest, affairs, unwanted pregnancies and births, mental illness in a family member, a gay or lesbian family member, legal or financial problems, suicides often become family secrets. Family secrets block the flow of communication in families and allow chronic anxiety to flourish unabated (Friedman, 1985).

High anxiety can become part of a family's homeostasis. Secrets also create unhealthy triangles. Self-differentiation becomes less likely in a highly anxious system because the homeostasis requires each family member to clone the family identity. Edwin Friedman identifies four negative effects of secrets that he calls "specific and predictable." Secrets divide families, create estrangement and false companionship, distort perceptions, and increase chronic anxiety which serves to worsen other family pathology (Friedman, 1985).

Friedman tells the story of the minister who was directed to keep secret the death of a brother from the four sisters who were in a car accident with him. The minister spent so much time thinking about how to avoid questions about the brother that he could not act genuinely and spontaneously. In other words, he could not be himself and he could not be effective. Families develop similar anxieties and rigid behaviors when secret keeping is practiced over a long time. They lose their spontaneity.

Complicated grief grows in an atmosphere of secrets. Lydia's husband of fifty-five years died. She went into a deep depression about ten months later. While in treatment she disclosed that she had kept secret the alcoholism and related problems of her husband's brother. She had served as the brother's supportive counselor over many years, but when her husband died, the brother would not even come to the funeral. She had wanted to protect her husband from the pain of knowing his brother was an alcoholic and abusive to his own wife.

Lydia's grief was delayed in part because her brother-in-law had distanced himself from the family after her husband died. She was able to see the triangle she had helped create and the secrets she had kept from the family. She felt abandoned by her brother-in-law and saddened that her secret keeping had unnecessarily distanced her from the rest of her family. Her depression deepened as the pain of the truth hit home. Her brother-in-law was a worse drinker than ever. She had no emotional support from him now that she was no longer needed to protect him from her husband's likely criticisms.

Among other interventions used in her grief counseling was explaining and identifying triangles and family secrets. These concepts helped make sense of her confusion over the behavior of her husband's brother. At first her pain and her depression deepened. She decided to confront her brother-in-law about his behavior, including his abandoning the family (especially her). Following the confrontation, Lydia began completing the tasks of mourning and her debilitating depression began to lift.

In addition, she decided that the family tradition of avoiding the open expression of deep feelings (a form of secret keeping) was over. She insisted that the family go on the traditional summer retreat as they had when her husband was alive. She took the lead in creating a service of remembrance for her deceased husband during the week's retreat. Three generations shed unexpected tears and shared in good-natured laughter as they recalled good times with her husband. Each family member found or made a symbol of their relationship to her deceased husband. These were explained during the service. She regarded that family experience, eighteen months after her husband's funeral, her real "good-bye." At last she was able to mourn.

The summer vacation turned into a true memorial service. It allowed a new and different way to structure the family memory of her husband and their relationship to each other. As Esther Shapiro (1994) points out, ". . . systemically informed grief therapy recognizes that the restructuring of family relationship patterns needs to take place in a way that fully recognizes and includes the family's emotional perspective."

IMPLICATIONS FOR CARE PROVIDERS

For the systems oriented care provider, the family is the unit of treatment. Whenever possible, all available family members should participate in bereavement programs and/or treatment. The care provider will gain much information from the family members and how they interact in classes or counseling sessions.

It is important to assess for and identify triangles. Counselors can support open communication and telling the truth as each person experiences it. Therapists encourage self-differentiation by creating a safe environment for people to share their feelings and opinions openly even if that process proves uncomfortable for others in the family.

Displaced family anger, fear, and anxiety can lead to a symptom-bearer, or an identified patient (IP). Counselors can help the IP clarify his or her values, feelings, and opinions, and teach and model assertion skills for telling the truth in a firm but respectful manner. All care providers can direct a family to look at itself as a whole and achieve a balance without finding an identified patient to blame. Shapiro (1994) puts it nicely, "A family that achieves an inclusive balance of self-with-others recognizes both similarities and differences and permits family members to feel fully included in a differentiated and authentic, rather than 'pseudomutual,' family cohesiveness."

It is critical to normalize the expression of intense emotions by asking family members to share feelings about the deceased in family sessions. An effective therapist will boldly go where perhaps no one in the family wants to go. The counselor must enter this process with genuineness and spontaneity. If the counselor is real, it will help the family members to be more authentic and spontaneous also.

Bereavement counselors can support telling the truth in families and educate them about the role of secrets. It is important to emphasize the healing consequences of telling the truth, as opposed to keeping secrets. When secrets are revealed, ". . . despite the fact that family members might at first be upset (either over the information or the fact that the secret is out), the anxiety level of the family generally decreases" (Friedman, 1985). Family members often say they want to "spare" someone's feelings, but that is usually a cover for self-protection. "Few of us are irreparably hurt by upset. Chronic anxiety, on the other hand, kills" (Friedman, 1985). Once the truth becomes a valued family tradition, temporary upset can replace chronic and debilitating anxiety.

Finally, each treatment provider must work on his or her own self-differentiation. Herz (1989) notes that the care provider or family therapist needs to remain calm, emotionally non-reactive, and well grounded. The family's intense emotional stress and reactivity can overwhelm a therapist who is unprepared, less mature in his or her own family of origin. It is easy to get overwhelmed by the family system, its temptations to join triangles and become emotionally over-reactive to perceived pain and problems in the family. Altruistic motives can go awry if not grounded in self-differentiation.

Family systems concepts enhance the potential effectiveness of every kind of care provider. All grief work is challenging and rewarding, requiring many resources and the most thoughtful and compassionate helpers. Family systems concepts provide such helpers a dynamic model for empowering individuals and families to heal the hurts of the most complicated grief.

REFERENCES

Bowen, M. (1976). Family reactions in death. In P. Guerin (Ed.), *Family therapy* (pp. 335-348). New York: Harper & Row.

Bowen, M. (1978). *Family therapy in clinical practice*. New York: Aronson

Bowlby-West, L. (1983). The impact of death on the family system. *Journal of Family Therapy, 5,* 279-294.

Crosby, J., & Jose, N. (1983). Death: Family adjustment to loss. In C. Figley & H. McCubbin (Eds.), *Stress and the family: Vol. 2. Coping with catastrophe* (pp. 76-89). New York: Brunner/Mazel.

Davies, B., Spinetta, J., Martinson, I., & Kulenkamp, E. (1986). Manifestations of levels of functioning in grieving families. *Journal of Family Issues, 7,* 297-313.

Friedman, E. H. (1985). *Generation to generation: Family process in church and synagogue*. New York: Guilford Press.

Herz, F. (1989). The impact of death and serious illness on the family life cycle. In B. Carter & M. McGoldrick (Eds.), *The changing family life cycle: A framework for family therapy* (2nd ed., pp. 457-482). Boston: Allyn & Bacon.

McGoldrick, M., & Gerson, R. (1985). *Genograms in family assessment*. New York: Norton.

Olson, D. (1988). Family types, family stress, and family satisfaction: A family developmental perspective. In C. J. Falicov (Ed.), *Family transitions: Continuity and change over the life cycle* (pp. 55-80). New York: Guilford Press.

Rando, T. (1998). *The interface of complicated and uncomplicated mourning: Conceptual and clinical issues*. Paper presented at the meeting of the King's College International Conference on Death and Bereavement, London, Ontario, Canada.

Spark, G. M., & Browdy, E. M. (1972). The aged are family members. In C. Sager & H. Kaplan (Eds.), *Progress in group and family therapy*. New York: Brunner/Mazel.

Shapiro, E. (1994). *Grief as a family process: A developmental approach to clinical practice*. New York: Guilford Press.

Silverman, P. (1998, May). *All grief is complicated*. Paper presented at the meeting of the King's College International Conference on Death and Bereavement, London, Ontario, Canada.

Sugarman, S. (1986). *The interface of individual and family therapy*. Rockville, MD: Aspen.

Wachtel, E. F., & Wachtel, P. L. (1985). *Family dynamics in individual psychotherapy: A guide to clinical strategies*. New York: Guilford Press.

Walsh, F., & McGoldrick, M. (Eds.) (1991). *Living beyond loss*. New York: Norton.
Worden, W. (1991). *Grief counseling and grief therapy: A handbook for the mental health practitioner* (2nd ed.). New York: Springer.

CHAPTER 21
Dying and Bereaved Children and the Arts, Humor, and Music

Gerry R. Cox

Like adults, children experience the death of people whom they love, respond to those losses, and sooner or later face their own deaths. Like adults, children may suffer from complicated grief. Perhaps, all grief is complicated at some level. Individuals suffering from complicated grief typically feel overwhelmed, unable to adapt, engage in behavior that is repetitive, or experience extensive interruptions of the healing process that abnormally lengthens their grieving. For children, complicated grief may be presented by the complete absence of grief reactions. Generally, the absence of grief reactions is associated with the broken heart syndrome and masked grief reactions (Marrone, 1997, p. 134). Humor, art, music, and other art forms may be used to aid children who are grieving or facing their own death to unmask their grief reactions.

Children may not be able to express their understanding of death in words or even be able to communicate their feelings with words. Children often make a conscious effort to keep their feelings and other responses secret in an attempt to protect their parents (Robinson & Mahon, 1997, p. 479). It is not from lack of knowledge that children are silent. Very young dying children do exhibit certain behaviors which indicate that a child is aware that he or she is dying and what dying means and like dying adults, dying children are most fearful of being abandoned or rejected during their dying (Marrone, 1997, p. 159). Like adults, children have needs that are often not met. Children may be more likely than adults to suffer from complicated grief because they are often excluded from the normal family coping rituals. These same children observe, overhear, and see sadness in the same adults that they are looking to for support and care. Children who lack the experience and knowledge of how to cope are often insulated from the very adults who could help them learn to cope. The child is often left to grieve without family support, which can lead to loneliness. Loneliness is inversely related to self esteem (Rokach & Brock, 1998, p. 107). The family that fails to provide the necessary social support to the grieving child may further complicate the child's grieving by helping to foster loneliness and the resulting loss of self-esteem. All people, including children, look to others for social information and engage in sociocultural modeling (Wellman, 1998, p. 36). If the adults do not provide a healthy model for children, how can they learn to manage their grief? Children can mourn successfully if supported. Silverstein and Bengtson (1997) found that kinship attachment is important in crisis. Parents and other adults have their own grief to attend to, but they also need to help support children who are grieving. Giving aid to children is typically helpful to the adults who are assisting the children. Various alternatives exist that can help heal children. Cultural beliefs have staying power. Magic works in the healing process while seemingly unexplained, is a form of social support (Coe, 1997, p. 3). Parents and other adults need to use strategies with children that will provide social support in a non-threatening manner. Coping and support processes do not change dramatically with age (Ptacek et al., 1997, p. 434). Support strategies that are non-threatening to children might include the use of humor, story-telling, literature, art, and music.

HUMOR AND SOCIAL SUPPORT

Humor is more than the absence of sadness. Neither life nor death are diseases. Most people have more vitality and courage than they themselves imagine and more than others would expect (Husebo, 1998, p. 44). This very courage and vitality makes humor possible. Just as food and medicine help heal, so, too, does humor. Norman Cousins suggests that humor was medicine for Albert Schweitzer when he lacked traditional medicines (Cousins, 1979, p. 82). Humor helps healing in many ways. Those who are facing death enjoy being able to laugh at their plight, as those who are grieving also need to be able to laugh. Speigel (1998) indicates that even those who were grieving and dying themselves lived an average of eighteen months longer if they were happy and that happiness is integral to good health even in dying people. Dame Cicely Saunders reports that three-fourths of the hospice patients and half of their relatives reported being happy in a recent study of hospice patients (Saunders, 1995-96, p. 1). Humor not only aids the survivors, but it also aids their families. Robert E. Neale suggests that we are all victims, and so we must laugh for the sake of humanity, and that by laughing together, we all become victors (Neale, 1993, p. 330). Humor is a form of social support. Glennys Howarth indicates that people in Western society have a proclivity to laugh at things which disturb and/or frighten in some way

(Howarth, 1996, p. 84). She further suggests that humor is a way of identifying common ground and nurturing friendship (Howarth, 1996, p. 91). Those who are dying and/or bereaved need a common ground on which to face their trials. As a grief educator, I have found that story-telling leads to humor in grief situations. I typically ask students or those in bereavement groups to tell stories about the deceased. It is not necessary to ask them to relate humorous stories. As with wakes, humorous stories emerge on their own. The use of humor allows children to express their feelings and to even laugh about their feelings. Other emotions are able to be expressed because of the use of humor.

Emotions of sadness, self-directed hostility, anger, fear, shame, guilt, and low levels of enjoyment are all significant in predicting depression (Carey et al., 1997, p. 27). Social support can allow a person to avoid depression and its precursors. If one can laugh with another person, one is able to share with that person in ways that open up other forms of communication and sharing. Guilt, shame, lack of enjoyment, sadness, self-directed hostility, and fear can all be addressed through sharing with another. Humor can open the doors to such sharing. By taking our situations too seriously, life can become unbearable. Rohde, Seeley, and Mace (1997) report that stressful life events, loneliness, low social support, current depression, and younger age are highly correlated with suicidal behavior. Humor generally allows one to take oneself and one's situations less seriously.

Children like to deal in abstractions. They also tend to take things seriously. Children will discuss anything. No subject is too painful or forbidden to them. Children tend to fuse together fantasy and reality. Fantasy never diminishes for children. Fairy tales and children's stories provide a social context that can provide insights that are invaluable for children (Lau, 1996, p. 241). There are literally hundreds of wonderful stories available for children that present a positive understanding of dying and death. Stories and folklore can provide a perspective, knowledge, and relationships (Bauman, 1996, p. 19).

Adults develop memories and learned responsibilities while children develop anxieties that are often peculiar to the young. Children often develop separation anxiety that may arise from basic physical needs such as feeding and protection. Children often have a sense of purpose, but it is often vague and may make them feel dwarfed by it all. Most children seem to keep their distance and fail to come to grips with their fears. Scenes remain ingrained in their memories. Intensity of fear may be inverse to the amount of danger. In the face of these reactions, children who are grieving often attempt to keep their feelings and other responses secret in order to protect their parents who are also grieving (Robinson & Mahon, 1997, p. 479).

Thomas Moore (1992) indicates that our habit of viewing our bodies as machines keeps us from attending to the beauty, the poetry, and the expressiveness of our bodies (Moore, 1992, p. 172). Secrets keep us from laughing. Having no taboo topics allows children to face reality. Children and adults who inhibit or hide emotions do not feel better. Suppression of emotions when facing sadness or other negative emotions does not provide relief from that emotion (Gross & Levenson, 1997, p. 102). Social support is an independent variable that affects people's physical and mental health (Palfai & Hart, 1997, p. 405). All children, including females, need that support.

Females generally are more likely to feel loved than males (Meyers, 1997, p. 353). This may effect their grief. They may feel more responsibility to manage their own grief to spare the parent or parents who love them. While we assume females to be more expressive than males, and because they are generally more mature, most parents are less concerned with their adjustment to grief. Because they appear to be "handling their grief," females often do not get the assistance that they need. Females may be better at "masking" their grief. They, too, suffer from complicated grief. By age six, females are twice as likely to experience anxiety disorders as males (Lewinsohn, 1998, p. 109). Perhaps because females are generally more mature and responsible than males as children, we tend to focus upon the grief disorders of males. All children need the help of adults when facing grief.

Even comic strips are able to make the point that children should be included and that they grieve. Sarah Brabant (1997-98), in her study of death and grief in comic strips suggests that even in comics the "ordinariness" of death affirms the impact of death on survivors, the uniqueness of the grieving process for each person, and the variation in time and intensity of the grief process (Brabant, 1997-98, p. 43). All who are grieving need social support. Humor, even gallows humor, can provide a sense of social support.

Steve Lipman (1991) wrote *Laughter in Hell: The Use of Humor during the Holocaust*, which demonstrates the use of humor in death camps. Humor is a reaction to oppressive conditions (Bauman, 1996, p. 157). Social support does aid coping behavior.

Social support can be exhibited in many ways. Certainly, if one is able to share humor with another, that person is exhibiting social support. When one is grieving, one is also typically more sensitive to the reactions of others. If one is secure enough to share humor and to laugh with another person, that person can be trusted to provide social support. Laughter gives the child and the adult something else to think about. Rather than thinking about the disease or the loss, the individuals involved can forget their pain for a few moments when given a reason to laugh. Laughter does promote confidence and hope. Humor conveys messages, facilitates social relationships, diverts aggression, and manages "touchy" situations by producing feelings of social support and social solidarity. Jokes allow a major tension shift (Thomas, 1997, p. 307).

Grieving creates tension for children. Grief makes life seem to be without purpose.

Loss or separation is a blow to a child's sense of being and purpose. One's health and well-being can be threatened by crisis and loss. Good health and well-being are the core features of life. Leading a life with a purpose, quality interactions with others, self-regard, and mastery lead to positive human health (Ryff, 1998, p. 28). Bereavement itself can have health consequences severe enough to require professional intervention (Schut et al., 1997, p. 63). Children who may already have difficulty expressing emotion, may have the problem compounded if the person who died was the very person who listened to them (Schut et al., 1997, p. 70). To help a child who has difficulty expressing emotions, adults can use several approaches. One approach is to use humor.

Not everyone will be able to use humor successfully. Humor is less likely to be used by adults who develop a pattern of keeping family secrets. Keeping secrets is a form of information control (Vangelesti & Caughlin, 1997, p. 680). Humor and laughter are the opposite of secrets. In a healthy relationship, acts that might be secret become sentimentalized and the object of laughter and joking. To laugh together is a positive form of sharing and social support. Humor is social. We rarely laugh alone (Morreall, 1983, p. 114). Death, itself, can be a welcome end to worldly injustice, tyranny, and pomp. Death is not always a great leveler. Laughter can tip the balance in favor of the formerly disadvantaged (Glasgow, 1997, p. 141). Sharing humor makes everyone relax. Not only is laughter contagious, but it also has a cohesive effect (Morreall, 1983, p. 115).

What better way to give social support to others than by laughing at one's own condition. Sharing is healing. Children and many adults tend to take themselves, their situations, and life far too seriously. The serious person is solemn and anxious. The humorous person is more relaxed (Morreall, 1983, p. 122). Seriousness can drive one to despair. By being too serious, we can make work of parties, vacations, and even making love. Acts that should provide joy can become a burden if they are viewed as all-important (Mindess, 1971, p. 122). Humor provides order to disorder (Lefcourt and Martin, 1986: 126).

Humor also facilitates social support. Those who can laugh together are viewed as caring and supportive. Those who do not find social support turn to isolation as a way to reduce pain (Rokach & Brock, 1998, p. 121). Humor is a shared activity. It is much harder to find joy or humor unless it is shared. Sometimes, we imagine how others would react, and we can smile and even laugh by ourselves. It is important to understand that just as laughter is beneficial for all parties who are sharing the laughter, social support is beneficial for not only the recipient, but it is also beneficial for those who are giving the social support to others (Jung, 1997, p. 77). Komproe et al. (1997) found that social support had a direct effect on depression and aided coping behavior. Aken and Asendorpf (1997) found that low social support by the mother provided the greatest risk of low general self-worth and that low social support by one parent could only be compensated for by social support by the other parent. Aken and Asendorpf also concluded that family support was strongly related to self-esteem (Aken & Asendorpf, 1997, p. 91). Social support networks are important to the psychological well-being of children (Allgood et al., 1997, p. 111). One method of opening the door for humor within the family might be to ask the children to offer their forms of social support to other families. Generally, girls provide emotional assistance, daily care-giving, and social services while sons typically offer advice (Goldsmith & Dun, 1997, p. 321). Any of these scenarios could offer the opportunity for a humorous situation that would allow the sharing of laughter and the diffusing of the seriousness of the situation. As adults, it is important to consider what kinds of humor, music, art, or whatever might help the children.

ART, LITERATURE, MUSIC, AND EXPRESSING GRIEF

Seemingly, all children like to draw and to express themselves in pictures. Christine Liddell suggests that children in all parts of the world are taught how to interpret pictures (Liddell, 1997, p. 269). All children offer pictures to adults to display in the home in a special place such as on the refrigerator or other prominent places. As children develop their oral abilities, they seem to draw less and less pictures. No matter what the level of oral fluency, pictures are a bridge to expression. For children of all ages, pictures hold a special significance (Liddell, 1997, p. 267).

In working with schools when a death has occurred, I typically ask the students to draw their feelings, their view of what occurred, their view of the death, or some other beginning question to get the drawings started. I may ask them to draw the animal that best expresses the person who died. The questions vary depending upon the age, event, and skills of the students involved. The medium used also varies. Crayons, paints, watercolors, clay, sand, or any other form of expression can be used. During the Gulf War, I asked students to illustrate their view of the war, what their family members might be doing in the war, and their views of war. These were all elementary school children. While some students may be slow to begin or require more patience, all students have been able to draw something which allowed them to express their feelings.

Literature offers adults a chance to relate to children in a way that is unparalleled. When an adult reads a story to a child, the child has the adult's undivided attention. Most adults find reading to children to be a pleasant experience. Children also find the experience to be quite pleasing. Clearly, adults often read stories to children that they themselves enjoy. As purchases of books are made, adults can choose to buy stories that they desire to read. As the child matures, the adult can continue to guide the literary taste of the child. If the adult continues to give this undivided attention to the child, the relationship will continue to grow. If the child wants to talk, the adult could turn off the television or put down the book or stop writing and listen to the child. The child must also learn to give his/her undivided attention to the adult when requested. Children learn what they live. If we read, they will read. If we give them respect, they will give us respect. If we trust their judgment, they will trust ours. The problem of finding books that will help the child of any age to learn about dying, death, and grief is no longer a problem. Hundreds of excellent books now exist for readers of all ages. Any dying and death textbook will typically contain many suggestions and bibliographies. On at least a weekly basis, I provide books and other reading material to many different audiences. While my own books often fail to return, the benefits are tremendous.

Music, like art, is another form of expression that does not require oral fluency. The effects of music are greater than the effects of silence (Wilson & Brown, 1997, p. 368). Music is a therapeutic tool. Norman Cousins suggests that humor was such an artistic act for Albert Schweitzer that he regarded it as being like a musical instrument (Cousins, 1979, p. 82). Humor, like music, has timing, flow, voice movements, and clarity. Like humor, music can change the mood of the individual. One does not need musical talent to benefit from music. A religious attitude can be understood or adopted through music. Music has been used throughout history to promote spiritual development (Lowis & Hughes, 1997, p. 47). An eleven year old dying of cancer who was creatively gifted applied his creative skills using music to control his pain and give meaning and understanding to his dying (Marrone, 1997, p. 87). Pain can be controlled by the mind. If one is playing a game that is both important to the player and is close in the score, the player will often not notice injuries or pains. Most marathoners want to finish the race. Various pains will come and go during the race. The pain is often forgotten with the elation of completing the marathon. When one has time to sit around and think about the pain, the pain will return. Creativity, like competition, gives the creative person something other than pain to concentrate upon. Creativity is more important to the creative person than the pain. Just as a child will put himself/herself into a drawing, a child can put himself/herself into music or any other creative endeavor. I have also found that music is a quite practical approach with children. I ask them what song reminds you of the deceased? What song represents the deceased? Or, perhaps, what song brings the deceased back to you? In the more than thirty years that I have been working with children both as students and as bereaved individuals, I have never found one that did not relate to some form of music including developmentally disabled children.

Children, like adults, are always learning, growing, and developing. Their knowledge, understanding, and reactions to illness, crisis, and loss are also constantly developing and changing. Natural or expressive therapies such as music, art, play, dance, or drama allow the child to be expressive in a less threatening fashion than talking one-on-one with an adult (Doka, 1995, p. xii). Children can be asked to relive and revisit through guided imagery, to examine their memories of the person who died and to test them with reality, to list and face anxieties or fears, to engage in fantasy and imagination exercises which might improve coping skills, or to engage in therapeutic rituals which focus on specific behaviors or activities which develop coping skills. Guided drawings are not intended to stifle creativity, but rather are designed to improve the drawing capacity and self-expression of children (Shatil, 1995, p. 130). Competition can be a problem depending upon the culture.

In urban U.S. schools, children are rewarded for competitive behavior more than in rural schools (Eisenberg & Mussen, 1989, p. 48). No only do children learn different styles of competition, but they also will exhibit different coping skills, artistic interest, and styles of responding. No list or single description of activities will ever suffice. Each caregiver must try to determine what kinds of music, art, humor, or literature might be useful for a child. While clearly not true of all children, there are patterns of differences between male and female children. Males like to give advice or tell others what they might do while females like to provide emotional assistance and care-giving services (Goldsmith & Dun, 1997, p. 321). The male child might be asked to draw a picture to aid another child who is having difficulty managing grief. Since you are an intelligent child, what would you say to another child who is having difficulty? The female child might be asked to indicate what kind of care she would give to another who was suffering. Generally, each child will address his or her own needs in reaching out to others. Those who give support to others benefit themselves from giving that support (Jung, 1997, p. 77).

As adults, there is a strong temptation for us to interpret all drawings, songs, and emotional statements of children. Certainly some aspects of artistic expression do seem to be universal. Cross-cultural studies do seem to show that fear is often expressed by the color black, envy by red, and anger by both black and red (Hupka et al., 1997, p. 165). Children all over the world draw pictures and attach meaning to their pictures. Pictures are a bridge to literacy. Pictures allow those who do not have the words to be able to express themselves (Liddell, 1997, p. 271). For adults, the problem is what do these pictures mean.

Certainly some expressions can easily be interpreted. Cox (1995), in a study of the effects of the Gulf War on children, used drawings and writings of grade school children to uncover their deepest fears and beliefs about the war (Cox et al., 1995, p. 115). While the differences increased with age and ability to express verbally, females tended to identify with people and emotions while males displayed more aggressiveness (Cox et al., 1995, p. 113). Care needs to be taken to not read too much into the drawings of children. It is not wise to create problems if none exist. Jonathan Shatil (1995) suggests that the art work of children should not be judged or be competitive and that it must instead be light, playful, and tranquil with no comparisons or saying what it should or should not mean. Many art forms exist for working with children of all ages. For children of all ages, fears get worse if nothing is done or attempts are made to overprotect the children (Sarefino, 1986, p. 81). Drawings and other art forms can be used to aid children.

For an excellent demonstration of using drawings with children see Nancy Boyd Webb (1993), *Helping Bereaved Children: A Handbook for Practitioners.* Another excellent text would be Linda Goldman (1996), *Breaking the Silence: A Guide to Help Children with Complicated Grief: Suicide, Homicide, AIDS, Violence, and Abuse.* Goldman discusses the use of visualization, photography, artwork, clay, toy figures, punching bags, tape recordings, and storytelling (Goldman, 1996, pp. 117-141). For younger children, the use of sandbox, dolls, doll houses, drawing materials, and other play materials. For older children, fantasy and play creative activities involving more words are more useful (Dyregrov, 1990, p. 107). Children may want to play funeral, to act out the ceremony with their peers. Children may want to communicate and share about the deceased, draw a picture, write a story, to leave a special gift in the casket (Worden, 1996, p. 144). Children may want to make a memorial book, to remember anniversaries, special days or some other means of expressing their grief and remembrance (Pennells & Smith, 1995, pp. 34-35). Children need to be encouraged to express their feelings in some form to help manage their grief. A family might create a book with pages for each month which can list by day the births and deaths of deceased family and/or friends on anniversaries of their deaths. Prayers, rituals, or other forms of ceremonies can be developed for these special days. A simple reading of the names of deceased family members who died on this day can give a new perspective on death to children. Those who have kept track of deaths over many years have a genealogical record of their family history that can become part of the family heritage. The book itself can assume symbolic significance.

Like art, music is also an excellent form of self expression. Music effects one's mind and body. Joyful music can elevate one's mood and encourage laughter. Deanna Edwards (1993) indicates that music is not just entertainment, but it is also a powerful therapy and teaching tool. Music is more than just sound. It has atmosphere and to some degree dramatic action. As a painter uses physical paints and the sculptor uses clay, the musician uses his or her voice, singing ability, words, message, attitudes, adaptation, and musical ability to provide a musical message for the listener. The listener brings a capacity for hearing, interpreting, and reliving the musical emotions of the creator. For most music, there is an intimate relationship between music and words. The nature of beauty in music does not need words, but the use of words can be powerful. For music to have a message, it needs to reach the listener with feeling, impulse, craving, wishing, inspiration, and ideation.

APPLICATION OF CREATIVE EXPERIENCES FOR CHILDREN

Hundreds of techniques exist to aid dying and grieving children. As an educator, I have used many, many techniques for children of all ages. For very young children who lack verbal skills and even skills necessary to draw or engage in other more traditional forms of creative expression, puppets, story-telling, and other forms of play seem to work best. As with any age, these children need holding, nurturing, and physical contact. Hold them as older children act out a story. Games like marshmallow charades may be helpful. Children playing funeral, wake, or vigil services may allow the small child to express his/her feelings. Puppets and story-telling seem to work best for very small children. A specific technique that has worked with many children is to use a specific animal with the child. A teddy bear, dragon, doll, or puppet that the child can hold, carry, or talk to will open up children of all ages. Even adults respond to such techniques. A slight variation is to ask the child to pick an animal that best represents the person who has died or is dying. A doll, blanket, or other objects can be used to give security to the child.

For the slightly older preschool child, play seems to be the major pattern. I would have these children engage in the same activities as younger children, but the emphasis seems to be on doing. If a death occurs, include them in planning the rituals and even taking part in the rituals. By this age of development, the adult can model by telling the child of his/her experiences with dying and death as a child. Again, dolls, puppets, and even dress-ups are useful. At this point, children are likely to ask far more questions than most adults can answer. Do your best to answer their questions and be honest in your answers.

The elementary school child has better self-expression skills. While using the above techniques, one can now focus more on creative expression of the arts. Drawings that answer adults' questions work well. What do you feel? What is death to you? Why is your teacher no longer here? Each situation will require different questions, but I have found that asking children to respond to questions with drawings works quite well. With older children, I ask them what song best expresses your feelings. As they mature, I ask them to read, tell stories, write journals, and make collages that express their feelings. With all ages, the child needs to feel safe to express his/her feelings, fears, questions, and concerns. As adults, our job is to aid them as best as we can. Children seem to be excellent at helping each other.

Not only are children aided through their grief by expression, children who are free to express their own emotions are more apt than other children to approach and assist others who are in need (Eisenberg & Mussen, 1989, p. 61). The use of art, music, and humor allows children to remove the sense of distance between themselves and others; to find relief for depression; to enhance their self-esteem; to lower anxiety, fear, and other feelings of grief; and to achieve a safe level of acceptance of reality. It is not necessary to flood the child with reality, but it is important to support and encourage a reasonable view of what actually occurred (Hemmings, 1995, p. 21).

CONCLUSIONS

Using humor, music, and art are effective ways to provide social support for children who are experiencing complicated grief. Various techniques ranging from story-telling to humor exist for aiding children who are grieving. Support from adults is required for children to maintain their self-esteem and to manage loss. Children need help to make choices. Children need to say good-bye by writing a letter, making a picture, sending up a balloon with a message to their loved one. Adults need to support their efforts. Humor, art, music, and other art forms are not "cures" for grief and bereavement, but they are helpful aids for dying and grieving children.

REFERENCES

Allgood, S. M., Crane, D. R., & Agee, L. (1997, Summer). Social support: Distinguishing clinical and volunteer couples. *The American Journal of Family Therapy, 25*(2), 111-119.

Bauman, R. (1996). Folklore as transdisciplinary dialogue. *Journal of Folklore Research, 33*(1), 15-20.

Brabant, S. (1997-98). Death and grief in the family comics. *Omega: Journal of Death and Dying, 36*(1), 33-44.

Carey, T. C., Carey, M. P., & Kelley, M. L. (1997). Differential emotions theory: Relative contribution of emotion, cognition, and behavior to the prediction of depressive symptomatology in non-referred adolescents. *Journal of Clinical Psychology, 53*(1), 25-34.

Coe, R. M. (1997, March). The magic of science and the science of magic: An essay on the process of healing. *Journal of Health and Social Behavior, 38*, 1-8.

Cousins, N. (1979). *Anatomy of an illness as perceived by the patient.* New York: Bantam Books.

Cox, G. R., Vanden Berk, B. J., Fundis, R. J., & McGinnis, P. J. (1995). American children and Desert Storm: Impressions of the Gulf conflict. In D. W. Adams &

E. J. Deveau (Eds.), *Beyond the innocence of childhood: Factors influencing children and adolescents' perceptions and attitudes toward death* (Vol. 1, pp. 109-121). Amityville, NY: Baywood.

Doka, K. J. (Ed.) (1995). *Children mourning: Mourning children.* Washington, DC: Hospice Foundation of America.

Dyregrov, A. (1990). *Grief in children: A handbook for adults.* London: Jessica Kingsley.

Edwards, D. (1993). Grieving: The pain and the promise. In J. D. Morgan (Ed.), *Personal care in an impersonal world: A multidimensional look at bereavement.* Amityville, NY: Baywood.

Eisenberg, N., & Mussen, P. H. (1989). *The roots of prosocial behavior in children.* Cambridge: Cambridge University Press.

Glasgow, R. D. V. (1997). *Split down the sides: On the subject of laughter.* New York: University Press of America.

Goldman, L. (1996). *Breaking the silence: A guide to help children with complicated grief: Suicide, homicide, AIDs, violence and abuse.* London: Taylor and Francis.

Goldman, D. J., & Dun, S. A. (1997). Sex differences and similarities in the communication of social support. *Journal of Social and Personal Relationships, 14*(3), 317-337.

Gross, J. J., & Levenson, R. W. (1997). Hiding feelings: The acute effects of inhibiting negative and positive emotion. *Journal of Abnormal Psychology, 106*(1), 95-103.

Hemmings, P. (1995). Communications with children through play. In S. C. Smith & M. Pennells (Eds.), *Interventions with bereaved children,* London: Jessica Kingsley Publishers.

Howarth, G. (1996). *Last rights: The work of the modern funeral director.* Amityville, NY: Baywood.

Hupka, R. B., Saleski, Z., Otto, J., Reidl, L., & Tarabrina, N. V. (1997, March). The colors of anger, envy, fear, and jealousy: A cross-cultural study. *Journal of Cross- Cultural Psychology, 28*(2), 156-171.

Husebo, S. (1998, Spring). Is there hope, doctor. *Journal of Palliative Care, 14*(1), 43-48.

Jung, J. (1997). Balance and source of social support in relation to well-being. *Journal of General Psychology, 124*(1), 77-90.

Komproe, I. V., Rijken, M., Ros, W. J. G., Winnubst, J. A. M., & Hart, H. (1997). Available support and received support: Different effects under stressful circumstances. *Journal of Social and Personal Relationships, 14*(1), 59-77.

Lau, K. J. (1996, Spring). Social structure, society, and symbolism: Toward a holistic interpretation of fairy tales. *Western Folklore, 55,* 233-244.

Lefcourt, H. M., & Martin, R. A. (1986). *Humor, life, and stress: Antidote to adversity.* New York: Springer-Verlag.

Lewinsohn, P. M., Lewinsohn, M., Gotlib, I. H., Seeley, J. R., & Allen, N. B. (1998). Gender differences in anxiety disorders and anxiety symptoms in adolescents. *Journal of Abnormal Psychology, 107*(1), 109-117.

Liddell, C. (1997, May). Every picture tells a story—Or does it? Young South African children interpreting pictures. *Journal of Cross-Cultural Psychology, 28*(3), 266-283.

Lipman, S. (1991). *Laughter in hell: The use of humor during the holocaust.* Northvale, NJ: Jason Aronson.

Lowis, M. J., & Hughes, J. (1957). A comparison of the effects of sacred and secular music on elderly people. *Journal of Psychology, 131*(1), 45-55.

Marrone, R. (1997). *Death, mourning, and caring.* Pacific Grove, CA: Brooks/Cole.

Meyers, S. A. (1997, April). The language of love: The difference a preposition makes. *Personality and Social Psychology Bulletin, 23*(4), 347-362.

Mindess, H. (1971). *Laughter and liberation.* Los Angeles: Nash.

Moore, T. (1992). *Care of the soul: A guide for cultivating depth and sacredness in everyday life.* New York: HarperCollins.

Morreall, J. (1983). *Taking laughter seriously.* Albany, NY: SUNY Press.

Neale, R. E. (1993). Joking with death. In K. J. Doka & J. D. Morgan (Eds.), *Death and spirituality* (pp. 323-331). Amityville, NY: Baywood.

Palfai, T. P., & Hart, K. E. (1997). Anger coping styles and perceived social support. *The Journal of Social Psychology, 137*(4), 405-411.

Pennells, M., & Smith, S. C. (1995). *The forgotten mourners: Guidelines for working with bereaved children.* London: Jessica Kingsley Publishers.

Ptacek, J. T., Pierce, G. R., Dodge, K. L., & Ptacek, J. J. (1997, December). Social support in spouses of cancer patients: What do they get and to what end? *Personal Relationships, 4*(4), 431-449.

Robinson, L., & Mahon, M. M. (1997). Sibling bereavement: A conceptual analysis. *Death Studies, 21,* 477-499.

Rohde, P., Seeley, J. R., & Mace, D. E. (1997, Summer). Correlates of suicidal behavior in a juvenile detention population. *Suicide and Life-Threatening Behavior, 27*(2), 164-175.

Rokach, A., & Brock, H. (1998). Coping with loneliness. *Journal of Psychology, 132*(1), 107-127.

Ryff, C. D., & Singer, B. (1998). The contours of positive human health. *Psychological Inquiry, 9*(1), 1-28.

Sarafino, E. P. (1986). *The fears of childhood: A guide to recognizing and reducing fearful states in children.* New York: Human Science Press.

Saunders, Dame C. (1995-96). A response to Logue's "Where hospice fails—The limits of palliative care". *Omega: Journal of Death and Dying, 32*(1), 1-5.

Schut, H. A. W., Stroebe, M. S., & Van Den Bout, J. (1997). Intervention for the bereaved: Gender difference in the efficacy of two counselling programmes. *British Journal of Clinical Psychology, 36,* 63-72.

Shatil, J. (1995). *The psychography of the child: Development of the psychographic capacity from drawings to writing, and the means for improvement.* New York: University Press of America.

Silverstein, M., & Bengstson, V. L. (1997, September). Intergenerational solidarity and the structure of adult child-parent relationships in American families. *American Journal of Sociology, 103*(2), 429-460.

Spiegel, D. (1998). Getting there is half the fun: Relating happiness to health. *Psychological Inquiry, 9*(1), 66-68.

Thomas, J. B. (1997). Dumb blondes, Dan Quayle, and Hillary Clinton: Gender, sexuality, and stupidity in jokes. *Journal of American Folklore, 110*(437), 277-313.

Van Aken, M. A. G., & Asendorpf, J. B. (1997). Support by parents, classmates, friends, and siblings in preadolescence: Covariation and compensation across relationships. *Journal of Social and Personal relationships, 14*(1), 79-93.

Vangelesti, A. L., & Caughlin, J. P. (1997). Revealing family secrets: The influence of topic, function, and relationship. *Journal of Social and Personal Relationships, 14*(5), 679-705.

Webb, N. B. (1993). Traumatic death of friend/peer: Case of Susan, age 9. In N. B. Webb (Ed.), *Helping bereaved children: A handbook for practitioners.* New York: Guilford Press.

Wellman, H. M. (1998). Culture, variation, and levels of analysis in folk psychologies: Comment on Lillard. *Psychological Bulletin, 123*(1), 33-36.

Wilson, T. L., & Brown, T. L. (1997). Reexamination of the effect of Mozart's music on spatial-task performance. *The Journal of Psychology, 131*(4), 365-370.

Worden, J. W. (1996). *Children and Grief: When a parent dies.* New York: Guilford Press.

Contributors

DAVID W. ADAMS, M.S.W., C.S.W., is Professor Department of Psychiatry and Behavioural Neurosciences, McMaster University, Faculty of Health Sciences and Executive Director, Hurst Place: The Employee Assistance Program. He has an extensive background as a clinician and educator and is especially noted for his work with ill and bereaved children, adolescents, and their families. He is a certified grief therapist and a certified death educator. He is co-editor of *Beyond the Innocence of Childhood,* a three volume series related to understanding of death, life-threatening illness, palliative care, and bereavement in childhood and adolescence. He is also co-author of *Coping with Childhood Cancer: Where Do We Go from Here?* And is internationally known as a workshop facilitator and lecturer. He is past chair of the International Work Group on Death, Dying, and Bereavement (IWG) and is a member of the CHIPPS Psychosocial/Spiritual/Bereavement Group of the National Hospice Organization.

THOMAS ATTIG, Ph.D., is the author of *How We Grieve: Relearning the World* (Oxford, 1996) and *The Heart of Grief: The Desire for Lasting Love* (Oxford, 2000). He is former president of the Association for Death Education and Counseling (ADEC) and currently Vice Chair of the International Work Group on Death, Dying, and Bereavement (IWG). Dr. Attig is professor emeritus and chair of the department of philosophy at Bowling Green State University in Ohio. He currently resides in San Francisco.

ROBERT A. BENDIKSEN, Ph.D., is professor of sociology and director of the Center for Death Education & Bioethics at the University of Wisconsin-La Crosse. He serves as the Secretariat of the International Work Group on Death, Dying, and Bereavement, as well as editor of *ILLNESS, CRISIS & LOSS* (Sage Publications) and coeditor of *THE*

MIDWEST SOCIOLOGIST (with G. Cox). He co-edited *Death and Identity,* Third Edition (with R. Fulton) and *Death, Dying & Bioethics* (with G. Cox). The Wisconsin Sociological Association awarded Dr. Bendiksen the 1999 George Floro Award for Outstanding Service to the Discipline of Sociology. E-mail: RBendiksen@aol.com.

KERRY CAVANAGH is a psychologist with the Marion Regional Team of The Child and Adolescent Mental Health Service, a community outreach program of Flinders Medical Centre in Oaklands Park, South Australia.

PAUL T. CLEMENTS Jr. is the Director of Operations for Public Health Services for the City of Philadelphia Department of Public Health. Paul is a Forensic Psychiatric Nurse, with a National Board Certification for Advanced Practice in Child, Adolescent, and Family Mental Health Nursing. Paul specializes in providing therapy to children who have been exposed to murder and other violent deaths.

GERRY R. COX, Ph.D., is an associate professor of sociology and associate with the Center for Death Education & Bioethics at the University of Wisconsin-La Crosse. He is a member of the International Work Group on Death, Dying, and Bereavement, as well as co-editor of *THE MIDWEST SOCIOLOGIST* (with B. Bendiksen). He has taught death and dying courses, trained hospice volunteers, facilitated bereavement groups, and has lectured and conducted workshops. He has edited, co-edited, and authored seven books and over forty articles and chapters in books and journals including *Death, Dying & Bioethics* (with B. Bendiksen). E-mail: Cox.Gerr@uwlax.edu

LARRY R. DARRAH is a Death Educator, certified by the Association of Death Education and Counseling. He is a Retired Air Force Major and Pediatric Nurse Practitioner, working with four pediatricians in a private practice where he counsels bereaved children in addition to his regular duties as a PNP. He is a hospice volunteer and has conducted numerous workshops and seminars to professional and lay audiences alike.

THE REVEREND RICHARD B. GILBERT, D.Min., BCC, is executive director of The World Pastoral Care Center and founding director of Connections—Spiritual Links. He has presented extensively on bereavement, spirituality, pastoral care, and health care, bringing his experience as a Board Certified Chaplain to his programs. Extensively published, he has contributed to six books and has three books of his ownnow available. His fourth book, also with Baywood, discussing spirituality and health care, is in final editing. He developed "Resources Hotline," providing reviews and resource information to over 600 people via email.

TONI GRIFFITH, MSA, MSW is a licensed social worker and executive director of Continuing Support Services, Inc. which is a non-profit organization dedicated to serving the community with loss, grief, and transition management, as well as HIV/AIDS prevention education, in Marlton, New Jersey.

PIPPA HALL received her MD from the University of Saskatchewan in 1983 and completed a Family Medicine Residency. After working in urban and rural communities for nine years, she completed a Fellowship in Palliative Care with the University of Ottawa in 1995. She has just completed her MEd from the University of Toronto. Dr. Hall is Assistant Professor in Family Medicine with the University of Ottawa Institute of Palliative Care.

CHRISTINE HODGSON began her social work career in England and later gained her MSW from McGill University. She practiced in several different areas, primarily in child welfare and adoption, before entering the field of health care. In 1991 she became the social worker and bereavement coordinator at the Ottawa Regional Palliative Care Unit, providing grief counseling and education to the families of patients both before and after the death.

STEPHEN J. HOOGERBRUGGE, Ph.D., a Presbyterian minister (retired), conducts family therapy and teaches in the Master of Science in Clinical Psychology program at Vanguard University of Southern California. He also supervises clinicians for Star View Community Services and conducts seminars on Grief and Loss issues from a Family Systems perspective.

JANIS L. KEYSER, Ph.D., is the Director of The Center for Grieving Children, Teens & Families in Philadelphia, Pennsylvania. She is also the Executive Director of UNITE, Inc. which offers grief support after the death of a baby. She holds dual certification as a Death Educator and Grief Counselor from the Association for Death Education and Counseling (ADEC). Janis came to this work after the birth/death of her daughter Jessica Brooke on January 15, 1980.

ANTOON A. LEENAARS, Ph.D., C.Psych., is a clinical psychologist in private practice in Windsor, Canada, and a member of the faculty at the

University of Leiden, The Netherlands. He was the first Past President of the Canadian Association for Suicide Prevention (CASP), and is a past President of the American Association of Suicidology (AAS). He has published ten books, most recently, *Studies of Lives and Deaths: Selections from the Works of Edwin S. Shneidman,* and is Editor-in-Chief of *Archives of Suicide Research.* Dr. Leenaars has been an international volunteer in regions with the highest rates of suicide (e.g., Arctic, Lithuania).

LYNNE MARTINS, MSW, ACSW, is a clinical social worker and a grief therapist in private practice in Tacoma, Washington, where she specializes in delayed and complicated grief responses resulting from sudden death and loss. The author of numerous publications and video productions, she has been counseling, writing, and teaching for more than a decade throughout the United States, Canada, and Australia.

DIANE L. MIDLAND, BSW, MS, is a certified Independent Social Worker and currently works as a Bereavement Educator at Gundersen Lutheran Medical Center, Inc. in La Crosse, Wisconsin. In addition to assisting with staff development programs at Gundersen Lutheran, Diane also teaches the *RTS* perinatal loss course and the *Compassionate Bereavement Care* course nationally. She was instrumental in the development of a general bereavement program at Gundersen Lutheran and works with physicians in compassionate death notification training. Prior to her current position, Diane was a social worker in the Trauma and Emergency Center for approximately fifteen years. She remains active in local and state Critical Incident Management programs.

SUSAN K. PARKER is a graduate of the University of North Texas with a Masters of Education in Counseling. Sue is licensed as a Licensed Professional Counselor and a Licensed Marriage and Family Therapist. She has a private practice where she specializes in grief and loss, life transitions, relationships, and women's issues. Sue conducts workshops, seminars, and inservice presentations and has presented at King's College International Conference on Death and Bereavement in London, Ontario, Canada. In addition to private practice, Sue is the Administrator of Catholic Counseling Services, an Agency of Catholic Charities of Dallas, Inc. This agency offers family counseling, maternity and adoption services, and a teen substance abuse program.

RICHARD J. PAUL, B.A., B.Ed., ADEC Certified Death Educator is dedicated to both learning all he can about grief and to sharing this information to assist people growing through their losses. He has a special interest in the subject of anticipatory grief particularly as it relates to palliative care. He was director of the North Bay & Area Palliative Care Association and was also a founding director of the Near North Palliative Care Network. He is the incoming President of the Bereavement Ontario Network. He is a caregiver and a funeral director dedicated to the philosophy "Committed to making a Difference."

JANE POWELL has been a member of L'Arche for twenty years. She has shared her life, on a daily basis, with people with intellectual disabilities and their assistants. She is also interested in palliative care and grief issues. Her interests also lie in the areas of symbolism and ritual, and augmentative means of communication. This chapter combines her experience and interest in these different areas.

BOYD C. PURCELL, M.A., M.Div., Ph.D., is a Licensed Professional and National Board Certified Counselor who has a quarter of a century of experience as a therapist in an agency, pastoral counseling, psychiatric hospital, private practice in mental health settings. He is presently the chaplain of Kenawha Hospice Care in Dunbar, West Virginia. He is also an adjunct faculty instructor at Marshall University Graduate College. He has presented on the topic of "spiritual abuse" at various state and regional conferences. He has also presented on this topic at the National Conference of Catholic and Professional Chaplains as well as the International Conference on Death and Dying at King's College, London, Ontario, Canada.

CATHERINE ANNE QUINN is an Australian Social Worker, a graduate in Arts and Social Work from the University of Queensland, and a master in Theology from the Sydney College of Divinity. She has worked in community-based aged care services since 1973, and for nine years taught Pastoral Theology at a member institute of the Sydney College of Divinity. She has a special interest in the social, psychological, and spiritual issues arising from dementing illnesses and in the management of loss and grief. She works as a counselor of people with dementia.

HANNAH SHEREBRIN, RN, ATR, ICET-RS—Art therapist, formerly clinical supervisor for the Art Therapy program at the University of Western Ontario, Canada, and Director of the UWO Art Craft Studio. Originator of the City Art Centre for consumers of the mental health services in London, Canada. Sherebrin presented in a number of bereavement conferences and has several published articles as well as a chapter in *Grief and the Healing Arts—Creativity as Therapy* edited by Sandra L. Bertman. She is currently engaged in private practice dealing with loss and trauma, as well as training and supervising volunteers who visit disabled veterans and bereaved families in Karmiel, Israel. This volunteer program is operated by the rehabilitation branch of the Israel Defense Ministry.

ROBERT G. STEVENSON was a secondary school teacher/counselor for thirty years until his retirement in June of 1997. He taught a death education course of his own design for twenty-five of those years and helped found a bereavement counseling center (The Center For Help In Time of Loss). He was co-chairman of the Seminar on Death at Columbia University from 1984 through 1995. He is currently working in an alcohol/ drug rehabilitation program for adolescents and an adult reentry program for adult parolees. He teaches graduate counseling courses at Mercy College in New York. He has published over sixty articles on loss and grief in professional journals and texts and edited several books, including *Teaching Students About Death* (Charles Press, 1996) and *What Will We Do? Preparing a School Community to Deal with Crises* (Baywood, 1994). He is an active member of both the International Work Group on Death, Dying, and Bereavement (I.W.G.) and the Association for Death Education and Counseling (ADEC). He is a graduate of the College of the Holy Cross (B.A.) and holds master's degrees from Fairleigh Dickinson University (M.A.T.) and Montclair State University (M.A.) and a doctorate (Ed.D.) from Fairleigh Dickinson. He is nationally certified by the Association for Death Education and Counseling as both a professional death educator and a professional grief counselor, has served on their board of directors, as chairman of their Education Institute and sits on their board of certification review. Dr. Stevenson has written curricula for social studies, health and death education, and has been honored for his work as an educator and counselor by: The New Jersey Professional Counselors' Association, the New Jersey Governor's Office, Best Practice Awards of the N.J. Department of Education, N.J. School Boards'

Association, United States Chess Federation, and the National Council for the Social Studies. He is listed in Who's Who Among America's Teachers, Who's Who Among Human Service Professionals, and Who's Who Among International Authors. He was the recipient of the 1997 Wendel Williams Outstanding Teacher Award and the 1993 ADEC Death Educator Award for his contributions to those fields. He is also in charge of an education program for the 88th Brigade of the New York State Guard. He participates in Living History events and reenacts themes from the American Revolution and Civil War for students and their families.

LYNDA WEAVER finished her Masters of Health Administration from the University of Ottawa in 1994. She has worked in the field of health services research and evaluation since 1990, primarily with small community agencies and in nursing research. Lynda has been with the University of Ottawa Institute of Palliative Care since 1995, coordinating research, evaluation, and education projects. She is in the process of obtaining her Masters of Education from the University of Toronto.

Index